ALZHEIMER'S DISEASE
Targets for New Clinical Diagnostic and Therapeutic Strategies

FRONTIERS IN NEUROSCIENCE

Series Editors
Sidney A. Simon, Ph.D.
Miguel A.L. Nicolelis, M.D., Ph.D.

Published Titles

Apoptosis in Neurobiology
Yusuf A. Hannun, M.D., Professor of Biomedical Research and Chairman, Department of
Biochemistry and Molecular Biology, Medical University of South Carolina, Charleston,
South Carolina
Rose-Mary Boustany, M.D., tenured Associate Professor of Pediatrics and Neurobiology, Duke
University Medical Center, Durham, North Carolina

Neural Prostheses for Restoration of Sensory and Motor Function
John K. Chapin, Ph.D., Professor of Physiology and Pharmacology, State University of New York
Health Science Center, Brooklyn, New York
Karen A. Moxon, Ph.D., Assistant Professor, School of Biomedical Engineering, Science, and
Health Systems, Drexel University, Philadelphia, Pennsylvania

Computational Neuroscience: Realistic Modeling for Experimentalists
Eric DeSchutter, M.D., Ph.D., Professor, Department of Medicine, University of Antwerp,
Antwerp, Belgium

Methods in Pain Research
Lawrence Kruger, Ph.D., Professor of Neurobiology (Emeritus), UCLA School of Medicine and
Brain Research Institute, Los Angeles, California

Motor Neurobiology of the Spinal Cord
Timothy C. Cope, Ph.D., Professor of Physiology, Wright State University, Dayton, Ohio

Nicotinic Receptors in the Nervous System
Edward D. Levin, Ph.D., Associate Professor, Department of Psychiatry and Pharmacology and
Molecular Cancer Biology and Department of Psychiatry and Behavioral Sciences, Duke
University School of Medicine, Durham, North Carolina

Methods in Genomic Neuroscience
Helmin R. Chin, Ph.D., Genetics Research Branch, NIMH, NIH, Bethesda, Maryland
Steven O. Moldin, Ph.D., University of Southern California, Washington, D.C.

Methods in Chemosensory Research
Sidney A. Simon, Ph.D., Professor of Neurobiology, Biomedical Engineering, and Anesthesiology,
Duke University, Durham, North Carolina
Miguel A.L. Nicolelis, M.D., Ph.D., Professor of Neurobiology and Biomedical Engineering,
Duke University, Durham, North Carolina

The Somatosensory System: Deciphering the Brain's Own Body Image
Randall J. Nelson, Ph.D., Professor of Anatomy and Neurobiology,
University of Tennessee Health Sciences Center, Memphis, Tennessee

The Superior Colliculus: New Approaches for Studying Sensorimotor Integration
William C. Hall, Ph.D., Department of Neuroscience, Duke University, Durham, North Carolina
Adonis Moschovakis, Ph.D., Department of Basic Sciences, University of Crete, Heraklion, Greece

New Concepts in Cerebral Ischemia
Rick C.S. Lin, Ph.D., Professor of Anatomy, University of Mississippi Medical Center, Jackson, Mississippi

DNA Arrays: Technologies and Experimental Strategies
Elena Grigorenko, Ph.D., Technology Development Group, Millennium Pharmaceuticals, Cambridge, Massachusetts

Methods for Alcohol-Related Neuroscience Research
Yuan Liu, Ph.D., National Institute of Neurological Disorders and Stroke, National Institutes of Health, Bethesda, Maryland
David M. Lovinger, Ph.D., Laboratory of Integrative Neuroscience, NIAAA, Nashville, Tennessee

Primate Audition: Behavior and Neurobiology
Asif A. Ghazanfar, Ph.D., Princeton University, Princeton, New Jersey

Methods in Drug Abuse Research: Cellular and Circuit Level Analyses
Barry D. Waterhouse, Ph.D., MCP-Hahnemann University, Philadelphia, Pennsylvania

Functional and Neural Mechanisms of Interval Timing
Warren H. Meck, Ph.D., Professor of Psychology, Duke University, Durham, North Carolina

Biomedical Imaging in Experimental Neuroscience
Nick Van Bruggen, Ph.D., Department of Neuroscience Genentech, Inc.
Timothy P.L. Roberts, Ph.D., Associate Professor, University of Toronto, Canada

The Primate Visual System
John H. Kaas, Department of Psychology, Vanderbilt University, Nashville, Tennessee
Christine Collins, Department of Psychology, Vanderbilt University, Nashville, Tennessee

Neurosteroid Effects in the Central Nervous System
Sheryl S. Smith, Ph.D., Department of Physiology, SUNY Health Science Center, Brooklyn, New York

Modern Neurosurgery: Clinical Translation of Neuroscience Advances
Dennis A. Turner, Department of Surgery, Division of Neurosurgery, Duke University Medical Center, Durham, North Carolina

Sleep: Circuits and Functions
Pierre-Hervé Luppi, Université Claude Bernard, Lyon, France

Methods in Insect Sensory Neuroscience
Thomas A. Christensen, Arizona Research Laboratories, Division of Neurobiology, University of Arizona, Tuscon, Arizona

Motor Cortex in Voluntary Movements
Alexa Riehle, INCM-CNRS, Marseille, France
Eilon Vaadia, The Hebrew University, Jerusalem, Israel

Neural Plasticity in Adult Somatic Sensory-Motor Systems
Ford F. Ebner, Vanderbilt University, Nashville, Tennessee

Advances in Vagal Afferent Neurobiology
Bradley J. Undem, Johns Hopkins Asthma Center, Baltimore, Maryland
Daniel Weinreich, University of Maryland, Baltimore, Maryland

The Dynamic Synapse: Molecular Methods in Ionotropic Receptor Biology
Josef T. Kittler, University College, London, England
Stephen J. Moss, University College, London, England

Animal Models of Cognitive Impairment
Edward D. Levin, Duke University Medical Center, Durham, North Carolina
Jerry J. Buccafusco, Medical College of Georgia, Augusta, Georgia

The Role of the Nucleus of the Solitary Tract in Gustatory Processing
Robert M. Bradley, University of Michigan, Ann Arbor, Michigan

Brain Aging: Models, Methods, and Mechanisms
David R. Riddle, Wake Forest University, Winston-Salem, North Carolina

Neural Plasticity and Memory: From Genes to Brain Imaging
Frederico Bermudez-Rattoni, National University of Mexico, Mexico City, Mexico

Serotonin Receptors in Neurobiology
Amitabha Chattopadhyay, Center for Cellular and Molecular Biology, Hyderabad, India

TRP Ion Channel Function in Sensory Transduction and Cellular Signaling Cascades
Wolfgang B. Liedtke, M.D., Ph.D., Duke University Medical Center, Durham, North Carolina
Stefan Heller, Ph.D., Stanford University School of Medicine, Stanford, California

Methods for Neural Ensemble Recordings, Second Edition
Miguel A.L. Nicolelis, M.D., Ph.D., Professor of Neurobiology and Biomedical Engineering,
  Duke University Medical Center, Durham, North Carolina

Biology of the NMDA Receptor
Antonius M. VanDongen, Duke University Medical Center, Durham, North Carolina

Methods of Behavioral Analysis in Neuroscience
Jerry J. Buccafusco, Ph.D., Alzheimer's Research Center, Professor of Pharmacology and Toxicology,
  Professor of Psychiatry and Health Behavior, Medical College of Georgia, Augusta, Georgia

In Vivo Optical Imaging of Brain Function, Second Edition
Ron Frostig, Ph.D., Professor, Department of Neurobiology, University of California,
Irvine, California

Fat Detection: Taste, Texture, and Post Ingestive Effects
Jean-Pierre Montmayeur, Ph.D., Centre National de la Recherche Scientifique, Dijon, France
Johannes le Coutre, Ph.D., Nestlé Research Center, Lausanne, Switzerland

The Neurobiology of Olfaction
Anna Menini, Ph.D., Neurobiology Sector International School for Advanced Studies, (S.I.S.S.A.),
  Trieste, Italy

Neuroproteomics
Oscar Alzate, Ph.D., Department of Cell and Developmental Biology, University of North
  Carolina, Chapel Hill, North Carolina

Translational Pain Research: From Mouse to Man
Lawrence Kruger, Ph.D., Department of Neurobiology, UCLA School of Medicine, Los Angeles,
  California
Alan R. Light, Ph.D., Department of Anesthesiology, University of Utah, Salt Lake City, Utah

Advances in the Neuroscience of Addiction
Cynthia M. Kuhn, Duke University Medical Center, Durham, North Carolina
George F. Koob, The Scripps Research Institute, La Jolla, California

ALZHEIMER'S DISEASE
Targets for New Clinical Diagnostic and Therapeutic Strategies

Edited by

Renee D. Wegrzyn, PhD

Adlyfe, Inc.
Rockville, Maryland, USA

Alan S. Rudolph, PhD, MBA

Center for Neuroengineering
Duke University
Durham, North Carolina, USA

CRC CRC Press
Taylor & Francis Group
Boca Raton London New York

CRC Press is an imprint of the
Taylor & Francis Group, an **informa** business

CRC Press
Taylor & Francis Group
6000 Broken Sound Parkway NW, Suite 300
Boca Raton, FL 33487-2742

© 2012 by Taylor & Francis Group, LLC
CRC Press is an imprint of Taylor & Francis Group, an Informa business

No claim to original U.S. Government works

Printed in the United States of America on acid-free paper
Version Date: 20120301

International Standard Book Number: 978-1-4398-2708-6 (Hardback)

Library of Congress Cataloging-in-Publication Data

Alzheimer's disease : targets for new clinical diagnostic and therapeutic strategies /
    editors, Alan S. Rudolph, Renee D. Wegrzyn.
        p. ; cm. -- (Frontiers in neuroscience)
    Includes bibliographical references and index.
    ISBN 978-1-4398-2708-6 (hardcover : alk. paper)
    I. Rudolph, Alan S., 1954- II. Wegrzyn, Renee D. III. Series: Frontiers in neuroscience.
    [DNLM: 1. Alzheimer Disease--diagnosis. 2. Alzheimer Disease--therapy. 3.
Biological Markers. WT 155]

616.8'31--dc23   2012005188

Visit the Taylor & Francis Web site at
http://www.taylorandfrancis.com

and the CRC Press Web site at
http://www.crcpress.com

The editors would like to dedicate this work to all of the patients and caregivers around the world who are suffering under the burden of Alzheimer's disease.

Renee D. Wegrzyn would like to thank her parents, Jerry and Jessie, and her ever supportive and loving husband, Brandon.

Alan S. Rudolph also honors his grandmother, Pauline Schwartz, the first person in his life that he knew with Alzheimer's disease.

Contents

Preface

The manuscripts collected in this volume seek to not only summarize the current state of the art of diagnostics and therapeutics for Alzheimer's disease, but also identify emerging technologies and molecules that show promise as future candidates for the management and treatment of Alzheimer's disease. The authors for this text were invited to participate not only for their distinguished contributions to the field of Alzheimer's disease and other neurodegenerative disorders, but also for their representation of the internationally diverse community that is working to improve the quality of life of patients and caregivers around the globe. This volume aims to bring together insights from the unique perspectives offered by each contributor to provide a resource to the community that may supplement existing knowledge. As a cohesive whole, the makeup of the contributing authors faithfully represents the collective efforts of academia, clinical practice, and the biotechnology and pharmaceutical industries that are critical for the advancement of the field of Alzheimer's and related disorders toward definitive diagnostics and medical interventions that not only ease the symptoms of disease, but aim to halt and ultimately reverse the underlying pathology of the disease.

Renee D. Wegrzyn
September 2011

Frontiers in Neuroscience

Sidney A. Simon, Ph.D.

Miguel A. L. Nicolelis, M.D., Ph.D.

The Frontiers in Neuroscience Series presents the insights of experts on emerging experimental technologies and theoretical concepts that are, or will be, at the vanguard of neuroscience.

The books cover new and exciting multidisciplinary areas of brain research, and describe breakthroughs in fields like visual, gustatory, auditory, olfactory neuroscience, as well as aging biomedical imaging. Recent books cover the rapidly evolving fields of multisensory processing, depression, and different aspects of reward.

Each book is edited by experts and consists of chapters written by leaders in a particular field. Books are richly illustrated and contain comprehensive bibliographies. Chapters provide substantial background material relevant to the particular subject.

The goal is for these books to be the references every neuroscientist uses in order to acquaint themselves with new information and methodologies in brain research. We view our task as series editors to produce outstanding products that contribute to the broad field of neuroscience. Now that the chapters are available online, the effort put in by us, the publisher, the book editors, and individual authors will contribute to the further development of brain research. To the extent that you learn from these books, we will have succeeded.

About the Editors

Renee D. Wegrzyn obtained her PhD in applied biology from the Georgia Institute of Technology where she studied the propagation of prion proteins in model systems. Dr. Wegrzyn was awarded an Alexander von Humboldt Research Fellowship for her postdoctoral studies to investigate de novo protein folding at the ribosome. She applied her expertise in protein folding to the challenge of developing in vitro diagnostics for neurodegenerative diseases including Alzheimer's and prion diseases as a group leader at Adlyfe, Inc. She is currently a scientific and technical consultant for the Department of Defense.

Alan S. Rudolph is currently a member of the senior executive service and director of Biological and Chemical Technologies for the Defense Threat Reduction Agency. He was previously chief executive officer at Adlyfe, Inc., an amyloid diagnostic and biomarker company, chief of Biological Sciences at the Defense Advanced Research Projects Agency, and director of Research at the Naval Research Laboratory. He has over 90 publications in diverse areas in biophysics of cryobiology and anhydrobiosis, lipid and protein self-assembly, liposome science and technology, and tissue and cellular engineering. He has edited two books including *Red Blood Cell Substitutes* (CRC, 1997) and *Neurotechnology for Biomimetic Robots* (The MIT Press, 2002). He has a PhD in zoology from the University of California at Davis and an MBA from the George Washington University.

Contributors

Shiela Beroukhim
Department of Neurology
David Geffen School of Medicine at
  UCLA
Los Angeles, California, USA

Mark P. Burns, PhD
Laboratory for Brain Injury and
  Dementia
Department of Neuroscience
Georgetown University Medical Center
Washington, D.C., USA

Sarah A. Chau, B.Sc.
Neuropsychopharmacology Research
  Program
Sunnybrook Health Sciences Centre
University of Toronto
Toronto, Canada

Mei-Sha Chen
Department of Neurology
David Geffen School of Medicine at
  UCLA
Los Angeles, California, USA

**Giora Z. Feuerstein, MD, M.Sc.,
FAHA**
Adlyfe, Inc.
Rockville, Maryland, USA

Nathan Herrmann, MD, FRCP
Neuropsychopharmacology Research
  Program
Sunnybrook Health Sciences Centre
University of Toronto
Toronto, Canada

Tien-Phat Huynh
Department of Neurology
David Geffen School of Medicine at
  UCLA
Los Angeles, California, USA

Ida Kircanski
Neuropsychopharmacology Research
  Program
Sunnybrook Health Sciences Centre
University of Toronto
Toronto, Canada

Krista L. Lanctôt, PhD
Neuropsychopharmacology Research
  Program
Sunnybrook Health Sciences Centre
University of Toronto
Toronto, Canada

Harry LeVine III, PhD
Sanders-Brown Center on Aging
Department of Molecular & Cellular
  Biochemistry
University of Kentucky
Lexington, Kentucky, USA

Kangning Liu, PhD
Neurodegeneration Discovery
  Performance Unit
GlaxoSmithKline R&D China
Shanghai, China

Guhan Nagappan, PhD
Neurodegeneration Discovery
  Performance Unit
GlaxoSmithKline R&D China
Shanghai, China

Eric Pang, PhD
Department of Neurology
David Geffen School of Medicine at
    UCLA
Los Angeles, California, USA

Rebecca F. Rosen, PhD
Yerkes National Primate Research
    Center
Emory University
Atlanta, Georgia, USA

Robin Roychaudhuri, PhD
Department of Neurology
David Geffen School of Medicine at
    UCLA
Los Angeles, California, USA

Alan S. Rudolph, PhD, MBA
Center for Neuroengineering
Duke University
Durham, North Carolina, USA

Daniel M. Skovronsky, MD, PhD
Avid Radiopharmaceuticals, Inc.
Philadelphia, Pennsylvania, USA

David B. Teplow, PhD
Mary S. Easton Center for Alzheimer's
    Disease Research at UUA
Department of Neurology

David Geffen School of Medicine at
    UCLA
Los Angeles, California, USA

R. Scott Turner, MD, PhD
Department of Neurology
Georgetown University Medical Center
Washington, D.C., USA

Lary C. Walker, PhD
Yerkes National Primate Research
    Center
Department of Neurology and Center
    for Neurodegenerative Disease
Emory University
Atlanta, Georgia, USA

Renee D. Wegrzyn, PhD
Adlyfe, Inc.
Rockville, Maryland, USA

Mingfeng Yang, PhD
Department of Neurology
David Geffen School of Medicine at
    UCLA
Los Angeles, California, USA

Minhua Zhang, PhD
Neurodegeneration Discovery
    Performance Unit
GlaxoSmithKline R&D China
Shanghai, China

1 The Amyloid β-Protein and Alzheimer's Disease

David B. Teplow, Mingfeng Yang, Robin Roychaudhuri, Eric Pang, Tien-Phat Huynh, Mei-Sha Chen, and Shiela Beroukhim

CONTENTS

1.1   THE MOLECULAR BIOLOGY OF ALZHEIMER'S DISEASE (AD)

1.1.1   "ON AN UNUSUAL ILLNESS OF THE CEREBRAL CORTEX"

In 1906, at a meeting of the South West German Society of Alienists, Dr. Alois Alzheimer presented the case of Auguste D., a 51-year-old woman who had been admitted to a hospital in 1901 with an unusual cluster of symptoms that included reduced comprehension and memory, aphasia, disorientation, unpredictable behavior, paranoia, auditory hallucinations, and pronounced psychosocial impairment. When Dr. Alzheimer first observed her in 1903, Auguste D. was bedridden, incontinent, and was becoming increasingly disoriented, delusional, and incoherent. She eventually required assistance to be fed, was unable to speak, and was often hostile. She died on April 8, 1906. Alzheimer published this case report, entitled "On an Unusual Illness of the Cerebral Cortex," (Alzheimer et al., 1995). He reported brain atrophy and also wrote, "Distributed all over the cortex, but especially numerous in the upper layers, there are minute miliary foci which are caused by the deposition of a special substance in the cortex." This "special substance" comprises extracellular proteinaceous deposits (plaques) of the amyloid β-protein (Aβ) (Alzheimer et al., 1995; Masters et al., 1985). Plaques, and intracellular deposits of tau protein (neurofibrillary tangles [NFT]), have remained pathognomonic histopathologic features of AD since Emil Kraepelin named the disease in 1910 (Kraepelin Emil, 2007).

Plaques are complex, extracellular foci that can vary in size from 5–200 nm and can be divided on the basis of structural appearance into two general types, diffuse and neuritic. Diffuse plaques contain low amounts of fibrillar Aβ, and hence do not stain with the amyloidophilic dye Congo red, nor are they associated with significant neuritic dystrophy or glial infiltration (Duyckaerts and Dickson, 2003). Neuritic plaques are denser, often displaying prominent cores, and contain abundant accretions of Aβ fibrils, stain with Congo red, and are associated with dystrophic neurites and substantial glial cell infiltration. Although tau is the main proteinaceous component of the plaque, acetylcholinesterase, a1-antichymotrypsin, amyloid P component, complement components, apolipoproteins E and J, glycosaminoglycans, and many other macromolecules have been found in plaques (Ariga et al., 2010; Duyckaerts and Dickson, 2003).

Tau deposits are found in the perikarya of neurons and thus are substantially smaller than Aβ plaques. They stain with thioflavin S (an amyloidophilic fluorescent dye) and often appear as bundles of unbranched filaments of diameter 20 nm that are termed *paired helical filaments* (PHF) (Lee et al., 1991; Rubenstein et al., 1986). The helices have a pitch of ≈80 nm. Single filaments of 20–50 nm across also may be observed. The tau protein within NFTs is hyperphosphorylated (Allen and Dawbarn, 2001).

1.1.2 GENETICS AND CELLULAR BIOLOGY OF AD

The modern era of AD research began in 1984, when Glenner and Wong reported the partial amino acid sequence of a 4.2 kDa protein isolated from the cerebrovascular amyloid of an AD brain (Glenner and Wong, 1984b). In a subsequent paper, they reported that the sequence of this protein was homologous to that found in amyloid fibrils isolated from patients suffering from Down's syndrome, suggesting that Down's syndrome might be a model for AD and that the "genetic defect" responsible for AD might be located on chromosome 21 (the chromosome triplicated in Down's syndrome) (Glenner and Wong, 1984a). Glenner's prescience has proven to be accurate. In 1987, four groups cloned the gene encoding Aβ, the amyloid β-protein precursor (AβPP, usually referred to as APP) gene on chromosome 21 (Goldgaber et al., 1987; Kang et al., 1987; Robakis et al., 1987; Tanzi et al., 1987). Alternative splicing produces a number of transcripts, among which the predominant forms produce proteins containing 695, 751, or 770 amino acids. APP is a type I integral membrane glycoprotein. It is not fully understood, but it has been implicated in cell adhesion, neurite growth, synaptogenesis, and promoting cell survival (for a review, see Mattson, 1997).

Aβ is produced from APP through the sequential action of two endoproteolytic activities, β-secretase and γ-secretase, which produce the Aβ N-terminus and C-terminus, respectively (Selkoe et al., 1996) (Figures 1.1 and 1.2). APP also is cleaved intramolecularly, between K16 and L17, by α-secretase, followed by cleavage by γ-secretase. This precludes formation of full-length Aβ, instead producing an N-terminally truncated Aβ peptide, p3 (Haass et al., 1992; Price and Sisodia, 1994; Vassar, 2001). The initial β-secretase or α-secretase cleavage releases the "soluble" APP N-terminal fragments sAPP$_β$ and sAPP$_α$, respectively. sAPP$_β$ decreases cell adhesion and increases axon elongation. sAPP$_α$ may be cytoprotective by reducing the excitotoxic effects of molecules like Aβ and glutamate (Allen and Dawbarn, 2001; Chasseigneaux et al., 2011; St. George-Hyslop and Petit, 2005). γ-secretase action produces the APP intracellular domain (AICD) (Bergmans and De Strooper, 2010), which has been reported to transit to the nucleus and affect gene transcription (Muller et al., 2011). AICD also may affect Ca^{2+} homeostasis by regulating mitochondrial adenosine triphosphate (ATP) levels. A lack of AICD has been correlated with reduced levels of ATP and with hyperpolarization of the inner mitochondrial membrane (Hamid et al., 2007).

The recognition that AD involved a protein that is ubiquitously and continuously expressed in the body (Cai et al., 1993; Haass and Selkoe, 1993) led researchers to determine whether gene defects in APP, and in genes related to it, might cause AD. Indeed, a number of families have been identified in which missense mutations in

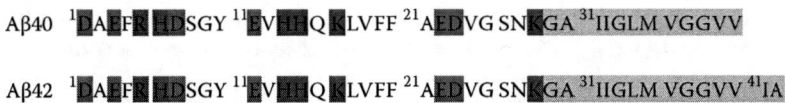

Aβ40 ^{1}DAEFR HDSGY ^{11}EVHHQ KLVFF ^{21}AEDVG SNKGA ^{31}IIGLM VGGVV

Aβ42 ^{1}DAEFR HDSGY ^{11}EVHHQ KLVFF ^{21}AEDVG SNKGA ^{31}IIGLM VGGVV ^{41}IA

FIGURE 1.1 (See color insert.) The primary structures of Aβ40 and Aβ42 are presented. Acidic residues are shaded red, basic residues are shaded blue, and the putative intramembrane peptide segments are shaded yellow.

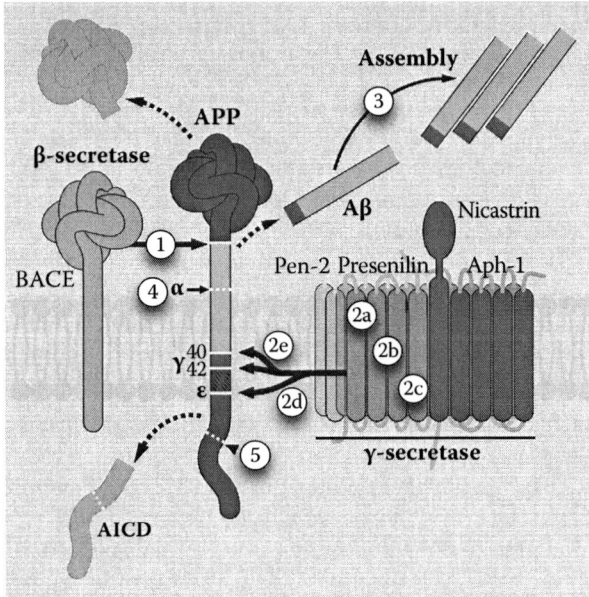

FIGURE 1.2 (See color insert.)   (1) β-secretase (BACE) cleavage of APP and (2) (a–e) by
a multisubunit γ-secretase complex (Nicastrin, Aph-1, Presenilin and Pen-2) to generate Aβ.
2a–2c refer to the active site, docking site and ATP binding site of γ-secretase. 2e refers to
the predilection of γ-secretase for γ or ε cleavage generating Aβ40 or Aβ42. (3) Production
and self-assembly of Aβ to toxic species. (4) APP cleavage by α-secretases (ADAM family
of proteins) precludes the production of Aβ. (5) Caspase cleavage of Aβ intracellular domain
(AICD) generates a C31 fragment that may affect toxicity by Aβ or an independent mechanism. (From E. D. Roberson et al., 2006. "100 Years and Counting: Prospects for Defeating
Alzheimer's Disease." *Science* 314 (5800): 781–784).

APP cause fully penetrant early-onset AD (EOAD) or late-onset AD (LOAD)
(Bertram et al., 2010). In 1994, specific apolipoprotein E (APOE)* alleles were linked
to AD risk (Saunders et al., 1993a; Saunders et al., 1993b; Strittmatter et al., 1993).
More recently, more than 100 highly penetrant mutations have been identified in APP,
PSEN1, and PSEN2 genes that cause EOAD (Tanzi and Bertram, 2001). APOE is the
single most important risk factor for AD (Bertram et al., 2010; Huang et al., 2001;
Tiraboschi et al., 2004). Genome-wide association studies (GWAS) have revealed
additional AD susceptibility loci, each of which may have a small effect on overall
risk for LOAD. These loci include *APOE* (apolipoprotein E), *CR1* (complement receptor 1), *CLU* (clusterin), *PICALM* (the phosphatidylinositol-binding clathrin assembly
protein), *BIN1* (the bridging integrator 1), *EPHA1* (ephrin receptor A1), *MS4A* (membrane spanning 4A), *CD33* (Siglec-3), *CD2AP* (CD2-associated protein), and *ABCA7*
(ATP binding cassette subfamily A, member 7) (Hollingworth et al., 2010; Naj et al.,
2010). *CLU, CR1, ABCA7, CD33,* and *EPHA1* have putative functions in the immune

---

* Genes are noted in all capital letters. The protein products therefrom are indicated by a combination
  of capital and lower case letters.

system. *PICALM, BIN1, CD33*, and *CD2AP* are involved in cell membrane processes and endocytosis. *APOE, CLU*, and *ABCA7* are involved in lipid processing.

1.1.3 THE AMYLOID CASCADE HYPOTHESIS

The extensive and invariant deposition of Aβ in the brain during the progression of AD, along with early studies of familial AD (FAD) that showed that mutations in APP caused autosomal dominant forms of the disease, led Hardy and Higgins in 1992 to propose the *amyloid cascade hypothesis* (Hardy and Higgins, 1992). This hypothesis posited that Aβ deposition was the seminal event in AD pathogenesis. This deposition resulted in a cascade of pathologic events, including NFT formation, cell loss, vascular damage, and dementia. In addition, the hypothesis stated that Aβ, or APP cleavage products were neurotoxic. The fact that autosomal dominant forms of AD are caused by mutations in APP, or in genes affecting Aβ metabolism, support an Aβ-centric view of disease causation.

Until recently, the amyloid cascade hypothesis had been the predominant working hypothesis for AD pathogenesis. However, this hypothesis has been supplanted by what some have called the *oligomer cascade hypothesis*, which posits that Aβ oligomers, rather than fibrils, are the proximate neurotoxic agents in AD (Ono et al., 2009). This new hypothesis arose because testing of the amyloid cascade hypothesis produced an increasing number of inconsistencies. A correlation between the appearance, distribution, and number of amyloid plaques (amyloid load) in the brain and neurodegeneration or synaptic loss has not been established (Arriagada et al., 1992; Bishop and Robinson, 2002; Terry et al., 1991). In contrast, a strong correlation exists between the numbers of NFTs in the cortex and dementia. In addition, the brains of nondemented, cognitively normal elderly individuals can show levels of cortical amyloid deposition as high as those in AD patients (Arriagada et al., 1992).

The development of mouse models of AD has yielded a wealth of information about AD pathobiology and the involvement of Aβ in it. Initial models revealed an obvious correlation between amyloid deposition and neurological status. However, limitations of these mouse models are becoming increasingly clear (Phinney et al., 2003; Radde et al., 2008). Most mouse models expressing FAD mutations develop plaques and exhibit memory deficits from 2–20 months of age, but none display tau tangle pathology or neurodegeneration, the two hallmarks of human AD. Transgenic mice can, however, be "forced" to display tau tangles by inclusion of additional genetic changes. Deletion of the p73 gene (tumor protein 73, a member of the p53 family of tumor suppressors, which is found in the nervous system and postulated to prevent neurodegeneration) (Wetzel et al., 2008) or simultaneously expressing APP and PS1 mutations, as in a 5X (APP K670N/M671L [Swedish]; I716V [Florida]; V717I [London]; PS1 M146L + L286V) FAD mouse model (Oakley et al., 2006), results in animals that rapidly accumulate massive levels of Aβ42 in the brain. These mice display very early amyloid deposition, gliosis, neuron loss, and spatial memory deficits.

The observation that APP-alone mouse models do not show tau pathology or neurodegeneration has led many to classify them as models of amyloidosis rather than AD. In addition, the rates of plaque deposition, as well as deficits in memory, are critically dependent on the mouse strain used and exhibit significant interstrain variations

(Brown and Wong, 2007; Crabbe et al., 1999; Wahlsten et al., 2003; Wolfer et al., 1998). Cheng et al. (Cheng et al., 2007) have shown, in APP transgenic mice carrying mutations adjacent to the Aβ region, that the addition of the Arctic mutation (Glu22Gly; Aβ numbering) markedly enhanced the formation of neuritic plaques but reduced the relative abundance of a 56-kDa, neurotoxic Aβ assembly (Aβ*56). Mice overexpressing the Arctic mutation, or even wild type Aβ, had similar behavioral and neuronal deficits when matched for Aβ*56 levels but had vastly different plaque loads. Thus, Aβ*56 was a likelier determinant of functional deficits in APP mice than were fibrillar Aβ deposits.

In vitro data also have shown that Aβ oligomers are more toxic than fibrils (Dahlgren et al., 2002; Jan et al., 2011; Ono et al., 2009; Sandberg et al., 2010; Shankar et al., 2008). In situ experiments performed in brains of living rats support the hypothesis that oligomers of Aβ have profound electrophysiological effects and may initiate synaptic dysfunction, an early event in AD (Klyubin et al., 2005; Shankar et al., 2007; Townsend et al., 2006). Additional evidence for the role of small, nonfibrillar assemblies has came from studies of the Arctic mutation in AD (Lam et al., 2008; Paivio et al., 2004; Whalen et al., 2005). Roychaudhuri et al. recently reviewed the broad class prefibrillar Aβ assemblies (Roychaudhuri et al., 2009).

1.1.4 PROTEIN COFACTORS IN AD PATHOGENESIS

1.1.4.1 Presenilin

Genetic studies of EOAD kindreds have revealed an important gene causing dominantly inherited FAD, presenilin (PSEN). *PSEN* exists in two forms, *PSEN1* and *PSEN2,* which reside on chromosomes 14 and 1, respectively (Rogaev et al., 1995; Sherrington et al., 1995). Both genes encode novel integral membrane proteins with 67% identity and 84% similarity (Levy-Lahad et al., 1995; Sherrington et al., 1995). The presenilin genes belong to a family of genes with high conservation among species. The human proteins are almost identical with their rat counterparts and show a high degree of similarity with *C. elegans* homologs *sel-12* and *spe-4* (Levitan et al., 1995; Sherrington et al., 1995). The *PSEN1* locus is ≈75 kb in size and comprises 12 exons, of which exons 3–12 constitute the protein open reading frame. *PSEN2* comprises 10 exons within an ≈90 kb gene locus. PS1 (Presenilin 1) and PS2 (Presenilin 2), the cognate proteins, are expressed in most tissues (Rogaev et al., 1995; Sherrington et al., 1995), including brain (primarily in neurons; see Kovacs et al., 1996), heart, liver, pancreas, spleen, kidney, and testis. *PSEN* mutations cause the majority of FAD, as evidenced by the >160 mutations in *PSEN1* and 10 mutations in *PSEN2* that have been identified in autosomal dominant AD kindreds. Most PS1 mutations are simple missense mutations that result in single amino acid substitutions in PS1 (De Strooper, 2007). *PSEN1* mutations are highly penetrant and cause aggressive forms of AD. The PS2 mutations N141I, M239V, and R62H display greater variability in penetrance and age of onset (Sherrington et al., 1996). In addition to missense mutations, a deletion mutant has been identified in which exon 9 (DE9) is missing (Crook et al., 1998). Mutations in either presenilin or APP increase the relative ratio between Aβ42/Aβ40 (De Strooper, 2007).

The PS holopresenilins are ≈50 kDa in molecular mass, but are processed post-translationally to yield an amino terminal fragment of ≈27–30 kDa and a carboxyl terminal fragment of ≈16–18 kDa (Wolfe, 2010). The PS proteins possess nine transmembrane peptide segments (Bergmans and De Strooper, 2010; Wakabayashi et al., 2008). PS is an aspartyl protease that acts within a heterotetramer comprising PS, nicastrin, Aph1 and Pen2, which together form a barrel-like structure in the membrane. Nicastrin is a 130-kDa type I integral membrane glycoprotein. Aph1 is a 25-kDa, seven-segment transmembrane protein. Pen 2 is a small hairpin-like protein with a molecular weight of ≈12kDa.

Recent data suggest that Aph1 contributes directly to the proteolytic activity of the complex by influencing the catalytic subunit of PS1 (Serneels et al., 2009). Cysteine scanning experiments have shown that the substrate binding site in PS1 lies in transmembrane domain 9. Alternative splicing of the different subunit genes results in heterogeneity of the enzyme complex. Data extant suggest that these altered complexes have quite different physiological properties. g-secretase, in addition to its role in producing Aβ, is a central effector of regulated intramembrane proteolysis (RIP) (Wolfe and Kopan, 2004), a process common to many proteins, including N-cadherin, E-cadherin, the neurotrophin receptor p75, the regulated β2 subunit of voltage-gated sodium channels, the axon guidance molecule DCC, and neuregulin (Bergmans and De Strooper, 2010). The central role of γ-secretase in Notch signaling in *Drosophila* and *C. elegans* has been unequivocally demonstrated. A PS cleavage mechanism has been proposed in which the substrate docks on the outer surface of the complex and then is transported to the active site cleft for hydrolysis (De Strooper and Annaert, 2010). The enzyme cuts APP initially at the ε-site and then progressively removes C-terminal residues until the g-cleavage site has been reached. Molecular weight estimates of the γ-secretase complex have been highly divergent, ranging from 250 to >2,000 kDa.

PS1 has been shown to be essential in mouse embryonic development. Its function in adult animals remains unknown. PS1$^{-/-}$ mice exhibit premature death, with embryos exhibiting abnormal patterning of the axial skeleton and spinal ganglia (Allen and Dawbarn, 2001). PS2 is a proapototic factor (Vito et al., 1996). PS2$^{-/-}$ mice display mild, transient apoptosis in lungs and mild pulmonary fibrosis (Herreman et al., 1999). Overexpression of PS2 in nerve growth factor (NGF)-differentiated PC12 cells enhances apoptosis upon NGF withdrawal (Wolozin et al., 1996). Recent data have revealed that the function of the presenilins extends beyond their functions as γ-secretases. Presenilins may constitute calcium leak channels in the endoplasmic reticulum (Nelson et al., 2007) and affect the regulation of ryanodine receptors and inositol 1,4,5-triphosphate receptors, resulting in increased accumulation of Ca^{2+} in the endoplasmic reticulum (Bergmans and De Strooper, 2010; Kovacs et al., 2010). Presenilin interacts with β-catenin and members of the *armadillo* family in regulating phosphorylation by protein kinase A and glycogen synthase kinase 3β (GSK-3β) followed by proteasomal degradation.

A presenilin hypothesis of AD suggests that partial loss of PS function might underlie impairment of memory and cause neurodegeneration in AD, and that Aβ42 may act primarily to antagonize PS-dependent functions by acting as an active site inhibitor of γ-secretase (Shen and Kelleher, 2007).

1.1.4.2 Apolipoprotein E

ApoE is a 34 kDa glycoprotein (Mahley 1988). ApoE is involved in the mobilization and redistribution of cholesterol in the turnover of myelin and neuronal membranes during development or after injury in the peripheral nervous system (Boyles et al.,

1990; Boyles et al., 1989; Ignatius et al., 1987; Poirier et al., 1991). In the central nervous system (CNS), ApoE, in combination with ApoJ and ApoC1, plays an important role in cholesterol delivery during membrane remodeling in synaptic turnover and dendritic reorganization (Leduc et al., 2010). Three isoforms exist in humans, ApoE2, ApoE3, and ApoE4, which are encoded by the cognate genes *APOE-ε2, APOE-ε3*, and *APOE-ε4* (Mahley 1988). These isoforms differ from each other only at amino acids 112 and 158. Apo3, the most common isoform, contains C112, R158, whereas apoE2 and apoE4 contain C112, C158 or R112, R158, respectively.

The ε4 allele of *APOE* is a major risk factor for AD and affects disease pathogenesis (Bertram et al., 2010; Roses et al., 1995; Saunders et al., 1993a; Strittmatter et al., 1993). The potential involvement of cholesterol transporters in APP metabolism and the role of ApoE come from initial observations made by Sparks (Leduc et al., 2010; Sparks et al., 2000; Sparks et al., 1995). Cholesterol transporters, like ApoE, ApoC1, and ApoJ, are major risk factors in AD (Hollingworth et al., 2010; Naj et al., 2010). *APOE-ε4* carriers account for 65–80% of all AD cases. Lowering cholesterol levels apparently decreases Aβ production (Huang 2010). Exposure to cholesterol-lowering agents such as probucol and the statins reduces the amyloid load in cultured cells and in murine models of AD (Champagne et al., 2003; Poirier 2003).

Progressive deterioration in cholesterol homeostasis correlates with AD progression (Sparks et al., 2000; Sparks et al., 1995). Specifically, ApoE4 inhibits tubulin polymerization in neurons (Holtzman et al., 1995; Nathan et al., 1995). It also impairs synaptogenesis in *APOE* transgenic mice and gene-targeted mice, and in primary neuronal cultures (Dumanis et al., 2009; Ji et al., 2003). Increased plaque and tangle load has been observed in AD cases expressing the *APOE-ε4* allele (Small and Duff, 2008; Tiraboschi et al., 2004). Cerebrospinal fluid (CSF) studies also have shown an association between *APOE-ε4*, Aβ, and phospho-tau levels (Glodzik-Sobanska et al., 2009). The involvement of *APOE* in disease pathogenesis also has come from a host of cell and animal models showing that allele type affects both Aβ and plaque accumulation (Bales et al., 2002; Demattos et al., 2004; Dodart et al., 2005). In addition, and importantly, the data suggest that ApoE affects Aβ and tau through independent mechanisms.

It has been suggested that ApoE released from astroglia clears Aβ from the brain parenchyma, but that ApoE4 is relatively ineffective (Bales et al., 2002; Demattos et al., 2004). The exact clearance mechanism is unknown, although isoform-dependent modulation of the local steady-state levels of ApoE is an attractive hypothesis because plasma ApoE concentrations have been reported to display the following rank order (highest to lowest) ApoE2 > ApoE3 > ApoE4 (Bales et al., 2009; Poirier 2008). Numerous in vitro studies have shown that human ApoE facilitates cellular Aβ uptake and degradation. ApoE promotes brain-to-blood removal of Aβ by transport across the blood–brain barrier, and as above, the efficiency of this process follows the rank order ApoE2 > ApoE3 > ApoE4 (Bales et al., 2009).

ApoE also may be involved in tau hyperphosphorylation. ApoE has been shown to activate GSK-3β (Hoe et al., 2006; Ohkubo et al., 2003). ApoE4 has the greatest activating activity and has the least affinity for tau at its GSK-3β binding site (Cedazo-Minguez et al., 2003; Gibb et al., 2000). It is also possible that ApoE binds tau, directly blocking access to the GSK-3β phosphorylation site (Huang et al., 1995). ApoE4 may also bind tau less avidly, increasing the likelihood of GSK-3β-mediated hyperphosphorylation (Gibb et al., 2000; Strittmatter and Roses, 1995). A compelling mechanism linking ApoE, GSK-3β, and tau phosphorylation does not require direct interaction with tau, but rather involves the low-density lipoprotein (LDL) receptor-related protein (LRP) that binds ApoE. LRP5 and LRP6 are the LRPs most directly involved in regulating GSK-3β as a part of the *wnt* signaling pathway (Caruso et al., 2006). LRP5 and LRP6, along with the *frizzled* family proteins, comprise a complex to which *wnt* can bind (De Ferrari and Moon, 2006; Halleskog et al., 2011). ApoE has been shown to inhibit this pathway by causing up-regulation of GSK-3β activity (Caruso et al., 2006). A genetic study in late-onset patients also has shown a link between ApoE and LRP6, suggesting that the identified LRP6 genetic variant affects *wnt* signaling, which is mediated by increased GSK-3β activity (De Ferrari et al., 2007). Indirect evidence for the ApoE:GSK-3β mechanism has been provided in gene expression studies in the entorhinal cortex, which is the site of initiation of tau pathology (Liang et al., 2007). Although studies in the in vitro models show an interaction among ApoE, tau, and GSK-3β, and *APOE-ε4* mice show some degree of tau hyperphosphorylation, these data should be interpreted cautiously because evidence for these interactions in vivo is still lacking.

Although the role of ApoE in Aβ metabolism is widely accepted, its role in influencing Aβ aggregation is controversial. In vitro studies show that ApoE isoforms affect Aβ aggregation by interfering with the nucleation step of aggregation, with ApoE4 being least effective (Evans et al., 1995; Ladu et al., 1995). These in vitro data contrast with in vivo data that show that *APOE* gene knockdown in mice significantly decreases Aβ deposition and thioflavin-S positive plaques (Holtzman et al., 2000). However, transgenic mice expressing human ApoE also show a decrease in Aβ deposition and plaque formation (Leduc et al., 2010).

ApoE also has Aβ-independent effects. In the absence of Aβ accumulation in transgenic mice overexpressing C-terminally truncated (D272-299) ApoE4, neuronal and behavioral deficits are observed (Harris et al., 2003). Mice expressing ApoE4 in astrocytes have impaired working memory compared with mice expressing ApoE3 (Hartman et al., 2001). In mouse organotypic hippocampal slice cultures, ApoE3 stimulates, but ApoE4 inhibits, neuronal sprouting (Teter et al., 2002). ApoE4 also inhibits tubulin polymerization in neuronal cells by the HSPG–LRP pathway (Holtzman et al., 1995; Nathan et al., 1995). ApoE receptors mediate neurite outgrowth by activating the *Erk* pathway in primary neuronal cultures. In rat primary cortical neuronal cultures, the addition of exogenous ApoE4, or a proteolytic fragment thereof, decreases the density of dendritic spines (Harris et al., 2003). Neuronal ApoE4 is more susceptible to proteolytic cleavage than neuronal ApoE3 (Huang et al., 2001). The ApoE4 fragments are present at much higher levels in the AD brain compared to age- and sex-matched controls (Harris et al., 2003; Huang et al., 2001). C-terminally truncated ApoE4 also has been found to be neurotoxic in vivo in transgenic mice and leads to AD-like neurodegeneration and behavioral deficits (Huang et al., 2001). In addition, ApoE4, but not ApoE2 or ApoE3, stimulates tau phosphorylation and formation of intracellular NFT-like inclusions in transgenic mice. ApoE4 fragments also target neuronal mitochondria leading to mitochondrial dysfunction and neurotoxicity (Chang et al., 2005; Huang 2010). In humans, both the Aβ-independent and Aβ-dependent effects of ApoE4 may act synergistically to produce the AD phenotype.

1.1.4.3 Tau

Tau protein is an important structural component of microtubules (Friedhoff et al., 1998; Giasson et al., 2003; Revesz and Holton, 2003). It is involved in microtubule stabilization, which is critical to normal neuronal function (Duyckaerts and Dickson, 2003). The gene encoding tau is located on chromosome 17 and has four 31–32 amino acid C-terminal tandem repeats (Goedert 2003). The gene is composed of 16 exons, 11 of which are expressed in the central nervous system, and the pre-mRNA undergoes alternative splicing of exons 2, 3, and 10. Exons 2 and 3 each encode 29 amino acids. The inclusion of exon 2 is coupled to exon 3 inclusion, but not vice versa. Exon 10 encodes the 31 amino acids comprising the second of the four microtubule-binding domains. Alternative splicing of exon 10 results in four-repeat (4R) tau or 3R tau. Tau thus may exist in humans in six different isoforms ([2N (both exons 2 and 3), 1N (exon 3 only), or 0N (neither)] ´ [3-repeat or 4-repeat]). Both the three- and four-repeat forms are equally expressed in the cortex (Cummings and Apostolova, 2007; Wolfe 2009).

Tau pathology is an invariant and pathognomonic feature of AD. This pathology comprises NFTs, neuropil threads, and dystrophic neurites. NFTs are composed of PHFs of tau that are 10–20 nm in width. Each paired helical filament nucleus is composed of 8–14 tau monomers (Cummings and Apostolova, 2007; Friedhoff et al., 1998). The tau comprising NFTs has been found to display truncation, phosphorylation, and glycation. Neuropil threads are commonly seen in AD and rarely identified in other kinds of tauopathies (Feany and Dickson, 1996). The threads are short, tortuous, thread-like structures that are found in dendrites (Duyckaerts and Dickson, 2003). Dystrophic neurites are dendritic structures that contain hyperphosphorylated tau and are seen in the periphery of the senile plaques (Baskakov, 2007). Dystrophic neurites appear swollen by abnormal accumulations of filaments, vesicles, tubules, and mitochondria (Fiala et al., 2007). NFTs accumulate initially in the transentorhinal area, layer II of the lateral entorhinal cortex, and the perirhinal cortex (Braak et al., 2000; Hof 1997; Van Hoesen et al., 2000). As the disease progresses, the NFTs affect layer II of the medial entorhinal cortex and the rest of the parahippocampal gyrus. In later stages, the tangles are seen in layer IV of entorhinal cortex (Van Hoesen et al., 2000). They spread to the hippocampus affecting the subiculum and the CA1 area, and later CA2, CA3, and CA4. The tangles then invade the temporal neocortex first on the medial and inferior and later on the lateral surface involving the parietal and frontal association cortices (Cummings and Apostolova, 2007). In the parahippocampal cortex of patients affected with NFT-predominant dementia, a subset of late onset dementia that is clinically different from traditional plaque and tangle AD, a higher frequency of "ghost tangles" is observed (Jellinger and Attems, 2007; Probst et al., 2007). *Ghost tangles are NFT that remain after neuron destruction. They display reduced basophilia.* During the progress of fibrillar tau inclusion maturation, tau fibrils are being formed, accumulate, and may be continuously modified (Mohorko et al., 2010). Biochemically, ghost tangles contain abnormally phosphorylated tau that is truncated both at the N- and C-terminus (Endoh et al., 1993).

A number of studies have suggested a link between Aβ and tau. Double transgenic mice expressing mutant APP and tau showed enhanced neurofibrillary tangle formation compared with single mutant tau mice (Lewis et al., 2001). Gotz et al. (Gotz et al., 2001) showed that injecting synthetic Aβ42 fibrils into the somatosensory cortex and the hippocampus of 5- to 6-month-old P301L tau transgenic mice significantly accelerated NFT formation. Neither Aβ, nor the mutant form of tau alone, was sufficient to produce large numbers of NFTs, suggesting that an increase in NFT pathology was a result of a tau–Aβ interaction. Support for tau–Aβ interactions also has come from studies showing that clearing Aβ by passive immunotherapy caused a reduction in preexisting tau pathology (Oddo et al., 2004). The clearance of intraneuronal Aβ led to a decrease in extracellular Aβ, and subsequently to a clearance of intracellular phospho-tau (Laferla 2010).

Another study by Oddo et al. (Oddo et al., 2007) also points to the lack of significant tauopathy in amyloid-only and tau-only mouse models. Their study shows that the tau–Aβ interaction is unidirectional, because genetically increasing tau levels and hyperphosphorylation in a triple (M146V PS1, Swedish APP, P301L tau) transgenic AD mouse model had no effect on the onset or progression of Aβ pathology (Oddo et al., 2007). A possible mechanistic explanation for the robust pathology in the bitransgenic models (V717 APP, P301L tau) and (GSK-3β, P301L tau) is that amyloid deposition increases GSK-3β and GSK-3α activity (Terwel et al., 2008), resulting in tau hyperphosphorylation.

Cognitive decline in AD and tauopathies correlates with the aggregation of Aβ and tau, respectively (Ashe and Zahs, 2010). In vivo data shows that these types of cognitive decline and neuropathology result from synergistic interactions among Aβ, tau, and even α-synuclein (Clinton et al., 2010). In a cellular model of memory measuring long-term potentiation (LTP), tau phosphorylation was a prerequisite for Aβ-induced impairment of synaptic plasticity in the hippocampus (Shipton et al., 2011). Recent data by Roberson et al. (2011) showed that tau reduction prevented cognitive decline due to the synergistic effects of Aβ and *Fyn*. Additional effects of tau reduction included lack of synaptic transmission, spontaneous epileptiform activity, and deficits in plasticity in multiple lines of hAPP mice. Reduction of tau also reduced the severity and spontaneity of chemically induced seizures in mice overexpressing both Aβ and *Fyn*. This suggests that Aβ, tau, and *Fyn* function jointly in disrupting synaptic and network function (Roberson et al., 2011).

An interaction between Aβ oligomers and tau has been shown in studies of the intracellular and extracellular clearance of Aβ deposits by Aβ-specific antibodies, which results in the subsequent disappearance of preexistent tau pathology, in neuronal protection, and in the reversal of memory deficits in a 3 × Tg-AD mouse model (Oddo et al., 2006). Rhein et al. (Rhein et al., 2009a), in another triple transgenic model (pR5 × APP/PS2), showed that 8-month-old mice had a reduction in mitochondrial membrane potential, but at 12 months of age, the effects were the strongest and affected oxidative phosphorylation and synthesis of ATP and reactive oxygen species, implying a molecular link between Aβ and tau in AD in vivo. In a separate study involving two transgenic mouse models (APPSw/NOS2$^{-/-}$ and APPSwD1/NOS2$^{-/-}$) that appear to model AD more closely, Wilcock et al. (Wilcock et al., 2009) showed that there was a 30% reduction in brain Aβ and a 35–45% reduction in hyperphosphorylated tau in Aβ42- or KLH-vaccinated APPSwD1/NOS2$^{-/-}$ mice. In APPSw/NOS2$^{-/-}$ animals, brain Aβ was reduced by 65–85% and hyperphosphorylated tau was reduced by 50–60%. These studies point to a link between Aβ and tau and the interdependence of the respective pathologies.

Aβ-mediated reduction in tau pathology could involve the C-terminus of heat shock protein 70 interacting protein (CHIP). CHIP is a tau ubiquitin ligase. Its deletion leads to tau accumulation (Dickey et al., 2006; Petrucelli et al., 2004). CHIP expression decreases as Aβ accumulates, and a concomitant increase in tau levels is then observed (Oddo et al., 2008). Increased CHIP expression has been shown to rescue the effects of Aβ on tau pathology. The fact that Aβ oligomers impair proteasome activity and contribute to the age-related pathological accumulation of Aβ and tau are consistent with this mechanism (Tseng et al., 2008).

Recently, an intriguing study suggested that tau might affect Aβ-mediated excitotoxic effects (Ittner et al., 2010). *Excitotoxicity* is a pathological process through which neurons are damaged or killed by excessive stimulation by neurotransmitters such as glutamate. Tau was shown to be involved in dendritic postsynaptic targeting of *Fyn*, thereby facilitating postsynaptic Aβ toxicity (Ittner et al., 2010). Consistent with this observation were prior studies demonstrating that reducing endogenous levels of tau protected against excitotoxicity and prevented behavioral deficits in transgenic mice expressing human APP (Roberson et al., 2007).

1.1.4.4   Prions

Prions are *pro*teinaceous *in*fectious agents that cause kuru, Creutzfeldt-Jakob disease (CJD), Gerstmann-Straussler-Scheinker (GSS) syndrome, and fatal familial insomnia (FFI) in humans (Hsiao et al., 1989; Masters et al., 1981; Prusiner, 1991). Prion diseases have sporadic, genetic, and infectious etiologies, which make these *prionoses* unique among human diseases (Masters et al., 1979). Prions belong to the disease class *transmissible spongiform encephalopathies* (TSE), which reflects one aspect of disease etiology (infectiousness) and one aspect of disease neuropathology (spongiform changes). Prions also cause scrapie (sheep), bovine spongiform encephalopathy (BSE), chronic wasting disease (white-tailed deer, mule deer, elk, and moose), transmissible mink encephalopathy, and feline spongiform encephalopathy (Prusiner, 2001).

The prion gene, *PRNP*, was cloned in 1985 (Oesch et al., 1985). *PRNP* encodes a protein, PrP, containing 254 amino acids in its nascent form. Post-translational processing results in removal of an N-terminal signal sequence of 22 amino acids as well as the C-terminal 23 amino acids (Bolton et al., 1987; Turk et al., 1988). This latter processing event allows creation of a glycosylphosphatidylinositol (GPI) anchor attached to Ser231 (Stahl et al., 1987). This normal cellular GPI-anchored form of PrP is referred to as PrP^c (cellular) (Basler et al., 1986). In addition to the GPI anchor, PrP contains a disulfide bridge between Cys179 and Cys214. PrP^c contains two N-linked glycosylation sites (Asn181 and Asn197 of human PrP; Asn180 and Asn196 of mouse PrP), to which high-mannose-type oligosaccharides are attached.

Insights into the effects of glycosylation have been obtained through studies using short synthetic PrP peptides. The unglycosylated form of a peptide derived from helix 2 of the prion protein (residues 175–195) was found to rapidly acquire β-sheet structure and form fibrils. However, the rate of fibril formation was significantly decelerated when the same peptide sequence was synthesized as a glycosylated peptide (Bosques and Imperiali, 2003). A similar effect was observed in the presence of O-linked sugars on PrP (108–144) (Chen et al., 2002). Although O-linked sugars have not been detected on PrP^c or PrP^{Sc}, these studies indicate that glycosylation can alter the equilibrium between monomeric PrP^c and an aggregated PrP form (Lawson et al., 2005).

The physiological roles of prions remain elusive. Prions are thought to be involved in controlling cellular oxidative stress and physical stresses. Nico et al. (Nico et al., 2005) have reported that PrP^c does not seem to be necessary for most behavioral functions in mice. However, they show that under situations that involve stress, the absence of PrP^c results in behavioral abnormalities. PrP^c has also been shown to exert a neuroprotective role against kainate (KA)-induced neurotoxicity, probably by regulating the expression of KA receptor subunits (Rangel et al., 2007).

Nuclear magnetic resonance (NMR) studies have shown that the normal protein fold is globular and comprises three helices and a short anti-parallel β-sheet (Riek et al., 1996). This normal structure converts into a form that causes disease, PrP^{Sc} (PrP scrapie), so designated because of the original linkage of prion diseases to scrapie in sheep. The PrP^C→PrP^{Sc} conversion involves a conformational change of α-helix into β-sheet (Pan et al., 1993). NMR studies of Syrian hamster PrP (23–231) (Tycko et al., 2010) show that PrP fibrils are in-register parallel β-sheets and includes the C-terminal region in the structurally ordered fibril cores. The C-terminal region includes residues 175–225 that form the second and third α-helices of monomeric PrP.

One of the most interesting aspects of prion biology is that pathogenetic characteristics, including species barriers, incubation time, and neuropathology, are "encoded" in the structure of the prion, not in its cognate structural gene (Prusiner, 1991). Different prions structures produce different characteristics of disease that are subsumed under the rubric of prion "strains" (Dickinson et al., 1968). Strain characteristics are propagated autocatalytically from existing PrP^{Sc} to nascent PrP^C proteins.

Similarities exist between the prionoses and AD. Both involve aberrant protein folding and amyloid deposition (Wisniewski et al., 1998). AD, variant CJD (vCJD), and GSS are associated with tau pathology, albeit the levels of tau are lower in the prion diseases (Giaccone et al., 2008). The *APOE-ε4* allele is a risk factor for both AD and CJD. Individuals expressing *APOE-ε4* have an increased risk of dementia after acute head injury or stroke, along with increased susceptibility to Parkinson's disease, multiple sclerosis, amyotrophic lateral sclerosis, human immunodeficiency virus, and herpes simplex virus (Bales et al., 2009). *APOE-e2* lowers the risk of AD and CJD (Gunther and Strittmatter, 2010). Interestingly, it has been reported that oligomeric Aβ also possesses infectious prion-like propagation characteristics (Meyer-Luehmann et al., 2006).

Intriguing experimental evidence suggests that PrP may be a pathogenetic cofactor of Aβ in AD. PrP^c has been found to colocalize with Aβ in plaques (Ikeda et al., 1994;

Miyazono et al., 1992), and conversely, AD-type pathology has been observed in CJD patients (Debatin et al., 2008). Recent genetic studies have suggested that *PRNP* is an AD susceptibility gene (Kellett and Hooper, 2009). In addition, a Met129Val polymorphism in *PRNP* may also predispose to early onset AD (Del Bo et al., 2006; Dermaut et al., 2003; Riemenschneider et al., 2004).

One mechanism responsible for an Aβ:PrP linkage would be direct physical interactions among PrP, Aβ, or APP. Expression cloning experiments recently identified the PrP^c region between amino acids 95–110 as a high-affinity and high-selectivity Aβ42 oligomer binding site (Lauren et al., 2009; Nygaard and Strittmatter, 2009). Site-directed spin labeling and surface plasmon resonance studies have confirmed this result and demonstrated that an additional, highly basic, binding region, 23–27, is critical to the interaction of PrP with Aβ42 oligomers (Chen et al., 2010). Deletion experiments suggested that the PrP(95–110) and PrP(23–27) act in concert. Recombinant PrP^c interacted with Aβ42 oligomers in "pull-down" assays and binding of synthetic Aβ42 oligomers to neurons was decreased in PrP$^{-/-}$ mice. Studies on hippocampal slices from these PrP null mice showed that LTP was not affected by addition of Aβ assemblies, whereas the opposite was true in wild-type slices. It thus was hypothesized that PrP^c acts as a receptor for Aβ42 oligomers. The authors did note, however, that other Aβ receptors also may exist, including APLP1, 30B, and the receptor for advanced glycation end products (RAGE).

These studies raised important questions, including: (1) what is the structural relationship between the synthetic Aβ oligomers used in the study and those produced naturally in the brains? (2) how do the Aβ-induced effects on LTP observed in the brain slices relate to the impairment in cognitive abilities in AD? and (3) how does the binding of Aβ to PrP^c affect neuronal plasticity (Cisse and Mucke, 2009)?

It should be noted that some have failed to reproduce the findings discussed above. For example, Kessels et al. showed that PrP^c was *not* required for Aβ-induced synaptic deficits, reduction in spine density, or diminished LTP (Kessels et al., 2010). Using Sindbis virus–infected organotypic hippocampal slice cultures expressing a C-terminal of APP construct (C100), Kessels et al. showed that increased expression and secretion of Aβ does not affect the function of neurons in electrophysiological studies. Exogenous application of synthetic Aβ42 oligomers showed no difference in loss of dendritic spines in wild-type or PrP$^{-/-}$ mice, indicating that PrP^c did not mediate the effect of Aβ42 on spine density. LTP induction by theta burst stimulation of hippocampal slices in wild-type and PrP$^{c-/-}$ mice showed similar levels of inhibition by Aβ42 in both genotypes. These studies suggest that although Aβ may bind to PrP^c, the latter protein does not seem to be the receptor responsible for synaptic and neurological deficits. Lauren et al. suggested that the viral expression system used in the Kessel study likely produced monomeric Aβ, which would have low binding affinity for PrP^c, and that the Aβ42 oligomer concentrations were an order of magnitude higher than the original study, thus likely producing PrP^c-independent effects (Kessels et al., 2010). Most recently, Balducci et al. (2010) reported that intracerebroventricular injections of synthetic Aβ42 oligomers, but not fibrils, into 7- to 8-week-old normal C57BL/6 male mice, impaired consolidation of long-term memory. Although the oligomers bound PrP^c with high affinity, the two proteins did not act together to induce memory derangement. Gimbel et al.

reported that PrP and Aβ were required for the induction of cognitive deficits, but not behavioral changes, in an AD mouse model (Gimbel et al., 2010). It appears that the PrP:Aβ question remains unanswered, but the question certainly is worthy of additional study.

Intriguingly, in addition to Aβ, PrP^c may interact with β-secretase (Parkin et al., 2007), inhibiting the β-secretase cleavage of APP and thus regulating the production of Aβ. This interaction results in a reduction of Aβ levels in human neuroblastoma N2a cells and in PrP^-/- mice. The regulatory role of PrP^c on β-secretase cleavage of APP required the localization of PrP^c to lipid rafts and was shown to be mediated by the N-terminal region of PrP^c through glycosaminoglycans (GAGs). A possible mechanism by which PrP^c regulates the cleavage of APP by β-secretase is by the N-terminus of PrP^c interacting via GAGs with one or more heparin binding sites on β-secretase within a subset of lipid rafts, thereby providing restricted access of β-secretase to APP (Parkin et al., 2007). PrP thus may regulate Aβ production, suggesting that it is protective in AD.

A key issue in the interpretation of data produced in the studies discussed previously, and in all Aβ studies, is the heterogeneity of Aβ assemblies and their transient nature (Teplow, 2006). Characterization of the different Aβ assembly states is key in studies that seek to eventually identify a therapeutic target for AD and in future studies that point to the involvement of Aβ in AD pathogenesis.

1.2   THE STRUCTURAL BIOLOGY OF Aβ ASSEMBLIES

The historical working hypothesis for Aβ and AD, the *amyloid cascade hypothesis*, posited that fibril formation is the seminal pathologic process (Haass and Selkoe, 2007). For this reason, a tremendous amount of work has focused on elucidating pathways of fibril assembly, the goal being to identify targets for inhibitors of this process. The importance of this goal was strengthened by early results suggesting that Aβ fibril formation was required for neurotoxicity (Haass and Selkoe, 2007). Since that time, a myriad of different neurotoxic Aβ assemblies have been reported, ranging in size from dimers to fibrils and other polymer types (for a recent review, see Roychaudhuri et al., 2009). Interestingly, all of these assemblies are neurotoxic, suggesting that many potential therapeutic targets exist. We discuss here the structures and assembly dynamics of this interesting array of Aβ assemblies.

1.2.1   MONOMERS

Aβ monomers exist *in vivo* predominately in two forms, Aβ40 and Aβ42, which contain 40 or 42 amino acids, respectively (Figure 1.1). The Aβ sequence is amphipathic in nature. The N-terminal 28 residues comprise both hydrophilic and hydrophobic groups, whereas the C-terminal 12–14 residues are all uncharged and largely apolar. In aqueous solution, Aβ is largely disordered, comprising a series of loops and turns (Hou et al., 2004; Zhang et al., 2000), and tends to aggregate rapidly, making structural determination studies difficult (Teplow, 2006). In water–alcohol mixtures or micellar solutions, Aβ possesses substantial α-helical conformation, with two helical segments connected by a flexible kink region (Coles et al., 1998; Crescenzi et al., 2002; Sticht et al., 1995; Tomaselli et al., 2006). The Aβ(21–30) segment is resistant to protease digestion, and nuclear magnetic resonance (NMR) analysis and computer simulations suggest this region exists as a turn structure that is stabilized by hydrophobic interaction between Val24 and Lys28 and by salt-bridge interactions between Glu22/Asp23 and Lys28 (Baumketner et al., 2006; Borreguero et al., 2005; Chen et al., 2006; Cruz et al., 2005; Fawzi et al., 2008; Grant et al., 2007; Krone et al., 2008; Lazo et al., 2005; Murray et al., 2009; Tarus et al., 2008). These turn characteristics have led to the hypothesis that this turn nucleates Aβ monomer folding (Lazo et al., 2005).

Although Aβ42 has only two additional amino acids at its C-terminus, Ile-Ala, it has significantly greater aggregation propensity and neurotoxicity than does Aβ40 (Dahlgren et al., 2002; Walsh et al., 1999). NMR studies, however, reveal little structural difference between the two peptides at the monomer level, other than the C-terminus of Aβ42 being "more rigid" than that of Aβ40 (Hou and Zagorski, 2006; Yan and Wang, 2006; Yang and Teplow, 2008). In silico studies of Aβ monomer conformational dynamics suggest that this increased rigidity may be due to the formation of a C-terminal β-hairpin-like structure that promotes Aβ42 aggregation (Yang and Teplow, 2008).

1.2.2 Low-Order Oligomers

Aβ oligomer structures are relatively poorly defined. The metrics used in the definitions are more descriptive than atomic, including oligomer order (such as monomer, dimer, trimer), morphology, and molecular weight. Structural differences between monomers, oligomers, and fibrils have been probed using antibody-binding properties. Glabe produced two antibody preparations, the polyclonal serum A11 and the polyclonal OC, which were specific for oligomers and fibrils, respectively (Glabe, 2008). They found that there are two distinct types of oligomers: prefibrillar oligomers that are OC negative and A11 positive, and fibrillar oligomers that are OC positive and A11 negative. They suggest that in order for oligomers to transform into fibrils, a structural or conformational change is necessary on the transient intermediate level of oligomers. Once *prefibrillar oligomers* transform into *fibrillar oligomers*, fibrillar oligomers may act as nuclei to which monomers can add to form elongated fibrils.[*] It should be noted that the A11 antibody is not Aβ-specific, but rather oligomer-specific, as it can recognize oligomers from a-synuclein, islet amyloid polypeptide, polyglutamine peptides, lysozyme, human insulin, and prion peptides (Kayed et al., 2003).

Studies of chemically stabilized Aβ oligomers of specific order have revealed an order-dependent increase in β-strand content (Bitan et al., 2003; Bitan et al., 2001; Ono et al., 2009). This increase in structural order was paralleled by increases in fibril seeding activity and specific neurotoxic activity (Ono et al.,

---

[*] The terms **prefibrillar oligomers** and **fibrillar oligomers** illustrate the difficulty of defining oligomer structures accurately and unambiguously. The former term refers to the assembly pathway in which the oligomer exists, namely that of fibril formation, and not to assembly morphology per se. The latter term refers to the morphology of the assembly rather than to its aggregation number. The authors suggest that it would be beneficial to the field to develop an agreed-upon nomenclature that was less ambiguous and more informative.

2009). Interestingly, and importantly, the order dependence of these activities increased disproportionately with oligomer order. Dimers were ≈3-fold more toxic than monomers, whereas trimers and tetramers were ≈8- to 13-fold more toxic, respectively. Dimers were approximately one order of magnitude more efficient nucleators of fibril formation than were monomers, whereas trimers and tetramers were approximately two orders of magnitude more efficient (Ono et al., 2009).

These results have implications for the targeting of therapeutic agents to appropriate oligomer types. In particular, the data suggest that because higher-order oligomers are substantially more toxic than are lower-order oligomers, these should be primary therapeutic targets. However, medicinal chemists also must consider the relative abundance of each oligomer type. First principles, and experimental data on nucleation and polymerization parameters of the Aβ system (Lomakin et al., 1997; Lomakina et al., 1996), suggest that the most abundant oligomer species will be those of lowest order (Ono et al., 2009). A reasoned target decision thus must weight abundance versus neurotoxic activity.[*]

In silico studies of Aβ conformational dynamics have revealed that Aβ40 and Aβ42 have different oligomer distributions (Urbanc et al., 2004). Aβ42 forms greater numbers of high-order oligomers (pentamers, hexamers, dodecamers), whereas Aβ40 forms greater numbers of low-order oligomers (such as dimers, trimers, tetramers). Similar differences in Aβ40 and Aβ42 oligomer distributions have been observed experimentally using photochemical cross-linking methods (Bitan et al., 2003) and ion mobility spectrometry (IMS) (Bernstein et al., 2009). Simulations also revealed that Aβ42 oligomer formation proceeded predominantly through intermolecular interactions involving the C-terminus (I31– A42) and the central hydrophobic region, whereas the oligomerization of Aβ40 depended more on the interactions between the central hydrophobic region and the N-terminus (A2-F4).

The importance of the C-terminus of Aβ in controlling Aβ assembly has been revealed in systematic studies of the effects of C-terminal amino acid substitutions on oligomerization that were done using the technique of photo-induced cross-linking of unmodified amino acids (PICUP) (Bitan et al., 2001). PICUP is a "zero-length" photochemical cross-linking method that stabilizes Aβ oligomers, allowing their quantitation using sodium dodecyl sulfate polyacrylamide gel electrophoresis (SDS-PAGE) and silver staining. This approach provides a means of correlating primary structure modifications with assembly characteristics. PICUP studies of oligomerization of freshly prepared Aβ40 and Aβ42 have revealed that each peptide produces a distinct oligomer size distribution (Bitan et al., 2003). Unlike the equilibrium mixture of monomer, dimer, trimer, and tetramer formed by Aβ40, Aβ42 preferentially forms pentamer/hexamer units that self-associated into larger oligomers, including dodecamers and octadecamers. The term *paranucleus* was introduced to describe these pentamer/hexamer units, which appear to be the basic unit of the Aβ protofibril and to distinguish them from the Aβ monomer

---

[*] Neurotoxic activity in vivo depends on many factors. Considering only those factors of Aβ oligomer size i and abundance (frequency) f_i, if the neurotoxic activity (t) of each Aβ assembly is given as t_i, then the total neurotoxic activity $T = \sum_{i=1}^{n} f_i t_i$.

folding nucleus (see previous discussion) (Bernstein et al., 2009; Bitan et al., 2003). Ile41 was found to be important for paranucleus formation and for paranucleus self-association. Ala42, and its carboxyl end group, also mediated paranucleus self-association.

Studies of missense APP mutations that cause FAD or cerebral amyloid angiopathy (CAA) and alter the primary structure of Aβ, including Glu22→Gln, Glu22→Gly, Glu22→Lys, and Asp23→Asn, revealed that the amino acid substitutions resulted in oligomer distributions of Aβ40 in which average order shifted to higher values (Bitan and Teplow, 2004). However, these substitutions had little effect on Aβ42 oligomerization. N-terminal residues also influenced the oligomerization of Aβ40 in particular. The removal of N-terminal residues Asp1–Gly9 in Aβ42 had no effect on its oligomer size distribution, whereas truncation of either of the N-terminal two or four residues of Aβ40 produced higher-order oligomers (Bitan and Teplow, 2004).

1.2.3 Paranuclei and Dodecamers

Ahmed et al. prepared Aβ42 pentamers under low-temperature and low-salt conditions and found that the disc-shaped oligomeric species thus formed were substantially more toxic to neurons than were protofibrils and fibrils (Ahmed et al., 2010). Further structural analysis suggested that Aβ42 pentamers were composed of loosely aggregated strands with the peptide C-termini buried inside the aggregates, protected from solvent (Ahmed et al., 2010), which is consistent with results from computer simulation of oligomer formation (Urbanc et al., 2010; Urbanc et al., 2004). New computational and experimental studies on Aβ C-terminus organization have revealed that the C-terminus of Aβ42 may fold into a β-hairpin-like conformation that facilitates hexamer and dodecamer formation, while abolishing the formation of dimers, trimers, and tetramers (Yang et al., submitted). This discovery implies that lower-order Aβ oligomers (dimer, trimer, and tetramer) may be structurally different from paranuclei, and play different roles on the pathway of Aβ aggregation. This suggestion is supported by IMS studies of the oligomerization differences between Aβ40 and Aβ42 (Bernstein et al., 2009).

Other dodecameric structures also have been described, including Aβ-derived diffusible ligands (ADDLs) (Lambert et al., 1998), Aβ*56 (Lesne et al., 2006), and *globulomers* (Barghorn et al., 2005). ADDLs are dodecamers produced in vitro from Aβ42 cultivated in cold F12 medium or brain slice culture medium. ADDLs appear in atomic force microscopy (AFM) studies as globular structures with heights of 5–6 nm (Catalano et al., 2006; Klein, 2002; Lambert et al., 1998). Aβ*56 was identified in sodium dodecyl sulfate (SDS) extracts from brains of Tg2576 transgenic mice. The *56* refers to the molecular weight of the oligomer, which is consistent with that of a dodecamer. The morphology of Aβ*56 is a prolate ellipsoid (Lesne et al., 2006), a structure that had been reported earlier in small-angle neutron scattering experiments (Yong et al., 2002). Globulomers (from "globular oligomers") are formed by Aβ42 in the presence of SDS. Protease digestion, antibody binding, and mass spectrometry studies of globulomers suggest a structural model in which the hydrophobic C-terminus (residues 24–42) forms a stable core and the more hydrophilic N-terminus is on the surface (Barghorn et al., 2005). Although globulomers have substantial β-sheet content, presumably at the C-terminus, they do not form fibrils and thus may be considered "off-pathway" for fibril assembly. A larger species, the "Aβ oligomer," also has been produced in vitro (Deshpande et al., 2006). Its molecular weight (≈90,000) suggests that its assembly order is ~15–20, consistent with that of an octadecamer.

1.2.4 PROTOFIBRILS

Protofibrils were discovered in in vitro experiments simultaneously and independently by two groups seeking to elucidate pathways of Aβ assembly (Harper et al., 1997b; Walsh et al., 1997). Protofibrils appeared in electron micrographs of AFM images as flexible filaments, often with a beaded chain appearance. Each bead was ≈5 nm in diameter. The length of these structures rarely exceeded 150 nm and could be as short as ≈5 nm, suggesting that the oligomer comprising the 5-nm structure was the equivalent of a unit cell for protofibril formation. Protofibrils bound ThT and Congo red at levels similar to those exhibited by fibrils, suggesting a similar structural organization. In fact, CD (circular dichroism) studies of protofibrils demonstrated β-sheet content very similar to that of fibrils (Arimon et al., 2005; Harper et al., 1997a; Harper et al., 1997b, 1999; Hartley et al., 1999; Walsh et al., 1999; Walsh et al., 1997; Williams et al., 2005). Protofibrils exist in dynamic equilibrium with Aβ monomers and low-order oligomers. This suggests that protofibril growth may occur both by monomer addition and by association of smaller protofibrillar species (Harper et al., 1999). Kinetics and solution-phase AFM experiments showed that protofibrils matured into fibrils (Harper et al., 1997b; Walsh et al., 1999). Protofibrils thus are considered to be the penultimate structural precursors of fibrils.

Recent studies have revealed new details of Aβ protofibril structure. A study combining hydrogen-exchange and scanning proline mutagenesis of (CLC)-stabilized Aβ40 protofibrils has confirmed the structural similarity between protofibrils and fibrils (Kheterpal et al., 2006). Aβ appears to exist as two extended β-strands (residues 15–21 and 30–36) connected by a flexible loop comprising residues 22–29. The N-terminal 14 residues and C-terminal 3–4 residues are flexible (Kheterpal et al., 2006; Williams et al., 2005). A solid-state NMR study suggests similar structural features (Scheidt et al., 2011).

Protofibrils are neurotoxic and their neurotoxic activity exceeds significantly that of mature fibrils. Protofibrils have been found to disrupt the normal metabolism of cultured neurons and cause alterations in the electrical activity of cultured primary neurons (Hartley et al., 1999; Walsh et al., 1999; Ward et al., 2000; Ye et al., 2003). Protofibril toxicity appears to be relevant to AD (Harper et al., 1997b; Martins et al., 2008). A FAD mutation that causes a Glu22Gly amino acid substitution in Aβ that enhances protofibril formation has been found to cause the *Arctic* form of AD (Kamino et al., 1992; Nilsberth et al., 2001). Protofibril concentration is anti-correlated with spatial learning in Arctic mutation transgenic mice (Lord et al., 2009). Oxidative stress, postulated to be a factor in AD causation, has been found to promote protofibril formation while inhibiting fibril formation (Siegel et al., 2007).

1.2.5 Fibrils

The prevailing working hypothesis for AD causation posits a seminal role for Aβ oligomers (Kirkitadze et al., 2002). In fact, some suggest that the fibrillar constitution of amyloid deposits may be protective by acting as a sink for toxic oligomers (Kirkitadze et al., 2002) Nevertheless, soluble fibrils are neurotoxic (Kirkitadze et al., 2002). In addition, amyloid deposits may be a source of Aβ monomers or oligomers because fibrils, although highly stable, remain in equilibrium with nonfibrillar species (Figure 1.3) (Inayathullah and Teplow, 2011; O'Nuallain et al., 2005). For these reasons, the study of fibrils per se remains important. Fibrils also remain an important subject because an improved understanding of Aβ fibrils is likely to be relevant for understanding the structural biology of other amyloids, all of which have similar fibril core organization (see the following discussion).

Aβ fibrils generally are ~10 nm in diameter, are unbranched, and may be up to micrometers in length. They may appear monofilar or demonstrate obvious multifilament substructure (Makin and Serpell, 2005) with or without helical twisting (Sachse et al., 2006). Fibril morphology depends on a number of factors, including the method of peptide preparation, solvent formulation (salts, metals, detergents), temperature, and agitation (Fändrich 2007; Fändrich et al., 2011). Even if conditions are scrupulously controlled, Aβ fibril morphology may not be constant (Meinhardt et al., 2009).

Aβ fibrils, like all amyloid fibrils, have a cross-β structural organization (Astbury et al., 1935), so-called because the β-strands comprising the extended β-sheets forming the fibril core are aligned orthogonally (across) the fibril axis. In this arrangement, interstrand H bonds are parallel to the fibril axis. Although the cross-β organization of the fibril core is an invariant and well-studied feature of all amyloids, the structural organization of noncore elements of fibrils remains undefined for Aβ. This is a

$$\begin{array}{cccccccc} 5 & 10 & 15 & 20 & 25 & 30 & 35 & 40 \end{array}$$
$$DAEFRHDSGYEVHHQKLVFFAEDVGSNKGAIIGLMVGGVVIA$$

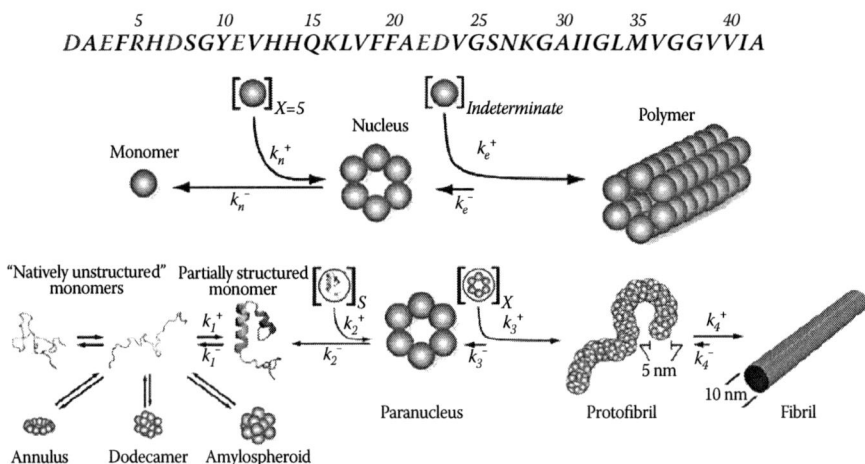

FIGURE 1.3 (See color insert.) Pathways of Aβ assembly. (From R. Roychaudhuri, M. Yang, M. M. Hoshi, and D. B. Teplow. "Amyloid β-Protein Assembly and Alzheimer Disease." 2009. *Journal of Biological Chemistry* 284: 4749–4753. With permission.)

result of the propensity of Aβ for fibril assembly and self-aggregation, as opposed to crystallization, which has precluded x-ray crystallographic analysis of full-length Aβ.

A technique that has provided detailed atomic resolution structural models of fibril core structure is solid-state NMR (Antzutkin et al., 2002; Tycko 2004). In combination with mass-per-unit length measurements from electron microscopy (EM) and site-directed spin labeling electron paramagnetic resonance (EPR) data, solid-state NMR has provided the most detailed model yet obtained of Aβ fibril core structure (Petkova et al., 2002). In this model, amino acids 12–24 and 30–40 comprise the two sides of a hairpin structure and amino acids 25–29 form the actual hairpin turn. This turn is stabilized by a salt-bridge interaction between Asp23 and Lys28. Each strand of the hairpin stacks with homologous neighbors arranged in parallel along the fibril axis to form extended, in-register, parallel β-strands. The β-sheet has two faces, one composed of hydrophobic residues and the other composed of charged and polar side chains and the N-terminus (Petkova et al., 2002). A similar parallel, in-register alignment of β-sheets has been found in Aβ42 fibrils. This alignment maximizes hydrophobic interactions (Antzutkin et al., 2002). Hydrogen–deuterium exchange (Kheterpal et al., 2006; Lührs et al., 2005) coupled with solution-state NMR revealed a similar Aβ fibril structure. This structure has β-strands at residues 18–26 and 31–42 with a turn region that is stabilized by Asp23 and Lys28 interaction (Figure 1.4). Although this interaction can occur intramolecularly, in fibrils, the Asp23 and Lys28 interaction likely is intermolecular (i.e., between sheets) (Lührs et al., 2005).

A complete determination of Aβ monomer structure within fibrils has not been achieved, but fragments of Aβ and other amyloid proteins can form microcrystals

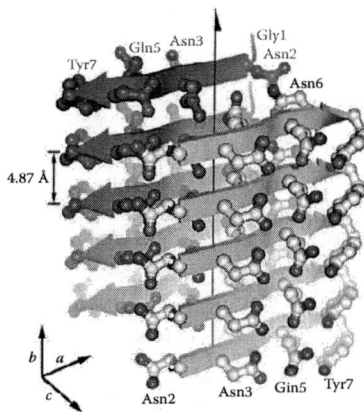

FIGURE 1.4 (See color insert.) "The pair-of-sheets structure, showing the backbone of each β-strand as an arrow, with side chains protruding. The dry interface is between the two sheets, with the wet interfaces on the outside surfaces. Side chains Asn 2, Gln 4 and Asn 6 point inwards, forming the dry interface. The 21 screw axis of the crystal is shown as the vertical line. It rotates one of the strands of the near sheet 180° about the axis and moves it up 4.87A°/2 so that it is superimposed on one of the strands of the far sheet." (From R. Nelson, M. R. Sawaya, M. Balbirnie, A. O. Madsen, C. Riekel, R. Grothe, and D. Eisenberg. "Structure of the Cross-β Spine of Amyloid-like Fibrils." 2005. *Nature* 435: 773–778. With permission.)

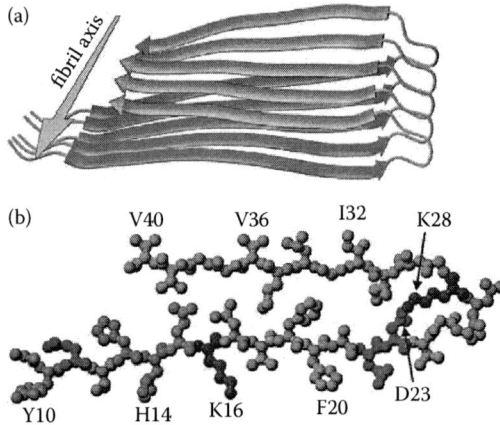

FIGURE 1.5 (See color insert.)   Structural model of Aβ40 fibrils.

that are amenable to x-ray crystallographic analysis. Analyses of a wide variety of amyloid peptides have revealed a *steric zipper* structure that comprises the fibril core (Nelson et al., 2005; Sawaya et al., 2007) (Figure 1.5). The "zipper" is formed through the interdigitation of the amino acid side chains of neighboring β-strands, like the teeth of a zipper. In many such structures, water is not present, and these anhydrous interfaces may be a common feature of amyloid fibril cores.

1.2.6 OTHER ASSEMBLIES

Nonfibrillar assemblies also are formed by Aβ. Annular structures with outside diameters of 8–12 nm and pore sizes of 2–2.5 nm have been described (Caughey and Lansbury, 2003; Haass and Selkoe, 2007; Kayed et al., 2009; Kokubo et al., 2009). These pore-like structures have been hypothesized to act as channels that alter membrane conductivity or create ion pores, disrupting normal cellular function (Kagan et al., 2002; Lashuel et al., 2002; Quist et al., 2005). Evidence suggests that Aβ pores may directly allow cellular Ca^{2+} influx or activate cell surface receptors coupled to calcium flux (Mattson and Chan, 2003; Smith et al., 2005).

The largest globular assemblies are amylospheroids (ASPDs) and β-amyloid balls (βamy balls). Amylospheroids are spheroidal structures with diameters of 10–15 nm that are formed by Aβ40 and Aβ42 (Hoshi et al., 2003). ASPDs can be found in vivo and has different surface tertiary structure from other smaller Aβ oligomers, because they do not bind to the A11 antibody (Noguchi et al., 2009). Further study revealed that ASPDs and fibrils are formed from independent pathways (Matsumura et al., 2011). βamy balls are very large (20–200 μm) spheroidal structures formed only by Aβ40 at high concentration (300–600 μM) (Westlind-Danielsson et al., 2001). Although these concentrations are nonphysiological, βamy balls may be an interesting model of amyloid plaques or of the inclusion bodies formed in Parkinson's and other diseases.

1.3 BIOLOGICAL MEDIATORS OF Aβ ASSEMBLY, ENVIRONMENTAL EFFECTS ON Aβ ASSEMBLY

Anfinsen hypothesized that the structure of a protein is encoded in its amino acid sequence (Anfinsen, 1973). However, an implicit assumption here is that the protein folds in a specific environment. Identical sequences can produce very different folds if their folding milieus differ. The milieu comprises not only solvent water, but also salts, metals, proteins, lipids, pH, and molecular crowding effects. We discuss here how these different factors may affect Aβ folding and assembly.

1.3.1 INTRACELLULAR Aβ ASSEMBLY

Aβ assembly has been likened to protein crystallization (Jarrett et al., 1993b), and although it is not identical, it does display nucleation dependence. The critical concentration for spontaneous aggregation of Aβ, and thus amyloid formation, is in the range of 6–40 μM (Harper et al., 1999; Lomakin et al., 1997). However, the average concentrations of Aβ in the cerebrospinal fluid (CSF) of AD patients are much lower, in the pM to nM range (Seubert et al., 1992; Strozyk et al., 2003). Several studies have shown an inverse correlation between CSF Aβ42 levels and cognitive function among patients with dementia (Andreasen et al., 1999b) or mild cognitive impairment (Gustafson et al., 2007). This suggests that the presence of Aβ assemblies within the CSF, and presumably in the extracellular spaces of the brain, is not obligatory for the neuronal toxicity and atrophy observed in AD. These observations have created what might be termed the *concentration conundrum*, that is, how can Aβ aggregation cause disease if the average Aβ concentration at the site of pathology is lower than the critical concentration, C_r, for peptide assembly? An answer may be that the average Aβ concentration does not reflect local concentrations in susceptible brain areas or cells.

The original amyloid cascade hypothesis proposed that the key pathological event in AD was the extracellular accumulation of insoluble, fibrillar Aβ. However, subsequent studies have revealed that an intracellular pool of Aβ exists in the brains of AD patients and in mouse models of AD (Laferla et al., 2007). Proposed sources for this intracellular pool of Aβ include normal APP processing within neurons or internalized extracellular Aβ (Mohamed and Posse De Chaves, 2011). In support of the latter mechanism, Hu et al. have shown that murine cortical neurons and neuroblastoma (SHSY5Y) cells can take up Aβ into late endosomes/lysosomes, where Aβ concentrations can reach the μM range (100-fold higher than the concentration of peptide added to the culture medium) (Hu et al., 2009). The resulting high concentrations lead to aggregation of Aβ into high molecular weight (HMW) species that can be released into the extracellular space, where they can seed amyloid formation in environments with average Aβ concentration < C_r (Hu et al., 2009). In the same study, the specific uptake of Aβ40 and Aβ42, but not scrambled Aβ, suggested that this uptake mechanism is receptor-specific and is thought to be the initial step in a pathway of intracellular Aβ degradation that removes Aβ from the extracellular space (Hu et al., 2009). Although Aβ clearance in late endosomes/lysosomes appears to be efficient, continuous exposure to extracellular Aβ eventually leads to accumulation of Aβ inside these vesicles, facilitating self-association (Hu et al., 2009). This hypothesis is supported by increased Aβ levels and plaque deposition in knockout mice that lack cathepsin B, a lysosomal protease known to degrade Aβ (Mueller-Steiner et al., 2006). Similarly, gene deletion of cystatin C, an endogenous inhibitor of cathepsin B, decreases the formation of plaques (Mi et al., 2007).

Intracellular Aβ also may be produced wherever APP, β-secretase, and γ-secretase colocalize. This includes the intramembranous compartments of the endoplasmic reticulum (ER) (Cook et al., 1997; Lee, 1998; Skovronsky et al., 1998; Wild-Bode et al., 1997), trans-Golgi network (TGN) (Hartmann et al., 1997), endosomes (including multivesicular bodies) (Kinoshita et al., 2003; Rogaeva et al., 2007; Takahashi et al., 2002), lysosomes (Langui et al., 2004), and mitochondria (Manczak et al., 2006) (Laferla et al., 2007). In the ER, retention of APP by Brefeldin A (BFA) treatment leads to continued production of intracellular Aβ42, but not Aβ40 (Cook et al., 1997). Preferential production of Aβ42 in the ER also is observed when APP is overexpressed (Wild-Bode et al., 1997), as determined by immunoelectron microscopy and cell fractionation experiments (Hartmann et al., 1997; Wild-Bode et al., 1997). In contrast, the production of Aβ40 appears to be favored in the TGN (Hartmann et al., 1997; Lee, 1998). It has been suggested that the greater thickness of Golgi membranes in the TGN promotes β-secretase cleavage at Val40, whereas the thinner ER membrane favors cleavage at Ala^{42} (Hartmann et al., 1997).

Interestingly, Aβ assembly may also occur in the mitochondria. Studies by Manczak et al. using oligomer-specific antibodies have indicated that there exist both monomers ($\approx$4 kDa) and oligomers (ranging from 15–50 kDa) within the mitochondria of neurons isolated from Tg2576 mice (Manczak et al., 2006). To explain this observation, the authors cite immunoelectron microscopic evidence showing that γ-secretase is found in mitochondria (Hansson et al., 2004). These in vitro findings are consistent with studies of human postmortem AD brains, in which accumulation of nonglycosylated APP is observed in mitochondrial import channels (Devi et al., 2006).

The data demonstrating proteolytic processing of APP within multiple organelles, or simply the presence there of Aβ40 or Aβ42, supports the contention that local Aβ concentrations may substantially exceed C_r (Jarrett et al., 1993a), allowing peptide oligomerization and higher-order aggregation that lead eventually to amyloid plaque formation. In this scenario, Aβ could be cytotoxic before being secreted extracellularly (Hartmann et al., 1997; Wild-Bode et al., 1997). Interestingly, intracellular sites of Aβ production seem to be exclusive to neurons, as no Aβ40 or Aβ42 production is detected in the corresponding compartments in non-neuronal cells (Hartmann et al., 1997).

1.3.2 pH

The role of pH in Aβ aggregation cannot be overemphasized. Aβ oligomerization is most efficient at pH 5, near its calculated isoelectric point (pI) of 5.5 (Wiesehan et al., 2007). Multiple studies have shown that as the pH approaches the Aβ pI, Aβ solubility decreases and protein aggregation occurs readily (Hortschansky et al., 2005; Sarell et al., 2010). However, specific charge–charge interactions between carboxylate groups and histidine residues have not been found to be essential for oligomerization (Hou et al., 2004; Kayed et al., 2003; Riek et al., 2001; Zhang et al., 2000).

Rather, compelling evidence suggests that repulsive electrostatic interactions can prevent aggregation and amyloid formation, as is the case in pH regimes distant from the Aβ pI (Calloni et al., 2005; Chiti et al., 2003; Guo et al., 2005).

At the molecular level, α-helical structure is favored at pH 1–4 and pH 7–10, whereas β-sheet conformations are favored at pH 4–7 (Barrow et al., 1992). In support of the amyloid cascade hypothesis, early studies showed that oligomeric Aβ assemblies possessed significant intermolecular β-sheet structure (maximally at pH 5.4), whereas monomers displayed much greater levels of α-helix (Barrow et al., 1992). Interestingly, Wood et al. reported that the aggregates produced at pH 5.8 bind less Congo Red and thioflavin T (ThT) than do aggregates formed in unstirred reactions at pH 7.4 (Wood et al., 1996), possibly due to differences in pH-dependent formation of oligomers versus fibrils. An alternate interpretation of these data would be that high aggregation propensity at pH 5.8 produces structures in which Congo Red or ThT binding sites are sequestered. These data are consistent with the aforementioned endosomal localization of Aβ aggregates, which would be expected due to the low endosomal pH and the concentration of solutes within the endosomal compartment (Burdick et al., 1997; Burdick et al., 1992; Liu et al., 2010).

1.3.3 CHOLESTEROL

Given that APP processing takes place in membranes, it is not surprising that lipids play a role in Aβ assembly (Grziwa et al., 2003). Indeed, Alois Alzheimer recorded the occurrence of "extraordinarily strong accumulation of lipoid material in the ganglion cells, glia and vascular wall cells, and the particularly numerous fibril-forming glia cells in the cortex and, indeed, in the entire central nervous system," and suggested these could play a role in the nature of presenile dementia, along with plaque formation (Alzheimer, 1907). However, this observation was largely ignored by early researchers, perhaps due to the limitations of analytical tools, when the available staining techniques were not sufficient for lipid granule studies, but rather favored a fibril-orientated approach (Di Paolo and Kim, 2011; Foley, 2010). We focus here on the role of lipids, particularly cholesterol, in mediating Aβ assembly.

Cholesterol levels and AD are correlated (Sjogren et al., 2006). The protein ApoE, in addition to playing central roles in plasma lipoprotein metabolism and cholesterol transport in various cell types of the body, is a central cholesterol transporter in the nervous system (Mahley, 1988; Weisgraber, 1994). Possession of one or two *APOE-ε4* alleles significantly increases ones risk for AD, an observation that supports a strong link between cholesterol and AD (Weisgraber and Mahley, 1996).

The cholesterol effect may involve lipid rafts. These are dynamic and highly ordered membrane microdomains that are rich in cholesterol and sphingolipids and are distinct from surrounding membranes containing unsaturated phospholipids (Simons and Toomre, 2000). It has been hypothesized that cholesterol, through its structural role in lipid raft formation, may directly affect β-secretase activity (Di Paolo and Kim, 2011). β-secretase is thought to be stabilized in lipid rafts enriched in ceramide, a central component in sphingolipid metabolism (ceramide serves as the backbone to generate sphingomyelin or more complex glycosphingolipids through the addition of phosphocholine or sugars) (Puglielli et al., 2003).

However, studies utilizing fluorescence lifetime imaging microscopy-Forster resonance energy transfer (FLIM-FRET) for visualization of the APP:β-secretase interaction found that increasing cholesterol concentration did not affect β-secretase activity per se, but rather increased the concentration of this enzyme in the lipid rafts (Marquer et al., 2011).

Due to the estimated small size (~20 nm) of lipid rafts (Pralle et al., 2000), which prevents direct conventional imaging, Marquer et al. also utilized fluorescence correlation spectroscopy (FCS) to gain molecular insight into the raft partitioning of APP and β-secretase in live primary neurons (Marquer et al., 2011). Previous studies in artificial membranes and cell lines demonstrated that FCS can differentiate between a liquid disordered (nonraft) phase, in which molecules diffuse faster, and a liquid ordered (raft) phase, in which molecules diffuse much slower. At the precise time of cholesterol exposure, FCS revealed the concomitant relocalization of APP from nonraft to raft domains at the membrane. In addition, because APP and β-secretase have similar membrane diffusion constants in lipid rafts, it was suggested that clustering in lipid rafts provides the enzyme ready access to its substrate, APP (Marquer et al., 2011). Membrane cholesterol loading induced increased production of Aβ thus may result from an increase in β-secretase accessibility to its substrate, APP, by clustering in lipid rafts. However, while β-secretase cleavage has been shown to occur late in the secretory pathway, after delivery to the cell surface, and during endocytosis (Daugherty and Green, 2001; Huse et al., 2000; Kamal et al., 2001; Koo and Squazzo, 1994; Perez et al., 1999), this process occurs mostly intracellularly, since inhibition of endocytosis greatly reduces the amount of Aβ produced (Ehehalt et al., 2003). Thus, the cleavage of APP by β-secretase seems to be endocytosis dependent.

Hypotheses have been proposed to explain the absence of β-secretase on the cell surface. Ehehalt et al. suggested that, despite the observation that both APP and β-secretase partition into lipid rafts in cellular membranes, and that amyloidogenic processing seems to be associated with rafts (Ehehalt et al., 2003; Vetrivel et al., 2005), surface APP and β-secretase are most likely present in separate rafts because these rafts are small and highly dispersed at the cell surface and contain only a subset of ~10–30 protein molecules (Pralle et al., 2000). For β-cleavage to occur, rafts would have to be clustered to get APP and β-secretase into the same raft platform, which can happen after endocytosis by clustering and coalescence of APP- or β-secretase-containing rafts within endosomes. Support for this hypothesis was provided by studies in which clustering of rafts was induced artificially by cross-linking of raft proteins with antibodies (Ehehalt et al., 2003). This system manipulation increased Aβ production. Interestingly, the amount of α-secretase processing of APP did not increase dramatically, probably due to extended raft association of APP (Ehehalt et al., 2003).

This finding has several important implications for providing mechanistic insights of how cholesterol affects Aβ production. While β- and γ-cleavages are part of the amyloidogenic pathway, the nonamyloidogenic pathway is mediated by α-secretase (localized mostly at the cell surface and out of lipid raft domains) (Haass et al., 1992; Parvathy et al., 1999) and is not affected by endocytosis inhibition (Ehehalt et al., 2003). In support of this hypothesis, studies on N2a and K269 cells, or on human AD brains, have suggested that cholesterol homeostasis is altered, resulting in higher β- and γ-secretase activity and total cholesterol levels (Ehehalt et al., 2003; Vetrivel et al., 2005; Xiong et al., 2008). As might be predicted from the results discussed, studies have shown that decreased Aβ levels are observed when cholesterol levels are low, a finding that may be due to altered association of the secretases to lipid rafts (Riddell et al., 2001; Vetrivel et al., 2005). In vitro experiments also show that cholesterol depletion shifts the partitioning of APP from lipid rafts to the surrounding lipid bilayer and leads to a decrease of β-secretase cleavage products and increases α-secretase cleavage (Ehehalt et al., 2003). Cholesterol also has been hypothesized to affect Aβ production by concentrating APP_β, a process that increases the substrate concentration for γ-secretase action and precludes release of $sAPP_\beta$ (Marquer et al., 2011; Marzolo and Bu, 2009). In the amyloidogenic pathway, β-secretase cleavage is followed by γ-secretase cleavage. It has been shown that all four components of the γ-secretase complex, namely presenilin 1 (PS1)-derived fragments, mature nicastrin, APH-1, and PEN-2, are associated with cholesterol-rich detergent insoluble membrane (DIM) domains in intracellular membranes of neurons that fulfill the criteria of lipid rafts (Spasic and Annaert, 2008; Vetrivel et al., 2004). The same study also showed that APP C-terminal fragments may be preferentially localized in lipid raft microdomains of post-Golgi and endocytic organelles (Vetrivel et al., 2004), allowing efficient processing by γ-secretase, which is also associated with lipid rafts (Spasic and Annaert, 2008). Relevant to this observation are the results of studies by Osenkowski et al. that show that cholesterol increases γ-secretase activity in various lipid mixtures (Osenkowski et al., 2008). Decreased γ-secretase activity and decreased Aβ generation also are observed when membrane cholesterol is depleted (Hartmann et al., 2007; Simons et al., 1998; Vetrivel and Thinakaran, 2010). In agreement with this model, cholesterol depletion disrupts β- and γ-secretase association to lipid rafts and causes a decrease in Aβ production (Cordy et al., 2003; Riddell et al., 2001; Vetrivel et al., 2005; Vetrivel et al., 2004), indicating again that lipid rafts are relevant sites for amyloidogenic processing of APP.

In vivo support for local concentration effects in lipid rafts has been provided by Kawarabayashi et al., who showed that Aβ dimers begin to accumulate in lipid rafts of Tg2576 mice at 6 months of age and accumulate by 24–28 months at levels 500-fold higher than those in young mice (Kawarabayashi et al., 2004). The same group found that the mice showed memory loss at times corresponding with the appearance of Aβ dimers (6 months). Because cholesterol is the main constituent of lipid rafts, alteration of cellular cholesterol concentration or localization has been an attractive potential therapeutic approach for manipulating Aβ production. Several studies have shown that the cholesterol-lowering drugs simvastatin and lovastatin reduce intracellular and extracellular levels of Aβ40 and Aβ42 in primary cultures of hippocampal neurons, CSF, and brain homogenates of guinea pigs, and in brain regions of transgenic mice (Fassbender et al., 2001). In contrast, a high-cholesterol diet induces an increase in Aβ production/accumulation, particularly amyloid load (% amyloid), deposit number, and size in the mouse model CNS (Refolo et al., 2001).

1.3.4 Effects of Metals on Aβ Assembly

Various metal ions, including Cu^{2+}, Fe^{3+}, and Zn^{2+}, are present in abnormally high levels in senile plaques (Bush et al., 1994). This observation has led many to explore connections between metals and Aβ-induced neuropathology. Aβ has a strong positive reduction potential and studies have shown that Aβ possesses high-affinity binding sites for the above-mentioned metal ions (Curtain et al., 2001; Danielsson et al., 2007; Garzon-Rodriguez et al., 1999; Kawahara et al., 1997; Syme et al., 2004).

The role of iron in Aβ toxicity, though still incompletely resolved, is nonetheless supported by experiments. For example, transgenic flies expressing Arctic Aβ42, and overexpressing ferritin heavy chain or light chain, displayed a 50–100% increase in median survival compared to controls not overexpressing ferritin (Rival et al., 2009). The ferritin effect likely is due to its sequestration of Fe^{2+} and Fe^{3+}. Similar results were obtained through treatment with the metal chelator clioquinol (Rival et al., 2009). Examination of Aβ42 levels in the Aβ42:ferritin double transgenic flies showed that Aβ levels actually increased. The effect of ferritin on Aβ toxicity thus may not be mediated by suppression of Aβ42 production (Rival et al., 2009). Instead, these effects may be through suppression of oxidative insults. Specifically, Rival et al. have shown that enhancing the activity of superoxide dismutase increases protein carbonyl levels in Arctic Aβ42 flies, suggesting that iron may mediate the generation of hydroxyl radicals through Aβ-mediated Fenton chemistry (Rival et al., 2009; Smith et al., 1997).

Circular dichroism measurements have revealed that Al^{3+} at alkaline pH is able to promote β-sheet formation in Aβ (Ricchelli et al., 2005). In the presence of Al^{3+}, Aβ forms fibrils faster and at much lower concentrations. Contradictory findings exist with respect to the effects of Cu^{2+} on Aβ aggregation. One study found that Cu^{2+}, similar to Al^{3+}, induces rapid Aβ fibril formation at alkaline pH and at similarly low Aβ concentrations (Sarell et al., 2010). Cu^{2+} appears to affect different steps in the aggregation processes of Aβ40 and Aβ42. The metal ion significantly reduces the lag time for Aβ40 nucleation, whereas its enhancement of elongation rates is more pronounced with Aβ42. Observations with transmission electron microscopy (TEM) confirmed the presence of fibrils in both cases. The same study found that these fibrils, like fibrils made in the absence of Cu^{2+}, can seed further fibril formation of metal-free Aβ.

As discussed in Section 1.3.2, Aβ aggregation is optimal at its pI. Sarell et al. have suggested that the coordination of Cu^{2+} to histidines may make the Aβ:metal complex more neutral, effectively producing the type of peptide behavior observed at its pI (Sarell et al., 2010). Consistent with the notion, other studies have found that Cu^{2+} accelerates Aβ aggregation into nonfibrillar aggregates (Chen et al., 2011). Of course, the conformational stabilization of the Aβ peptide within the Aβ:metal complex may also facilitate peptide self-association and assembly.

In vitro studies indicate that physiological concentrations of Zn^{2+} can accelerate Aβ aggregation (Crouch et al., 2008). Zn^{2+} binding appears to induce Aβ conformations in which substantial exposure of hydrophobic regions exists, resulting in accelerated self-association (Chen et al., 2011). NMR studies have shown that Zn binding involves histidine residues 6, 13, and 14, and the Aβ N-terminus (Danielsson et al., 2007; Liu et al., 1999). The study also found that Aβ has an affinity for Zn that is similar to its affinity for Cu, with which the peptide shares one of its two known binding sites. Metal binding affinities of Aβ(1–28), which contains the metal coordination center, were ≈0.4 μM for Cu^{2+} and ≈1.1 μM for Zn^{2+}. This information is in agreement with proton NMR data showing that Aβ has the same binding sites for copper and zinc (Syme et al., 2004).

1.3.5 INSULIN SIGNALING

Insulin and IGF-I (insulin-like growth factor I) belong to the same protein family (Mattson, 2002) and modulate brain function through, for instance, maintaining brain energy balance and modulating neuronal excitability and synaptic plasticity (Carro and Torres-Aleman, 2004). A number of studies have found abnormal levels of both proteins in the sera of AD patients (Carro and Torres-Aleman, 2004). Not surprisingly, studies also have identified diabetes mellitus as a risk for AD (Gotz et al., 2009).

There are currently several hypotheses about insulin's role in AD. There is direct and indirect evidence that insulin, overall, causes an increase in extracellular Aβ levels in the brain (Carro and Torres-Aleman, 2004). Mice completely lacking insulin-degrading enzyme (IDE; for which Aβ is a substrate), for instance, have increased cerebral Aβ levels as early as three months of age (Farris et al., 2004).

Studies have found that cardiovascular disease is a risk factor for AD (Martins et al., 2006). One possible hypothesis that hints at an indirect role for insulin in AD, is that cerebrovascular damage due to diabetes mellitus (DM) affects cognitive function (Takeda et al., 2011). The observation of Aβ deposition around cerebral blood vessels in diabetic AD mice suggests that vascular damage may contribute to AD pathogenesis (Takeda et al., 2011). Vascular inflammation and cerebral amyloid angiopathy also may be involved (Takeda et al., 2011). Hyperglycemia may also contribute to the vascular pathology of AD through oxidative stress or advanced glycation end products (Biessels and Kappelle, 2005).

A different, but related, mechanism explaining the correlation between AD and diabetes focuses on the presence of insulin resistance and hyperglycemia in both diseases. In diabetes, hyperglycemia triggers the release of additional insulin from the pancreas to stimulate glucose uptake by cells (Takeda et al., 2011). This gradually results in widespread cellular insulin resistance. Under normal conditions, insulin stimulates both the release and degradation of Aβ (Carro and Torres-Aleman, 2004). Increased insulin concentrations can further increase Aβ levels by increasing its release from neurons, modulating γ-secretase activity, or due to increase in its concentration competitively inhibiting IDE (Carro and Torres-Aleman, 2004; Takeda et al., 2011). The latter effect results in decreased degradation of Aβ and thus a subsequent rise in Aβ levels. Data showing that γ-secretase activity increases and IDE activity decreases in insulin-resistant AD transgenic mice support this hypothesis (Ho et al., 2004). Not surprisingly, the same study found increased Aβ generation and amyloid plaque burden in the brain.

A consensus on the role of insulin in AD remains elusive. Biessels and Kappelle, for example, label AD as insulin-resistant due to an apparent decrease in cerebral insulin levels in AD found in some studies (Biessels and Kappelle, 2005; Frolich et al., 1998). However, voluminous data demonstrate a positive correlation between diabetes, in which high blood glucose levels stimulate additional pancreatic insulin secretion, and the typical insulin-resistant state observed in AD (Takeda et al., 2011). This observation would seem to argue against the occurrence of lowered insulin levels in AD. Takeda et al., nonetheless, also report studies revealing lowered expression of insulin and insulin signaling pathway molecules in postmortem AD brains

(Takeda et al., 2011). It may be possible that insulin has alternative paths in its role in AD. Its increase can lead to increased levels of Aβ through the pathways mentioned previously, or its decrease can result in a disrupted insulin receptor signaling pathway that plays a role in the pathogenesis of AD.

The role of IGF-I in AD may be even less clear than that of insulin. Moloney et al. reported increased levels of IGF-I receptor (IGF-IR) in AD cases and increased IGF-I levels within and around Aβ plaques (Moloney et al., 2010). They also reported lowered expression of IGF-IR in neurons in AD, which may offer an explanation of earlier claims of an inverse relationship between serum levels of IGF-I and brain amyloid (Carro and Torres-Aleman, 2004).

Insulin and insulin signaling processes clearly correlate with disease state in AD, although a mechanistic elucidation of these roles remains a subject of debate. It is noteworthy, however, that AD incidence continues to rise, as does diabetes, and that both may be related to the well-known effects of diet on general health (Scarmeas et al., 2006). For a recent review on high-fat diets and sedentary lifestyles as disease risk factors, see Martins et al. (2006).

1.3.6 CELL CYCLE

The direction of AD research over the last century largely has been driven by the pathognomonic disease features, amyloid plaques and tangles, and the associated proteins Aβ and tau, respectively. However, other important areas of study exist, among them the role of cell cycle perturbation in AD neurons. After terminal differentiation, neurons are thought to lose their proliferative capacity, remaining as mitotically quiescent cells in the G_0 phase of the cell cycle. To validate this hypothesis and examine the effects of cell cycle perturbations in neurons, experiments have been done in which neuronal cell division was artificially induced either by the addition of an oncogene (SV40 Large T antigen) or a mutant tumor suppressor gene (pRb) to transgenic mice (Al-Ubaidi et al., 1992; Clarke et al., 1992; Feddersen et al., 1992; Jacks et al., 1992; Lee et al., 1992; Lee et al., 1994). Unlike other cell types, in which these genetic alterations would be expected to produce uncontrolled cellular proliferation, developing neuronal populations undergo substantial cell death. Herrup and Busser reported that the re-expression of cell cycle proteins and the incorporation of BrdU into DNA preceded target-related cell death of the granule cells of the cerebellar cortex and the neurons of the inferior olive (located on the ventral surface of the medulla oblongata), which has a developmental target dependency on the cerebellar Purkinje cells, similar to the granule cells (Herrup and Busser, 1995). Blocking the cell cycle with cyclin-dependent kinase inhibition could block neuronal cell death in culture (Copani et al., 1999; Copani et al., 2001; Herrup et al., 2004; Neve and McPhie, 2006; Park et al., 1996; Park et al., 1997; Pines, 1993; Van Den Heuvel and Harlow, 1993). It has been proposed that the activation of cell cycle proteins in neurons is necessary to carry out physiological processes such as synaptic reorganization in plastic regions of the adult brain, and failure to regulate such processes might lead to inappropriate cell cycle reentry (Ueberham and Arendt, 2005). In fact, inappropriate cell cycle reentry has been linked to neurodegeneration in diseases such as amyotrophic lateral sclerosis (Ranganathan and Bowser, 2003), Parkinson's disease

(Hoglinger et al., 2007; Jordan-Sciutto et al., 2003), ataxia telangiectasia (Yang and Herrup, 2005), stroke (Love, 2003), and some forms of encephalitis (Jordan-Sciutto et al., 2002; Jordan-Sciutto et al., 2000). In AD, aberrant expression of cell cycle proteins and DNA tetraploidy have been reported in neurons in pathologically affected regions of AD brain (Arendt et al., 1996; Busser et al., 1998; McShea et al., 1997; Nagy et al., 1997b; Vincent et al., 1997; Yang et al., 2001).

Neurons in AD brains have been found to move from G_0 to G_1 and to later cell cycle stages (McShea et al., 1997; Nagy et al., 1997a; Smith and Lippa, 1995). Though the exact mechanism responsible for this process is unclear, numerous cell cycle markers have been observed in regions of brains that are affected in AD, including cdc2, cdk4, p16, Ki-67, cyclin B1, and cyclin D (Neve and McPhie, 2006). It is possible that cell cycle reentry could involve genes known to be risk factors for AD, including APP, PS1, and PS2. These genes have been found to function in cell cycle regulation and have been shown to be mitogenic in vitro (Milward et al., 1992; Schubert et al., 1989). For example, APP has a role in the activation of neuronal cell cycle proteins such as APP-BP1 (Copani et al., 1999; Milward et al., 1992; Schubert et al., 1989). APP-BP1 is an adaptor protein involved in the cleavage of APP, but it also functions as a cell cycle protein that regulates mitotic transition from the S to M phase. Modest overexpression of APP leads to an increase of APP-BP1 in lipid rafts, along with the entry of neurons into S phase, ultimately leading to apoptosis (Bonda et al., 2010; Neve and McPhie, 2006). The interaction of APP with APP-BP1 activates a pathway leading to the conjugation of the protein NEDD8 to hUbc12, its target protein. NEDD8 functions as a ubiquitin-activating enzyme (E1) and hUba3 functions as a ubiquitin-conjugating enzyme (E2) (Kumar et al., 1993) and they co-function in a pathway that is analogous to ubiquitination called *neddylation* (Cope and Deshaies, 2003). After conjugation, Ubc12 directly transfers NEDD8 to its substrate, Cul1, which is a member of the Cullin family of ubiquitin ligase subunits. Cul1 is a subunit in a multisubunit complex called *SCF*, which belongs to a large class of enzymes known as E3 ubiquitin ligases (Deshaies, 1999). Despite the similarity to ubiquitination pathways, in which proteins conjugated to E3 complex are targeted for degradation, neddylation of Cul1 seems to enhance SCF's ability to ubiquitinate other proteins in vitro (Cope and Deshaies, 2003; Kipreos et al., 1996; Neve and McPhie, 2006; Podust et al., 2000; Read et al., 2000; Wu et al., 2000). The neddylation pathway has been shown to regulate protein degradation pathways participating in cell cycle progression, thus promoting APP-mediated cell cycle entry and apoptosis (Freed et al., 1999; Liakopoulos et al., 1999; Neve and McPhie, 2006; Podust et al., 2000; Tateishi et al., 2001).

PS1 and 2 have been shown to associate with the centrosome, nuclear membrane, and kinetochore antigens of dividing cells, and overexpression of the cognate genes induces cell cycle arrest in G_1, whereas lowering their expression accelerates the G_1 to S transition (Bonda et al., 2010; Li et al., 1997). Interestingly, analyses of hippocampal pyramidal and basal forebrain neurons in AD brains have shown that these neurons undergo either full or partial DNA replication and exit the S phase (Yang et al., 2001). However, these cells do not move from G_2 to M but rather undergo apoptosis (Hernandez-Ortega et al., 2007). It has been proposed that the resulting state of tetraploidy is lethal to neurons (Yang et al., 2001). More importantly, cell cycle events are associated not only with end-stage neuropathology, but also with the very earliest neuronal changes that occur in the disease, preceding gross cytopathological changes such as Aβ deposits and neurofibrillary tangles in some cases (Busser et al., 1998; McShea et al., 1997; Nagy et al., 1997a; Sheng et al., 2000; Vincent et al., 1998; Zhu et al., 2007). It is possible that the initiation of cell cycle reentry in neurons is an early sign of neuronal distress and that Aβ deposits are not necessary factors to induce cell cycle reentry, at least in APP transgenic mouse models (Lee et al., 2009). Zhu et al. proposed a two-hit hypothesis, according to which, either oxidative stress or abnormalities in mitotic signaling can independently serve as initiators of neuro-degeneration, but both processes are necessary to propagate disease pathogenesis (Zhu et al., 2007; Zhu et al., 2004).

Additional evidence for cell cycle involvement in AD has come from epide-miologic studies of individuals chronically taking large doses of nonsteroidal anti-inflammatory drugs (NSAIDs). These patients have been found to have a sig-nificantly reduced risk of developing AD (McGeer and McGeer, 1996; Stewart et al., 1997). In addition to their intended function of inhibiting cyclooxygenases, NSAIDs appear to activate the nuclear hormone receptor peroxisome proliferator-activated receptor γ (PPARγ). PPARγ has been proposed to modulate the APP-BP1 pathway that causes neurons to transit to the S phase, though the exact point of intervention is still unclear (Chen et al., 2000). PPARγ activation also appears to inhibit the gen-eration of proinflammatory and neurotoxic products in microglia and monocytes exposed to Aβ. PPARγ agonists decrease the secretion of Aβ (Sastre et al., 2003; Weggen et al., 2001; Weggen et al., 2003) and attenuate Aβ-mediated impairment of long-term potentiation (Costello et al., 2005).

Members of the serine/threonine cyclin-dependent kinase (cdk) family have been implicated in tau hyperphosphorylation and the consequent development of neurofi-brillary tangles in AD (Neve and McPhie, 2006; Vincent et al., 2003). Concomitant activation of cdc2, cdk4, and cdk5 in degenerating neurons has been described in AD (Herrup and Arendt, 2002; Monaco and Vallano, 2005; Vincent et al., 2003). The protein cdk5 has been subject to intense research due to its association with tau (Baumann et al., 1993; Kobayashi et al., 1993). However, cdk5 does not partici-pate directly in cell cycle reentry, but rather plays critical roles in CNS development (Fu et al., 2001; Gao et al., 1997), in the regulation of membrane transport (Floyd et al., 2001; Iijima et al., 2000; Rosales et al., 2000), neuronal migration (Gilmore et al., 1998; Ohshima et al., 1999; Ohshima et al., 1996), axon guidance (Connell-Crowley et al., 2000; Luo, 2000), myogenesis (Lazaro et al., 1997), actin dynamics (Connell-Crowley et al., 2000; Kato and Maeda, 1999; Nikolic et al., 1998), microtu-bule stability/transport (Paglini et al., 1998; Pigino et al., 1997), and synaptic struc-ture and plasticity (Dhavan and Tsai, 2001; Greengard et al., 1994; Humbert et al., 2000; Rosales et al., 2000). Like other cdk proteins, cdk5 shows no enzymatic activ-ity and requires association with a regulatory partner for activation. In the CNS, p35 was identified as a cdk5 binding partner in brain extracts, where it targets cdk5 to the membrane and phosphorylates several substrates (Dhavan and Tsai, 2001; Kusakawa et al., 2000; Lee et al., 2000; Nath et al., 2000; Van Den Haute et al., 2001). It has been proposed that exposure of neurons to oxidative stress, Aβ, or excitotoxic-ity activates the calcium-dependent protease calpain, which converts p35 into p25.

p25 lacks a myristoylation signal and is mislocalized to the cytoplasm, allowing cdk5 access to substrates in the cytoplasm. While p35 is short-lived and catabolized through ubiquitin-mediated proteolysis, p25 has a longer half-life and causes sustained activation of cdk5. Thus, conversion of p35 to p25 translates into elevated and mislocalized cdk5 activity, hyperphosphorylation of neurofilament and tau proteins, cytoskeletal disruption, and neuronal death (Ahlijanian et al., 2000; Busciglio et al., 1995; Dhavan and Tsai, 2001; Jeffrey et al., 1995; Patrick et al., 1999; Qi et al., 1995). The p25-cdk5 complex has been shown to efficiently generate AD-like tau that is phosphorylated at the same sites as tau present in paired helical filaments, the ultrastructural component of NFTs (Paudel et al., 1993). Expression of p25–cdk5 complexes in transfected cells results in increased AD-like tau phosphorylation, followed by morphological and cytoskeletal disruption and apoptosis (Patrick et al., 1999). In support of this hypothesis, concurrent p25 accumulation, cdk5 activation, and tau hyperphosphorylation were also observed in the postmortem brains of AD patients (Patrick et al., 1999; Pei et al., 1998; Tseng et al., 2002).

A significant body of evidence suggests that Aβ is mitogenic in vitro (McDonald et al., 1998; Pyo et al., 1998). To determine how cdk5 might be involved in triggering abortive cell cycle entry in AD, Lopes et al. examined the levels/activation of several cell cycle–associated proteins in cultured cortical neurons treated with Aβ40 (Lopes et al., 2009). Significant increases in cdk4, phosphorylated Rb, and proliferating cell nuclear antigen (PCNA) levels were observed. The proteins cdk2, 4, and 6 play vital roles in the G_1-to-S transition, and their activation by association with cyclin regulatory units leads to the phosphorylation of Rb (Copani et al., 1999; Kuan et al., 2004; Tannoch et al., 2000; Weinberg, 1995). When cortical neurons from E15 rat embryos are treated with Aβ, an increase in expression of cell cycle markers such as cyclin D1, phosphorylated Rb, activated cdk4 (events associated with mid-G_1 phase), and the induction of cyclin E and A (markers of late G_1 and S phase; Pines, 1993; Van Den Heuvel and Harlow, 1993), followed by cell death (Copani et al., 1999), was observed. Inactivation of cdk4 or cdk2 prevented both the entry into S phase and the development of apoptosis (Copani et al., 1999). These observations suggested an induced formation of functionally active cdk4/6-cyclin D1 complex leading to phosphorylation of Rb. Rb originally was identified as a tumor-suppressor gene that functions together with transcription factors such as E2F to prevent transcription of genes encoding proteins of importance in cell proliferation (Tannoch et al., 2000). Activation of Rb through phosphorylation causes it to dissociate from this transcription–repressor complex, which in turn leads to the transcription of several cell cycle proteins that drive the cell through the G_1-to-S transition (Copani et al., 1999; Kuan et al., 2004; Nath et al., 2000). While the neurons used in the experiments of Copani et al. did not progress beyond the S phase (Copani et al., 1999), the aberrant expression of cyclin-B1-cdc2 indicates that degenerating neurons in AD may reach the G_2 phase in some cases (Nagy et al., 1997b; Vincent et al., 1997). The absence of mitotic structures in neurons in these experiments suggested that there is a "mitotic catastrophe" (Bowen et al., 2002; Bowser and Smith, 2002; Ogawa et al., 2003), as indicated by the aberrant expression and localization of the cell cycle markers mentioned previously. All of this evidence points to an inadequate or failed control of the cell cycle in AD neurons.

Pin 1 (peptidyl-prolyl isomerase), a member of the parvulin subclass of the pep-
tidyl–prolyl cis/trans isomerases (PPIase) family also has been implicated in AD
(Butterfield et al., 2006). Pin1 catalyzes the isomerization of the peptide bond
between pSer/Thr-Pro in proteins and induces conformational change in its target
phosphoproteins (Lu et al., 1996). In dividing cells, Pin1 regulates the progression of
the cell cycle by interacting with a large number of mitosis-specific phosphoproteins,
including the cdk family (Butterfield et al., 2006; Lu et al., 1996; Shen et al., 1998;
Stukenberg and Kirschner, 2001; Zhou et al., 2000). Previous studies have shown
that Pin1 colocalizes with phosphorylated tau (Ramakrishnan et al., 2003). Pin1
conversion of phospho-Thr231 tau to the *trans* isomer both restores the ability of
phosphorylated tau to promote microtubule assembly (Andreasen et al., 1999a) and
also enables its dephosphorylation by PP2A (Zhou et al., 2000).

Despite knowledge of its molecular interactions, the role of Pin1 in AD is controversial. Initially it was thought that Pin1 facilitated the transition from G_0 to
G_1 in neurons by up-regulating expression of cyclin D1, which eventually leads to
neuronal dedifferentiation and apoptosis (Hamdane et al., 2002). However, other
studies suggested that Pin1 appears to protect against neurodegeneration. Liou
et al. reported that Pin1 knockout mice displayed age-dependent neuropathology
that included accumulation of abnormal and hyperphosphorylated tau, tau filaments, and neurodegeneration (Liou et al., 2003). This inverse association of Pin1
and tau accumulation was confirmed in another study done on AD brains, in which
neurofibrillary tangles were absent in neurons containing high Pin1 accumulations
(Holzer et al., 2002). It has been argued that because improper activation of mitotic
events may contribute to the hyperphosphorylation of tau, that subsequent isomerization and dephosphorylation of tau mediated in part by Pin1 are able to restore
the function and conformation of phosphorylated tau, thereby regulating mitotic
events (Butterfield et al., 2006). This proposition is supported by in vivo studies
in which Pin1 was found to be oxidatively modified and showed reduced activity
and decreased expression in hippocampi from mild cognitive impairment (MCI)
and AD patients (Butterfield et al., 2006; Sultana et al., 2006a; Sultana et al.,
2006b). Pin1 thus may play a role in the transition from G_0 to G_1 (cell cycle check-
points) in neurons, leading eventually to neuronal dedifferentiation and apoptosis
(Butterfield et al., 2006).

Though Pin1 has been suggested as a therapeutic target, more research is needed
to establish the protein's connection to AD. Identification of additional cellular targets besides tau and cdks will provide more insight into how Pin1 is involved in
different processes in neurons.

1.4 MECHANISMS OF TOXICITY

1.4.1 EFFECTS OF Aβ ON MEMBRANES

Amyloidogenic proteins can interact with membranes in a number of ways. Some
membranes bind amyloidogenic proteins, promoting amyloid misfolding and aggregation (Chi et al., 2008). Amyloidogenic proteins themselves can increase membrane
conductivity (Sokolov et al., 2006) and mediate membrane permeabilization (Kayed

et al., 2004), allowing small molecules and ions to transit the membrane in an unregulated manner. This latter effect often leads to cellular dysfunction and death.

To elucidate mechanisms of peptide:membrane interactions, model membranes that duplicate important features of cellular membrane composition have been studied. Natural membranes comprise a lipid bilayer containing a variety of specialized lipids, glycolipids, and proteins. Model membranes generally lack protein components, which may affect the experimental results, but model membranes are highly amenable to experimental manipulation and possess properties that are reproducible, facilitating interpretation of experimental results (Butterfield et al., 2010). Model membranes may comprise glycerophospholipids, including phosphatidylserine, phosphatidylinositol, and phosphatidylcthanolamine (Vestergaard et al., 2008). These membranes may be planar or vesicular in nature. Planar membranes include monolayers and bilayers (Richter et al., 2006; Rossi and Chopineau, 2007). Vesicles include small unilamellar vesicles (SUVs, 20–50 nm diameter), large unilamellar vesicles (LUVs, >>100 nm), and giant unilamellar vesicles (GUVs, 1–10 mm) (Chan and Boxer, 2007; Maler and Graslund, 2009).

Aβ toxicity has been correlated with its ability to disrupt membrane function and ionic homeostasis (Lashuel and Lansbury, 2006; Quist et al., 2005). Arispe et al. proposed that the toxicity of Aβ results from formation of ion channels, which induce Ca^{2+} leakage (Arispe et al., 1993a, 1993b, 1996). Aβ pores also may activate cell surface receptors coupled to calcium flux (Mattson and Chan, 2003; Smith et al., 2005). The breakdown of Ca^{2+} ion homeostasis is one characteristic of neurodegenerative diseases like AD and Parkinson's disease (PD), which is consistent with ion channel mechanisms (Hajieva et al., 2009; Mattson and Chan, 2001). Jang et al. used molecular dynamics (MD) simulation to examine the biophysical properties of Aβ peptide fragments 9–42 and 17–42 (Jang et al., 2010). They observed that these peptides formed ion channels. Experimental studies using AFM and single-channel conductance measurements verified the biological relevance of the simulations. Other morphologic studies using AFM, and EM, also revealed pore formation (Dzwolak et al., 2005; Kagan et al., 2002, 2004; Lashuel and Lansbury, 2006), providing additional support for the "channel hypothesis."

It has been reported that membrane disruption is related to phospholipids, gangliosides (McLaurin and Chakrabartty, 1996), and membrane leakage and dissolution (Ambroggio et al., 2005; Sparr et al., 2004). However, Aβ has been reported to bind to the basement membrane and induce the expression of membrane components such as laminin or collagen IV (Misumi et al., 2009). Aβ may also cause membrane lipid peroxidation, resulting in the perturbation of glucose transport and consequent neuronal degeneration (Mark et al., 1997). In vitro studies have shown that lipids can be oxidized by Aβ in the presence of low concentrations of ascorbate and copper (Murray et al., 2005). Furthermore, amyloid fibril formation can increase 4-hydroxy-2-nonenal (HNE) levels that result in oxidative lipid damage and the covalent modification of His side chains of Aβ, which further accelerates membrane damage and fibril formation in a feed-forward loop (Murray et al., 2007).

Interestingly, the mechanism of action of many antimicrobial peptides also involves channels or pore formation (Butterfield and Lashuel, 2010; Melo et al., 2009). A key factor in this mechanism is the amphipathicity of the peptides, which allows insertion of hydrophobic surfaces into the membrane and the maintenance of a hydrophilic core. These peptides may serve as models for Aβ:membrane interactions due to the similar amphipathic organization of the Aβ peptide (Bechinger and Lohner, 2006; Butterfield and Lashuel, 2010).

In Section 1.3.4 we discussed the effects of metals on Aβ assembly. One by-product of metal effects on Aβ assembly per se is the biological activities of the resulting assemblies. Zn^{2+} and Cu^{2+} facilitate β-sheet to α-helix conformational changes in Aβ that are accompanied by membrane-penetrating ability (Curtain et al., 2001; Talmard et al., 2009). These effects do not appear to result from simple metal bridging of multiple Aβ monomers. Even at substoichiometric concentration, Cu^{2+} and Zn^{2+} ions can react with Aβ to produce Cu^{2+}:Aβ and Zn^{2+}:Aβ complexes, rather than ternary Cu^{2+}:Aβ:Cu^{2+} complexes (Talmard et al., 2007). Cu^{2+}:Aβ complexes aggregate on anionic membrane surfaces and can penetrate the membrane by forming small vesicles. This penetration enhancement effect increases the cytotoxicity of Aβ (see Section 1.4.1) (Curtain et al., 2001; Faller, 2009; Faller and Hureau, 2009; Gehman et al., 2008). In the presence of Zn^{2+} or Cu^{2+} ions, Aβ42 is able to penetrate into palmitoyloleoyl phosphatidylcholine/palmitoylolyl phosphatidylserine vesicles at pH 5.5–7.5, an effect correlated with the formation of α-helical structure. In contrast, in the absence of these metal ions, Aβ42 is only able to penetrate into the vesicles below pH 5.5. Metal ions thus could allow Aβ42 to become membrane active at physiologic pH (Curtain et al., 2003).

In addition to active effects of Aβ on cellular membranes, the membrane themselves may actively facilitate Aβ aggregation (Relini et al., 2009). Membrane binding may be initiated by electrostatic interactions between Aβ and phospholipids, after which Aβ can insert into the lipid bilayer, forming a nidus for further Aβ accumulation (Aisenbrey et al., 2008; Chi et al., 2008). Membrane binding facilitates conformational changes in Aβ that facilitate in situ fibril formation leading to higher cytotoxicity (Chi et al., 2008; Okada et al., 2007). The effectiveness of the membrane in this capacity depends on its composition (Kim et al., 2006) and chemical properties (Bokvist and Grobner, 2007; Kayed et al., 2004), which affect membrane fluidity and phase (Wong et al., 2009). Effectiveness also is affected by environment factors such as metal ions, pH, cholesterol, and peptide-to-lipid ratio (Barnham et al., 2003; Bystrom et al., 2008). Cell membrane ganglioside GM1 can accelerate Aβ fibril formation (Chi et al., 2007).

1.4.2 Aβ AND MITOCHONDRIA

The mitochondrion is the key source of cellular energy and participates in a variety of other cellular processes, including apoptosis. During the production of *adenosine triphosphate* (ATP), reactive oxygen species (ROS) may be formed as metabolic by-products. This may cause mitochondrial dysfunction that is relevant to normal cellular aging processes as well as to neurodegenerative diseases (Cardoso et al., 2004; Ohta and Ohsawa, 2006; Tillement et al., 2011).

Due to the crucial role of mitochondria in cellular energy metabolism, ROS production, and aging, interactions between Aβ and mitochondria may be relevant to the cellular toxicity and dysfunction observed in AD (Tillement et al., 2011).

Caspersen et al. found Aβ in mitochondria from postmortem brain specimens of AD patients and an accumulation of Aβ in the brain mitochondria of APP transgenic mice (Caspersen et al., 2005). Manczak et al. found Aβ monomers and oligomers in isolated mitochondria from the cerebral cortex of APP transgenic mice (Manczak et al., 2006). A variety of mechanisms have been postulated to explain Aβ-mediated mitochondrial toxicity.

The interaction of Aβ with mitochondria may involve mitochondrial penetration, which has been observed in human neuroblastoma cells (Tillement et al., 2006). Tillement et al. reported that Aβ42 fragments colocalize with complex II of the respiratory chain enzymes, which indicates that Aβ can penetrate both the outer and inner mitochondrial membranes. Penetration appears to involve the translocase of the outer membrane (TOM40) and the translocase of the inner membrane (TIM22) (Hansson Petersen et al., 2008). Moreover, the interaction between Aβ and the membrane permeability transition pore (MPTP), which is formed as a complex of a voltage-dependent anion channel (VDAC), adenine nucleotide translocase, and cyclophilin-D, can change the permeability of the mitochondrial membrane, induce mitochondrial swelling, change the mitochondrial membrane potential ($\Delta\Psi$), and lead to cellular apoptosis and neuronal degeneration (Du et al., 2008; Moreira et al., 2002).

Aβ binds to various molecules inside the mitochondrion. Aβ-binding alcohol dehydrogenase (ABAD), a multifunctional enzyme with 261 amino acid residues, is one such molecule. In the brain mitochondria of AD transgenic mice (i.e., mAPP/ABAD mice), ABAD can be overexpressed in the Aβ-rich environment and exacerbate Aβ-induced apoptosis (Lustbader et al., 2004). The interaction between Aβ and ABAD can inhibit the 4-hydroxynonenal (4-HNE) detoxification function of ABAD, allowing persistence of ROS and consequent mitochondrial dysfunction (Murakami et al., 2009).

Aβ has been reported to uncouple the mitochondrial respiratory chain and enhance MPTP opening, leading to mitochondrial dysfunction or cell death (Tillement et al., 2006). Aβ is able to stimulate cytochrome c reductase (complex III) and inhibit cytochrome c oxidase (complex IV) (Rhein et al., 2009b). The overactivation of complex III, reported as a locus for superoxide radical production, increases ROS generation and damages mitochondria (Turrens, 2003). The decrease of complex IV activity results in increased carbonylation of proteins and also increases ROS production (Manczak et al., 2006). It also has been suggested that Aβ interacts with ATP synthase subunit α, thus inhibiting ATP production (Schmidt et al., 2008).

Aβ can enhance nitric oxide (NO) production within mitochondria (Keil et al., 2004). NO functions as an important signaling molecule in mammals. The generation of NO results in ATP depletion, ROS production, inhibition of cytochrome oxidase, S-nitrosylation of dynamin-related protein 1 (Drp1), and MPTP opening, which in turn induces mitochondrial dysfunction and leads to neurodegeneration (Brown and Borutaite, 2002; Cho et al., 2009; Keil et al., 2004). Aβ also has been reported to increase hippocampal interleukin-1β (IL-1β) and trigger c-Jun N-terminal kinase activation in rat hippocampus, inhibiting long-term potentiation and leading to apoptosis (Minogue et al., 2003).

Interactions of Aβ with the endoplasmic reticulum (ER) can induce calcium release from ER stores. This release can affect mitochondrial metabolism, inducing mitochondrial-mediated apoptosis (Ferreiro et al., 2008; Supnet and Bezprozvanny, 2010). This breakdown of calcium homeostasis can decrease endogenous glutathione levels, increase ROS production, and thus further affect normal mitochondrial function (Ferreiro et al., 2008).

The dynamics of mitochondria is governed by the equilibrium between organelle fission and fusion (Wang et al., 2007). Wang et al. reported that Aβ can alter the fission–fusion equilibrium, resulting in mitochondrial fragmentation and exacerbating cellular dysfunction (Wang et al., 2008). Aβ-induced S-nitrosylation of Drp-1 may be involved (Cho et al., 2009). Aβ also can reduce mitochondrial density in the cell periphery of M17 cells or neuronal processes of primary neurons, an effect that has been related to the presence of ADDLs, and may lead to mitochondrial and synaptic dysfunction in AD brains (Wang et al., 2009).

One hypothesis that may explain the effect of aging on the development of AD is mitochondrial DNA damage (Mancuso et al., 2008). It has been reported that the accumulation of point mutations in mitochondrial DNA (mt DNA) can reduce the activity of complex IV (cytochrome c oxidase) of the respiratory chain in the AD brain (Davis et al., 1997). These effects of Aβ on mitochondrial DNA appear to be mainly indirect, that is, they are mediated by increased ROS production (Volicer and Crino, 1990). Such indirect mechanisms have been verified in PC12 cells, in which exposure to Aβ fragments induces oxidative damage of mitochondrial DNA (Bozner et al., 1997). Aβ-induced oxidative effects on mitochondrial RNA (mt RNA) also have been suggested (Nunomura et al., 2009).

1.4.3 Aβ EFFECTS ON NEURONAL NETWORKS

Synaptic loss is one of the pathological hallmarks of AD and is correlated significantly with cognitive impairment (Dekosky and Scheff, 1990; Terry et al., 1991). Aβ may function as a modulator of synaptic activity, as it can affect synaptic transmission for different neurotransmitter systems in key brain areas that regulate executive and cognitive functions (Mura et al., 2010). It is a positive regulator presynaptically and a negative regulator postsynaptically (Palop and Mucke, 2010). Chronic Aβ exposure in a hippocampal neuron network model produces network dysfunction and affects hippocampal oscillatory properties (Pena et al., 2010). Recent studies in vitro and in APP transgenic mice show that oligomeric Aβ contributes to the decrease of LTP and synaptic plasticity observed in AD neurons, which can lead to decreased glutamatergic synaptic transmission strength and to the triggering of aberrant neural network activity (Billings et al., 2005; Chapman et al., 1999; Cleary et al., 2005; Hsia et al., 1999; Walsh et al., 2002). Aβ can cause decreases in the numbers of 2-amino-3-(3-hydroxy-5-methylisoxazol-4-yl) propionic acid (AMPA), N-methyl-D-aspartate receptors (NMDA), and metabotropic glutamate receptors, an effect that is associated with the collapse of glutamatergic dendritic spines (Hsieh et al., 2006; Parameshwaran et al., 2008; Shankar et al., 2007). The dysfunction of synaptic transmission further contributes to the destabilization of the entire neural networks (Palop and Mucke, 2010).

Intriguingly, neurons themselves may regulate Aβ production and aggregation (Cirrito et al., 2005; Hsieh et al., 2006; Kamenetz et al., 2003). In normal brains, synaptically regulated Aβ production is mediated, in part, by clathrin-dependent endocytosis of surface APP at presynaptic terminals, endosomal proteolytic cleavage of APP, and also Aβ release at synaptic terminals (Cirrito et al., 2005).

A number of mechanisms have been proposed to explain Aβ-mediated effects on neuronal electrical activity. In hippocampal neurons, Aβ affects several different Ca^{2+}-regulated signaling pathways. Aβ is able to increase intracellular Ca^{2+} concentration by enhancing Ca^{2+} efflux from voltage-gated Ca^{2+} channels and nonselective cation channels, by promoting Ca^{2+} release from intracellular stores, and by reducing Ca^{2+} efflux through NMDA receptors. The change in Ca^{2+} signaling further inhibits protein kinases, including Ca^{2+}/calmodulin-dependent protein kinase II, protein kinase A, and extracellular regulated kinases (Erk). Affecting these multiple Ca^{2+}-regulated signaling pathways may lead to synaptic dysfunction (Xie, 2004).

It also has been reported that low-order Aβ oligomers species inhibit LTP, can decrease dendritic spine density in organotypic hippocampal slice cultures, and also impair learning of complex behavior in rats (Rowan et al., 2005; Selkoe, 2008). Aβ trimers may be more effective in inhibiting LTP in rodents than are dimers (Townsend et al., 2006). The ability of Aβ oligomers to affect neuronal activity has been observed consistently in transgenic mouse models of AD, and may explain why cognitive impairment appears earlier than does amyloid deposition (Chapman et al., 2001; Rovelet-Lecrux et al., 2006; Zerbinatti et al., 2004).

1.4.4 Aβ CHEMISTRY

We discussed the role of metals on Aβ aggregation per se in Section 1.3.4. The concentrations of metals such as copper, zinc, and iron can be high in amyloid plaques of AD brains (Lovell et al., 1998; Miller et al., 2006). In vitro work supports the hypothesis that these metals can promote Aβ aggregation and fibrillization (Atwood et al., 1998; Bush et al., 1994; Esler et al., 1996; Mantyh et al., 1993). Furthermore, at physiological concentrations (pM), Aβ does not appear to aggregate, indicating that metals may be necessary for Aβ aggregation (Atwood et al., 2000; House et al., 2004; Huang et al., 2004; Sengupta et al., 2003). We discuss here some of the chemical properties of the Aβ:metal system.

Metal concentrations and distributions usually are regulated stringently by metalloproteins such as plastocyanin, one of the families of blue copper proteins, and

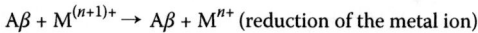

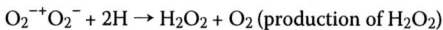

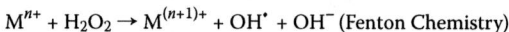

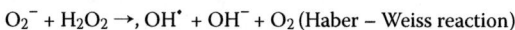

$$A\beta + M^{(n+1)+} \rightarrow A\beta + M^{n+} \text{ (reduction of the metal ion)}$$

$$M^{n+} + O_2 \rightarrow M^{n+1} + O_2^-$$

$$O_2^- {}^+ O_2^- + 2H \rightarrow H_2O_2 + O_2 \text{ (production of } H_2O_2)$$

$$M^{n+} + H_2O_2 \rightarrow M^{(n+1)+} + OH^\bullet + OH^- \text{ (Fenton Chemistry)}$$

$$O_2^- + H_2O_2 \rightarrow, OH^\bullet + OH^- + O_2 \text{ (Haber – Weiss reaction)}$$

FIGURE 1.6 Aβ in the Fenton and Haber-Weiss reactions. (From D. G. Smith, R. Cappai, and K. J. Barnham. "The Redox Chemistry of the Alzheimer's Disease Amyloid β Peptide." 2007. *Biochim Biophys Acta* 1768: 1976–1990. With permission from Elsevier).

ceruloplasmin, the major copper-carrying protein in the blood. However, metal homeostasis can be disrupted if the levels of certain metalloproteins decrease. For example, levels of metallothionein-3 (Zn_7MT-3), a metalloprotein that can regulate Cu^+ balance by capturing Cu^+ and forming a Cu^+-thiolate cluster, is down-regulated in AD brains (Meloni et al., 2008). The result of this down-regulation is the availability of copper for binding by Aβ, which binds Cu^+ with high affinity (Atwood et al., 2000; Opazo et al., 2002). The resultant Cu^+–Aβ complex induces oxidative damage and neuron degeneration through Fenton (Figure 1.6) chemistry and a Haber-Weiss reaction (Huang et al., 1999b; Smith et al., 2007). In AD brains, disruption of metal ion homeostasis may result in the overproduction of ROS. In vivo, *Drosophila* over-expressing wild-type Aβ42 were more likely to die given food with 10% (v/v) H_2O_2 than were nontransgenic control flies (Rival et al., 2009). Quantitative analysis of oxidative damage (carbonyl group levels) to brain proteins showed higher levels of carbonyls in transgenic flies (Rival et al., 2009). These results support a role for oxidative stress in AD-like brain pathology. In addition to the potential involvement of Fenton reactions in AD pathogenesis, glucose-6-phosphate dehydrogenase and heme oxygenase activities are increased, both of which can be related to oxidative stress. Increased ROS concentrations can further elevate the level of other toxic reactive compounds, such as HNE and malondialdehyde (Balazs and Leon, 1994; Martins et al., 1986; Schipper, 2004), which can attack lipids and organelles, leading to lipid peroxidation and organelle dysfunction (Markesbery and Lovell, 1998; Sayre et al., 1997; Williams et al., 2006). Several polyunsaturated fatty acids that constitute membrane phospholipids are particularly vulnerable to peroxidation (Nitsch et al., 1992). Furthermore, carbonyl derivatives can be generated by the ROS-mediated oxidation of protein side chains and introduced into proteins to form protein carbonyls through glycation and glycoxidation (Aksenov et al., 2001; Hensley et al., 1995; Lyras et al., 1997; Pamplona et al., 2005). Cellular damage such as this may lead to neuronal apoptosis and consequent brain dysfunction.

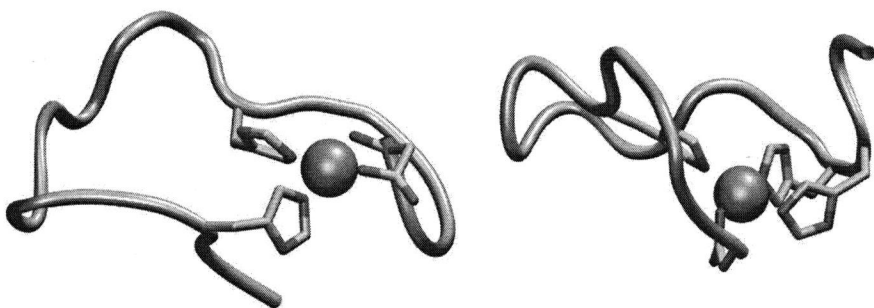

FIGURE 1.7A (See color insert.) Models of Cu(II) binding to Aβ: (N-term, His6, His13 or His14, Asp1-COO-) (left panel) and (Asp1-COO-, His6, His13, His14) (right panel). (From P. Faller. "Copper and Zinc Binding to Amyloid-Beta: Coordination, Dynamics, Aggregation, Reactivity and Metal-Ion Transfer." 2009. *Chembiochem* 10: 2837–2845; and P. Faller and C. Hureau. "Bioinorganic Chemistry of Copper and Zinc Ions Coordinated to Amyloid-β Peptide." 2009. *Dalton Trans* 1080–1094. With permission from John Wiley and Sons.)

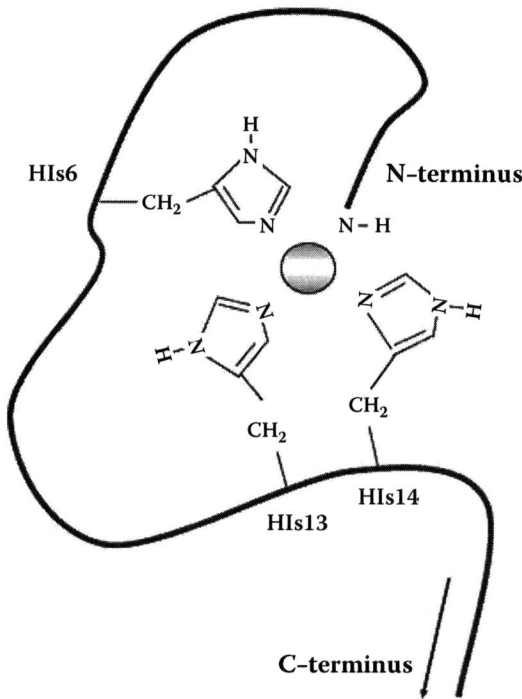

FIGURE 1.7B A model of Aβ bound to Zn2+. Three histidine residues and the N-terminus of Aβ coordinate the metal ion. Studies using various techniques, including signal intensity changes, relaxation data, and induced amide proton stability, suggest a turn at Glu3 and possibly at Gly9 and Gly25. (From J. Danielsson, R. Pierattelli, L. Banci, and A. Graslund. "High-Resolution NMR Studies of the Zinc-Binding Site of the Alzheimer's Amyloid β-Peptide." 2007. *FEBS* J 274: 46–59. With permission from John Wiley and Sons.)

Significant effort has been expended to understand the details of Aβ–metal coordination (Curtain et al., 2001; Dong et al., 2003; Karr and Szalai, 2008). It has been reported that Aβ can coordinate Cu^{2+} by forming ternary complexes involving the peptide N-terminus (Rozga et al., 2009). Depending on experimental conditions, the copper coordination center can be formed by Asp1-COO^-, N-term, His6, His13 (or His 14) or by Asp1-COO^-, His6, His13, and His14 (Figure 1.7a) (Drew et al., 2009; Faller, 2009; Kowalik-Jankowska et al., 2003).

The Cu^{2+} dissociation constant (K_d) has been determined using two general approaches: Cu^{2+} titration or competition of Cu^{2+} with His, Gly, and Phen Green ligands. In both approaches, K_d is determined by Tyr fluorescence, NMR, or isothermal titration calorimetry (ITC) (Faller and Hureau, 2009; Hatcher et al., 2008; Sokolowska and Bal, 2005). Table 1.1 summarizes results of these experiments (Faller, 2009). K_d values vary significantly (one or two orders of magnitude). It is likely that this variation reflects differences in experimental systems.

Fe^{3+} also has been implicated in Aβ-mediated toxicity through its catalytic role in Fenton chemistry, which results in the production of ROS such as $\cdot OH$ and $\cdot O_2^-$

TABLE 1.1
Dissociation Constants Reported for the Stoichiometric Coordination of Cu(II) to Aβ Peptides

Aβ Fragment	Kd/μM	Calculated Kd/nM	pH	Buffer/Competing Ligand	Experiments	Ref.	Kd (nM) Calculated According to:		
							(Hatcher, Hong et al. 2008)	(Tougu, Karafin et al. 2008)	(Sokolowska and Bal 2005)
1-16/28		0.21/0.024	7.4		Potentiometry	(Kowalik-Jankowska, Ruta et al. 2003)			
1-40/42	1.6–2.0		7.4	10mM Tris	Tyr fl.	(Garzon-Rodriguez, Yatsimirsky et al. 1999)	0.63	73–91	
1-16/28		100	7.8	Gly (His)	Tyr fl.	(Syme, Nadal et al. 2004)	0.4		
1-16/28/40	11–47		7.4	100mM Tris	Tyr fl.	(Karr, Akintoye et al. 2005)	~0.002	12–32	
1-16		10–100	7.8	Gly (His)	Tyr fl.	(Ma, Hu et al. 2006)	~0.4		
1-16/28		~100	7.4	Gly (His)	Tyr fl.	(Guilloreau, Damian et al. 2006)	~0.4		
1-40	8		7.2	50mM PO_4^-	Tyr fl.	(Raman, Ban et al. 2005)			
1-40	2.5		7.2	10mM Hepes	Tyr fl.	(Danielsson, Pierattelli et al. 2007)			300

Aβ		pH	Buffer	Method	Reference	Kd
1-40	0.4	7.2	10mM PO_4^-	Tyr fl.	(Danielsson, Pierattelli et al. 2007)	0.4/0.003/0.002
1-40	1.2/3.8/30	7.4	20/50/100mM Tris	Tyr fl.	(Tougu, Karafin et al. 2008)	35/24/54
1-40	0.6/0.9/2.5	7.4	20/50/100mM Hepes	Tyr fl.	(Tougu, Karafin et al. 2008)	24–36
1-16/28	0.1	7.4	50mM Hepes	ITC	(Guilloreau, Damian et al. 2006)	2.5
1-16	8	7.4	50mM Tris	ITC	(Faller and Hureau 2009)	0.006 / 50
1-40	16	7.3	5mM PO_4^- (at 4°)	NMR	(Hou and Zagorski 2006)	
1-16/40	0.4	7.4	Gly	ITC	(Hatcher, Hong et al. 2008)	
1-40	13[0.05][a]	7.4	Different chelator of known $^{c}K_d$	Chelator/Aβ separation	(Bush, Pettingell et al. 1994)	
1-42	5[6×10^{-9}][a]	7.4	Different chelator of known $^{c}K_d$	Chelator/Aβ separation	(Bush, Pettingell et al. 1994)	
1-40/42	4/0.3	7.4	20mM CH_3COO^-	Abs 214nm	(Atwood, Moir et al. 1998)	

[a] The number without brackets corresponds to the stoichiometric, but lower affinity binding site. The higher affinity value given in brackets was reported to correspond to substoichiometric metal content, and at least in case of Aβ42, to be an artifact of the measurement.

TABLE 1.2
Dissociation Constants Reported for the Stoichiometric Coordination of Zn(II) to Aβ Peptides

Aβ Fragment	Kd/μM	Kd/nM	pH	Buffer/Competing Ligand	Experiments	Ref.
1-40/42	300/57		7.4	10mM Tris	Tyr fl.	(Garzon-Rodriguez, Yatsimirsky et al. 1999)
1-16/28/40	22/10/7		7.4	Hepes and Tris	ITC	(Talmard, Bouzan et al. 2007)
Soluble 1-16/28/40/42		14/12/7/7	7.4	Hepes	Competition with Zincon	(Talmard, Bouzan et al. 2007)
Aggregated 1-40/42		3/3	7.4	Hepes	Competition with Zincon	(Talmard, Bouzan et al. 2007)
1-28	6.6		7.2	10mM Hepes	Tyr fl. of Zn/Cu competition NMR	(Danielsson, Pierattelli et al. 2007)
	1.2		7.2	10mM PO_4^-	Tyr fl. of Zn/Cu competition NMR	(Danielsson, Pierattelli et al. 2007)
1-40	1.1		7.2	10mM PO_4^-	Tyr fl. of Zn/Cu competition NMR	(Danielsson, Pierattelli et al. 2007)
1-40	60/184		7.4	10/100 mM Tris	Tyr fl.	(Tougu, Karafin et al. 2008)
	65		7.4	20mM Hepes	Tyr fl.	(Tougu, Karafin et al. 2008)
1-40/42		2	7.4	Zincon	Competition with Zincon after 30' incubation	(Tougu, Karafin et al. 2008)
		>11	7.4	Zincon	Before incubation	(Tougu, Karafin et al. 2008)
1-40	3.2		7.4	10mM Hepes or 10mM Tris	Displacement assay with cold and radioactive Zn	(Clements, Allsop et al. 1996)
	5[0.1][a]		7.4	20mM Tris	Displacement assay with cold and radioactive Zn	(Bush, Pettingell et al. 1994)
1-16/40/42	1–10		7.4	100mM Tris	Tyr fl.	(Ricchelli, Drago et al. 2005)

[a] For the Cu(II) ion, the number without brackets corresponds to the stoichiometric, but the number given in brackets corresponds to a substoichiometric binding of Zn(II) to Aβ40 with an apparent Kd of ~100 nM, which was determined by displacement assay with radioactive and cold Zn(II) binding to blotted peptide (Bush, Pettingell et al. 1994). However, in a subsequent study also using blotted peptide, but on a different membrane, no evidence was found for a sub-mM binding but confirmation of a Kd of ~5 mM for Aβ40 was given (Clements, Allsop et al. 1996).

(Huang et al., 1999a, 1999b; Liochev, 1999; Markesbery, 1997; Schubert and Chevion, 1995; Smith et al., 2007; Turnbull et al., 2001). In the AD brain, where metal ion homeostasis may be abnormal, high Fe^{3+} concentration can facilitate this chemistry, leading to structural modification of macromolecules (proteins, lipids, nucleic acids).

Zn^{2+} appears to have an effect opposite to those of Cu^{2+} and Fe^{3+}. By competing with Cu^{2+} or Fe^{3+} for binding to Aβ, Zn^{2+} can inhibit Aβ-mediated redox reactions, thereby reducing ROS production (Cuajungco et al., 2000) (Figure 1.7b). Zn^{2+} binding is followed by the deposition of Aβ into plaques, which many now argue are nontoxic (Smith et al., 2007). It has been reported that cells exposed to Aβ42 in the presence of both Cu^{2+} and Zn^{2+} display less injury than those treated with Cu^{2+} and Aβ42 alone, evidence of the aforementioned protective effect of Zn^{2+}. Zn^{2+} binding constants are summarized in Table 1.2 (Faller, 2009). As with Cu^{2+}, these values vary significantly depending on experimental conditions (Bush et al., 1994; Clements et al., 1996; Danielsson et al., 2007; Garzon-Rodriguez et al., 1999; Talmard et al., 2007). Nevertheless, comparing the Zn^{2+} and Cu^{2+} values, the K_d of Zn^{2+} is significantly higher than that of Cu^{2+} when using the same experimental system, which means Zn^{2+} binds less avidly to Aβ than does Cu^{2+}. Hence, the protective effect of Zn^{2+} is more limited.

Fundamental principles of chemical kinetics argue that if Aβ is involved in oxidation reactions, it also should be involved in reduction reactions, under appropriate system conditions. In fact, under certain conditions, Aβ does act as an antioxidant. In cerebrospinal fluid, Aβ, at concentrations between 0.1–1 nM, has antioxidant properties. However, at higher concentrations, pro-oxidant and cytotoxic activities are observed in vitro (Lee et al., 2005; Ueda et al., 1994). Aβ, in both oligomeric and fibrillar forms, can promote H_2O_2 generation at low Cu^{2+} concentration. However, inhibition of H_2O_2 generation occurs when the Cu^{2+} concentration increases (Fang et al., 2010). Functionally speaking, at nM concentration, Aβ may be neuroprotective (Smith et al., 2007; Whitson et al., 1989, 1990; Yankner et al., 1990), which is consistent with an antioxidant role. A full understanding of these concentration-dependent effects has not yet been achieved.

Aβ redox activity also is affected by ascorbic acid and α-tocopherol (vitamin E). Administration of these vitamins in combination decreases AD risk in elderly subjects (Zandi et al., 2004). Aβ-mediated release of free fatty acids can be inhibited by vitamin E (Koppal et al., 1998). However, α-lipoic acid has been reported to inhibit the activities of pyruvate dehydrogenase complex (PDHc). PDHc activity is reduced in AD brain and thus the functional and structural impairment of PDHc is believed to be related to AD. This further indicates that α-lipoic acid may facilitate AD development. Concomitant treatment of cultures with α-lipoic acid and Fe^{2+}/H_2O_2 significantly potentiated toxicity, promoting free radical production and oxidative stress (Lovell et al., 2003).

A substantial literature exists suggesting that Met35 is involved in redox chemistry and consequent Aβ toxicity (Butterfield and Boyd-Kimball, 2005; Clementi et al., 2006; Crouch et al., 2006). Met35 can be oxidized to methionine sulfoxide (MetO) or methionine sulfone $Met(O_2)$ (Moskovitz et al., 1999). Murakami et al., using site-directed spin labeling and electron spin resonance spectroscopy, found that the S-oxidized radical cation of Met35 could be produced in Aβ42 by the reduction of a Tyr10 radical that is brought into the proximity of Met35 by turn formation at residues 22 and 23 (Murakami et al., 2005, 2007). MetO can be reduced back to methionine by methionine sulfoxide reductase. However, methionine sulfone formation is irreversible in vivo. In AD brains, decreased methionine sulfoxide reductase activity has been detected, which is an observation consistent with a role for MetO in AD development (Gabbita et al., 1999; Lovell et al., 2000).

1.4.5 PROTEASOME EFFECTS

Proteasomes are large protein complexes, localized in the cytoplasm of eukaryotic cells, which function to degrade misfolded proteins and prevent accumulation of protein aggregates (Fratta et al., 2005; Peters et al., 1994). Proteins are tagged for proteasomal degradation by covalent addition of the small protein ubiquitin. Ubiquitinated proteins are quickly degraded by the 26S proteasome, the proteolytic component of the complex (Hegde, 2010). The ubiquitin–proteasome pathway is essential for cellular homeostasis. Dysfunction or disruption of the pathway is linked to neurodegeneration of the AD type.

In AD, Aβ can disrupt the degradation of ubiquitinated proteins by inhibiting proteasome activity. This can create a feed-forward cycle in which proteasome inhibition results in decreased Aβ degradation, allowing accumulation of Aβ that can further disrupt proteasome activity. The result is increased Aβ-induced toxicity. Aβ:proteasome interactions have been reported by many (Gregori et al., 1995, 1997). Based on these experiments, it was proposed that Aβ was a proteasome substrate and evidence demonstrating that Aβ42 aggregates are substrates for the chymotrypsin-like activity of the human 20S proteasome were published in 2010 (Zhao and Yang, 2010).

The interaction between Aβ and proteasomes may be relevant to other signaling pathways. For example, the intraneuronal Aβ42 accumulation occurring in multivesicular bodies (MVBs) is able to impair the MVB sorting pathway by inhibiting proteasome and de-ubiquitinating enzymes. Impairment of epidermal growth factor (EGF) signaling may occur due to abnormal ubiquitination and degradation of the epidermal growth factor receptor caused by intraneuronal Aβ aggregation (Almeida et al., 2006).

Aβ effects on proteasomes have been observed in vivo in the Tg2576 APP transgenic mice. Here, extracellular Aβ was found to enter neurons and inhibit proteasomal activity (Oh et al., 2005). In addition, in the triple-transgenic mouse model (3×Tg-AD), Aβ oligomers inhibited the chymotrypsin-like, trypsin-like, and postglutamyl peptide hydrolytic-like (also abbreviated as PGPH-like) activity of 20S proteasome in vitro. This inhibition produced a remarkable increase in Aβ and tau accumulation in these animals (Tseng et al., 2008).

As with other working hypotheses explaining the mechanism of Aβ toxicity, contrary opinions exist. This is the case with respect to proteasome effects as well. Antonella et al. reported that μM levels of Aβ40 could kill cortical neurons and induce the ubiquitination of several neuronal proteins (Favit et al., 2000). These results suggest that Aβ neurotoxicity occurs because the peptide activates the ubiquitin-proteasome pathway. In fact, Aβ toxicity can be blocked by preventing ubiquitination with Leu-Ala and inhibiting proteasome activity with lactacystin. Leu-Ala also can completely block Aβ-induced ubiquitination that is not lactacystin sensitive.

The effects of lactacystin are realized by blocking the activity of the proteasome downstream of ubiquitination (Favit et al., 2000; Obin et al., 1999). It also has been suggested that proteasome inhibition may decrease Aβ production by preventing β-secretase cleavage, without interfering with the PS1-dependent γ-secretase activity (McAlpine et al., 2009).

1.4.6 INFLAMMATORY EFFECTS

In the postmortem brains of AD patients, pro-inflammatory cytokines and chemokines, complement activation products, and oxygen radicals are observed (Akiyama et al., 2000; Heneka and O'Banion, 2007; McGeer and McGeer, 2003; Rojo et al., 2008). These molecules are produced by the innate immune system, which can be activated through pattern recognition receptors that recognize two types of molecular patterns, pathogen-associated molecular patterns (PAMPs), associated with microbial pathogens and cellular stress, and damage-associated molecular pattern (DAMP) molecules, associated with apoptotic and necrotic cells, protein aggregates, and aberrant cancer cell structures (Akira et al., 2006). Furthermore, cells under stress can secrete *alarmins*, such as HMGB1, S100, and HSPs that activate the immune system (Bianchi, 2007).

Aβ oligomers and fibrils not only induce neuron degeneration by direct cytotoxicity, but they also can trigger the innate immune system. This can result in astrocyte and microglial activation and the induction of NO production through an NF-kB-dependent mechanism (Akama et al., 1998; Hu and Van Eldik, 1999). Glial activation triggers the production of more DAMPs, creating a damaging cycle of inflammatory stimuli and neuropathogenesis (Hu and Van Eldik, 1999; Overmyer et al., 1999; Sheffield et al., 2000). The ability of Aβ to form membrane pores can activate the secretion of inflammasomes and IL-1β, which enhance neuronal kinase activity and result in the expression of hyperphosphorylated tau (Sheng et al., 2000). The hyperphosphorylation of tau can further lead to tangles of paired helical filaments and straight filaments, which are involved in the pathogenesis of Alzheimer's disease (Alonso et al., 2001).

It remains unclear precisely how Aβ activates glial cells, although NF-kB may be involved. NF-kB is a transcription factor that induces transcription of genes including IL-1β and inflammasomes. It has been reported that in primary rodent glial cultures, Aβ-induced increases in IL-1β secretion can be inhibited by antisense NF-kB (Bales et al., 2000). N-formyl peptide receptors and receptor for advanced glycation end products (RAGE), interacting with Aβ, also appear to contribute to NF-kB activation (Schmidt et al., 2001)

Another component of the innate immune response is macrophage phagocytosis of Aβ aggregates. A number of studies suggest that phagocytosis is defective in AD brains (Avagyan et al., 2009; Fiala et al., 2005, 2007; Masoumi et al., 2009; Zaghi et al., 2009). This defect leads to compensatory responses from the immune system, such as the overexpression of pro-inflammatory cytokines by neutrophils and monocytes. Furthermore, macrophages may migrate from the cerebral neuropil into vessels, causing vascular damage through apoptotic cell death and the release of Aβ aggregates that they could not digest.

1.5 CONCLUDING REMARKS

In his landmark work on the conduct of science, *The Structure of Scientific Revolutions*, Thomas S. Kuhn discussed how scientific revolutions involve periods during which myriad competing hypotheses exist, none of which achieve immediate supremacy over the others (Kuhn, 1962). As evidenced by the myriad hypotheses about the role of Aβ in AD, the AD field certainly must be considered to exist in this revolutionary state. The current AD "revolution" will end when a new paradigm emerges that provides better answers and predicts system behavior more accurately than do current paradigms. Prior to the late twentieth century, the AD field was guided by the amyloid cascade hypothesis, which argued the primacy of Aβ fibrils in disease causation. A minor revolution now has created a modified hypothesis in which Aβ oligomers are considered the key neurotoxic agents, and therefore the most important therapeutic targets. In the chapters that follow, discussions of diagnostic, prognostic, and therapeutic approaches toward AD are built, to a large degree, on the foundation of Aβ. Is this strategy reasonable? Will it be successful? At this point in time, no one can answer these questions.

For the reader who seeks a "take home message" or "the answer," the crisis state of the AD field may be disappointing. Scientific crises are resolved by the establishment of new, broad, and compelling experimental and theoretical paradigms. We hope that the reader, rather than being discouraged by what is unclear, will use the information provided here and in the following chapters as a basis for the development and testing of their own hypotheses about the etiology, pathogenesis, and treatment of AD, thereby accelerating progress toward a cure for this tragic disorder.

ACKNOWLEDGMENTS

This work was supported by grants AG027818 and NS038328 from the NIH, by the Jim Easton Consortium for Alzheimer's Disease Drug Discovery and Biomarkers at UCLA, and by grant #07-65806 from the State of California Alzheimer's Disease Research Fund.

REFERENCES

Ahlijanian, M. K., Barrezueta, N. X., Williams, R. D., Jakowski, A., Kowsz, K. P., McCarthy, S., Coskran, T., Carlo, A., Seymour, P. A., Burkhardt, J. E., Nelson, R. B., and McNeish, J. D. 2000. Hyperphosphorylated tau and neurofilament and cytoskeletal disruptions in mice overexpressing human p25, an activator of cdk5. *Proc Natl Acad Sci USA* 97: 2910–2915.

Ahmed, M., Davis, J., Aucoin, D., Sato, T., Ahuja, S., Aimoto, S., Elliott, J. I., Van Nostrand, W. E., and Smith, S. O. 2010. Structural conversion of neurotoxic amyloid-β(1-42) oligomers to fibrils. *Nat Struct Mol Biol* 17: 561–567.

Aisenbrey, C., Borowik, T., Bystrom, R., Bokvist, M., Lindstrom, F., Misiak, H., Sani, M. A., and Grobner, G. 2008. How is protein aggregation in amyloidogenic diseases modulated by biological membranes? *European Biophysics Journal with Biophysics Letters* 37: 247–255.

Akama, K. T., Albanese, C., Pestell, R. G., and Van Eldik, L. J. 1998. Amyloid β-peptide stimulates nitric oxide production in astrocytes through an NFκB-dependent mechanism. *Proc Natl Acad Sci USA* 95: 5795–5800.

Akira, S., Uematsu, S., and Takeuchi, O. 2006. Pathogen recognition and innate immunity. *Cell* 124: 783–801.

Akiyama, H., Barger, S., Barnum, S., Bradt, B., Bauer, J., Cole, G. M., Cooper, N. R., Eikelenboom, P., Emmerling, M., Fiebich, B. L., Finch, C. E., Frautschy, S., Griffin, W. S., Hampel, H., Hull, M., Landreth, G., Lue, L., Mrak, R., Mackenzie, I. R., McGeer, P. L., O'Banion, M. K., Pachter, J., Pasinetti, G., Plata-Salaman, C., Rogers, J., Rydel, R., Shen, Y., Streit, W., Strohmeyer, R., Tooyoma, I., Van Muiswinkel, F. L., Veerhuis, R., Walker, D., Webster, S., Wegrzyniak, B., Wenk, G., and Wyss-Coray, T. 2000. Inflammation and Alzheimer's disease. *Neurobiol Aging* 21: 383–421.

Aksenov, M. Y., Aksenova, M. V., Butterfield, D. A., Geddes, J. W., and Markesbery, W. R. 2001. Protein oxidation in the brain in Alzheimer's disease. *Neuroscience* 103: 373–383.

Allen, S. J., and Dawbarn, D., eds. 2001. *Neurobiology of Alzheimer's disease*, 2nd ed. Oxford: Oxford University Press.

Almeida, C. G., Takahashi, R. H., and Gouras, G. K. 2006. β-amyloid accumulation impairs multivesicular body sorting by inhibiting the ubiquitin-proteasome system. *J Neurosci* 26: 4277–4288.

Alonso, A., Zaidi, T., Novak, M., Grundke-Iqbal, I., and Iqbal, K. 2001. Hyperphosphorylation induces self-assembly of tau into tangles of paired helical filaments/straight filaments. *Proc Natl Acad Sci USA* 98: 6923–6928.

Al-Ubaidi, M. R., Hollyfield, J. G., Overbeek, P. A., and Baehr, W. 1992. Photoreceptor degeneration induced by the expression of simian virus 40 large tumor antigen in the retina of transgenic mice. *Proc Natl Acad Sci USA* 89: 1194–1198.

Alzheimer, A. Über eine eigenartige Erkrankung der Hirnrinde. 1907. *Allgemeine Z Psychiatrie Psychisch-Gerichtliche Med* 64: 146–148.

Alzheimer, A., Stelzmann, R. A., Schnitzlein, H. N., and Murtagh, F. R. 1995. An English translation of Alzheimer's 1907 paper, "Uber eine eigenartige Erkankung der Hirnrinde." *Clin Anat* 8: 429–431.

Ambroggio, E. E., Kim, D. H., Separovic, F., Barrow, C. J., Barnham, K. J., Bagatolli, L. A., and Fidelio, G. D. 2005. Surface behavior and lipid interaction of Alzheimer β-amyloid peptide 1-42: A membrane-disrupting peptide. *Biophys J* 88: 2706–2713.

Andreasen, N., Hesse, C., Davidsson, P., Minthon, L., Wallin, A., Winblad, B., Vanderstichele, H., Vanmechelen, E., and Blennow, K. . 1999a. Cerebrospinal fluid β-Amyloid(1-42) in Alzheimer disease: Differences between early- and late-onset alzheimer disease and stability during the course of disease. *Arch Neurol* 56: 673–680.

Andreasen, N., Minthon, L., Vanmechelen, E., Vanderstichele, H., Davidsson, P., Winblad, B., and Blennow, K. 1999b. Cerebrospinal fluid tau and Abeta42 as predictors of development of Alzheimer's disease in patients with mild cognitive impairment *Neuroscience Letters* 273: 5–8.

Anfinsen, C. B. 1973. Principles that govern the folding of protein chains. *Science* 181: 223–230.

Antzutkin, O. N., Leapman, R. D., Balbach, J. J., and Tycko, R. 2002. Supramolecular structural constraints on Alzheimer's β-amyloid fibrils from electron microscopy and solid-state nuclear magnetic resonance. *Biochemistry* 41: 15436–15450.

Arendt, T., Rodel, L., Gartner, U., and Holzer, M. 1996. Expression of the cyclin-dependent kinase inhibitor p16 in Alzheimer's disease. *Neuroreport* 7: 3047–3049.

Ariga, T., Miyatake, T., and Yu, R. K. 2010. Role of proteoglycans and glycosaminoglycans in the pathogenesis of Alzheimer's disease and related disorders: Amyloidogenesis and therapeutic strategies—A review. *J Neurosci Res* 88: 2303–2315.

Arimon, M., Diez-Perez, I., Kogan, M. J., Durany, N., Giralt, E., Sanz, F., and Fernandez-Busquets, X. 2005. Fine structure study of Aβ1-42 fibrillogenesis with atomic force microscopy. *FASEB J* 19: 1344–1346.

Arispe, N., Pollard, H. B., and Rojas, E. 1993a. Giant multilevel cation channels formed by Alzheimer disease amyloid β-protein [Aβ P-(1-40)] in bilayer membranes. *Proc Natl Acad Sci USA* 90: 10573–10577.

Arispe, N., Rojas, E., and Pollard, H. B. 1993b. Alzheimer disease amyloid β protein forms calcium channels in bilayer membranes: Blockade by tromethamine and aluminum. *Proc Natl Acad Sci USA* 90: 567–571.

Arispe, N., Pollard, H. B., and Rojas, E. 1996. Zn2+ interaction with Alzheimer amyloid beta protein calcium channels. *Proc Natl Acad Sci USA* 93: 1710–1715.

Arriagada, P. V., Marzloff, K., and Hyman, B. T. 1992. Distribution of Alzheimer-type pathologic changes in nondemented elderly individuals matches the pattern in Alzheimer's disease. *Neurology* 42: 1681–1688.

Ashe, K. H., and Zahs, K. R. 2010. Probing the biology of Alzheimer's disease in mice. *Neuron* 66: 631–645.

Astbury, W. T., and Dickinson, S. 1935. The x-ray interpretation of denaturation and the structure of the seed globulins. *The Biochemical Journal* 29: 2351–2360 2351.

Atwood, C. S., Moir, R. D., Huang, X., Scarpa, R. C., Bacarra, N. M., Romano, D. M., Hartshorn, M. A., Tanzi, R. E., and Bush, A. I. 1998. Dramatic aggregation of Alzheimer Aβ by Cu(II) is induced by conditions representing physiological acidosis. *J Biol Chem* 273: 12817–12826.

Atwood, C. S., Scarpa, R. C., Huang, X., Moir, R. D., Jones, W. D., Fairlie, D. P., Tanzi, R. E., and Bush, A. I. 2000. Characterization of copper interactions with Alzheimer amyloid β peptides: Identification of an attomolar-affinity copper binding site on amyloid beta1-42. *J Neurochem* 75: 1219–1233.

Avagyan, H., Goldenson, B., Tse, E., Masoumi, A., Porter, V., Wiedau-Pazos, M., Sayre, J., Ong, R., Mahanian, M., Koo, P., Bae, S., Micic, M., Liu, P. T., Rosenthal, M. J., and Fiala, M. 2009. Immune blood biomarkers of Alzheimer disease patients. *J Neuroimmunol* 210: 67–72.

Balazs, L., and Leon, M. 1994. Evidence of an oxidative challenge in the Alzheimer's brain. *Neurochem Res* 19: 1131–1137.

Balducci, C., Beeg, M., Stravalaci, M., Bastone, A., Sclip, A., Biasini, E., Tapella, L., Colombo, L., Manzoni, C., Borsello, T., Chiesa, R., Gobbi, M., Salmona, M., and Forloni, G. 2010. Synthetic amyloid-β oligomers impair long-term memory independently of cellular prion protein. *Proc Natl Acad Sci USA* 107: 2295–2300.

Bales, K. R., Dodart, J. C., Demattos, R. B., Holtzman, D. M., and Paul, S. M. 2002. Apolipoprotein E, amyloid, and Alzheimer disease. *Mol Interv* 2: 363–375, 339.

Bales, K. R., Du, Y., Holtzman, D., Cordell, B., and Paul, S. M. 2000. Neuroinflammation and Alzheimer's disease: Critical roles for cytokine/Aβ-induced glial activation, NF-κB, and apolipoprotein E. *Neurobiol Aging* 21: 427–432; discussion 451–423.

Bales, K. R., Liu, F., Wu, S., Lin, S., Koger, D., Delong, C., Hansen, J. C., Sullivan, P. M., and Paul, S. M. 2009. Human APOE isoform-dependent effects on brain β-amyloid levels in PDAPP transgenic mice. *J Neurosci* 29: 6771–6779.

Barghorn, S., Nimmrich, V., Striebinger, A., Krantz, C., Keller, P., Janson, B., Bahr, M., Schmidt, M., Bitner, R. S., Harlan, J., Barlow, E., Ebert, U., and Hillen, H. 2005. Globular amyloid β-peptide oligomer: A homogenous and stable neuropathological protein in Alzheimer's disease. *J Neurochem* 95: 834–847.

Barnham, K. J., Ciccotosto, G. D., Tickler, A. K., Ali, F. E., Smith, D. G., Williamson, N. A., Lam, Y. H., Carrington, D., Tew, D., Kocak, G., Volitakis, I., Separovic, F., Barrow, C. J., Wade, J. D., Masters, C. L., Cherny, R. A., Curtain, C. C., Bush, A. I., and Cappai, R. 2003. Neurotoxic, redox-competent Alzheimer's β-amyloid is released from lipid membrane by methionine oxidation. *J Biol Chem* 278: 42959–42965.

Barrow, C. J., Yasuda, A., Kenny, P. T., and Zagorski, M. G. 1992. Solution conformations and aggregational properties of synthetic amyloid β-peptides of Alzheimer's disease. Analysis of circular dichroism spectra. *J Mol Biol* 225: 1075–1093.

Baskakov, I. V., 2007. *Protein misfolding, aggregation, and conformational diseases.* New York: Springer.

Basler, K., Oesch, B., Scott, M., Westaway, D., Walchli, M., Groth, D. F., McKinley, M. P., Prusiner, S. B., and Weissmann, C. 1986. Scrapie and cellular PrP isoforms are encoded by the same chromosomal gene. *Cell* 46: 417–428.

Baumann, K., Mandelkow, E. M., Biernat, J., Piwnica-Worms, H., and Mandelkow, E. 1993. Abnormal Alzheimer-like phosphorylation of tau-protein by cyclin-dependent kinases cdk2 and cdk5. *FEBS Lett* 336: 417–424.

Baumketner, A., Bernstein, S. L., Wyttenbach, T., Lazo, N. D., Teplow, D. B., Bowers, M. T., and Shea, J. E. 2006. Structure of the 21-30 fragment of amyloid β-protein. *Protein Sci* 15: 1239–1247.

Bechinger, B., and Lohner, K. 2006. Detergent-like actions of linear amphipathic cationic antimicrobial peptides. *Biochim Biophys Acta* 1758: 1529–1539.

Bergmans, B. A., and De Strooper, B. 2010. γ-Secretases: From cell biology to therapeutic strategies. *Lancet Neurol* 9: 215–226.

Bernstein, S. L., Dupuis, N. F., Lazo, N. D., Wyttenbach, T., Condron, M. M., Bitan, G., Teplow, D. B., Shea, J.-E., Ruotolo, B. T., Robinson, C. V., and Bowers, M. T. 2009. Amyloid-β protein oligomerization and the importance of tetramers and dodecamers in the aetiology of Alzheimer's disease. *Nature Chemistry* 1: 326–331.

Bertram, L., Lill, C. M., and Tanzi, R. E. 2010. The genetics of Alzheimer disease: Back to the future. *Neuron* 68: 270–281.

Bianchi, M. E. 2007. DAMPs, PAMPs and alarmins: All we need to know about danger. *J Leukoc Biol* 81: 1–5.

Biessels, G. J., and Kappelle, L. J. 2005. Increased risk of Alzheimer's disease in Type II diabetes: Insulin resistance of the brain or insulin-induced amyloid pathology? *Biochem Soc Trans* 33: 1041–1044.

Billings, L. M., Oddo, S., Green, K. N., McGaugh, J. L., and Laferla, F. M. 2005. Intraneuronal Aβ causes the onset of early Alzheimer's disease-related cognitive deficits in transgenic mice. *Neuron* 45: 675–688.

Bishop, G. M., and Robinson, S. R. 2002. The amyloid hypothesis: Let sleeping dogmas lie? *Neurobiol Aging* 23: 1101–1105.

Bitan, G., Kirkitadze, M. D., Lomakin, A., Vollers, S. S., Benedek, G. B., and Teplow, D. B. 2003. Amyloid β-protein (Aβ) assembly: Aβ 40 and Aβ 42 oligomerize through distinct pathways. *Proc Natl Acad Sci USA* 100: 330–335.

Bitan, G., Lomakin, A., and Teplow, D. B. 2001. Amyloid β-protein oligomerization: Prenucleation interactions revealed by photo-induced cross-linking of unmodified proteins. *J Biol Chem* 276: 35176–35184.

Bitan, G., and Teplow, D. B. 2004. Rapid photochemical cross-linking: A new tool for studies of metastable, amyloidogenic protein assemblies. *Acc Chem Res* 37: 357–364.

Bokvist, M., and Grobner, G. 2007. Misfolding of amyloidogenic proteins at membrane surfaces: The impact of macromolecular crowding. *J Am Chem Soc* 129: 14848–14849.

Bolton, D. C., Bendheim, P. E., Marmorstein, A. D., and Potempska, A. 1987. Isolation and structural studies of the intact scrapie agent protein. *Arch Biochem Biophys* 258: 579–590.

Bonda, D. J., Lee, H. P., Kudo, W., Zhu, X., Smith, M. A., and Lee, H. G. 2010. Pathological implications of cell cycle re-entry in Alzheimer disease. *Expert Rev Mol Med* 12: e19.

Borreguero, J. M., Urbanc, B., Lazo, N. D., Buldyrev, S. V., Teplow, D. B., and Stanley, H. E. 2005. Folding events in the 21-30 region of amyloid β-protein (Aβ) studied in silico. *Proc Natl Acad Sci USA* 102: 6015–6020.

Bosques, C. J., and Imperiali, B. 2003. The interplay of glycosylation and disulfide formation influences fibrillization in a prion protein fragment. *Proc Natl Acad Sci USA* 100: 7593–7598.

Bowen, R. L., Smith, M. A., Harris, P. L., Kubat, Z., Martins, R. N., Castellani, R. J., Perry, G., and Atwood, C. S. 2002. Elevated luteinizing hormone expression colocalizes with neurons vulnerable to Alzheimer's disease pathology. *J Neurosci Res* 70: 514–518.

Bowser, R., and Smith, M. A. 2002. Cell cycle proteins in Alzheimer's disease: Plenty of wheels but no cycle. *Journal of Alzheimer's Disease: JAD* 4: 249–254.

Boyles, J. K., Notterpek, L. M., and Anderson, L. J. 1990. Accumulation of apolipoproteins in the regenerating and remyelinating mammalian peripheral nerve. Identification of apolipoprotein D, apolipoprotein A-IV, apolipoprotein E, and apolipoprotein A-I. *J Biol Chem* 265: 17805–17815.

Boyles, J. K., Zoellner, C. D., Anderson, L. J., Kosik, L. M., Pitas, R. E., Weisgraber, K. H., Hui, D. Y., Mahley, R. W., Gebicke-Haerter, P. J., Ignatius, M. J., et al. 1989. A role for apolipoprotein E, apolipoprotein A-I, and low density lipoprotein receptors in cholesterol transport during regeneration and remyelination of the rat sciatic nerve. *J Clin Invest* 83: 1015–1031.

Bozner, P., Grishko, V., Ledoux, S. P., Wilson, G. L., Chyan, Y. C., and Pappolla, M. A. 1997. The amyloid β protein induces oxidative damage of mitochondrial DNA. *J Neuropathol Exp Neurol* 56: 1356–1362.

Braak, H., Del Tredici, K., Schultz, C., and Braak, E. 2000. Vulnerability of select neuronal types to Alzheimer's disease. *Ann NY Acad Sci* 924: 53–61.

Brown, G. C., and Borutaite, V. 2002. Nitric oxide inhibition of mitochondrial respiration and its role in cell death. *Free Radic Biol Med* 33: 1440–1450.

Brown, R. E., and Wong, A. A. 2007. The influence of visual ability on learning and memory performance in 13 strains of mice. *Learn Mem* 14: 134–144.

Burdick, D., Kosmoski, J., Knauer, M. F., and Glabe, C. G. 1997. Preferential adsorption, internalization and resistance to degradation of the major isoform of the Alzheimer's amyloid peptide, Aβ 1-42, in differentiated PC12 cells. *Brain Res* 746: 275–284.

Burdick, D., Soreghan, B., Kwon, M., Kosmoski, J., Knauer, M., Henschen, A., Yates, J., Cotman, C., and Glabe, C. 1992. Assembly and aggregation properties of synthetic Alzheimer's A4/β amyloid peptide analogs. *J Biol Chem* 267: 546–554.

Busciglio, J., Lorenzo, A., Yeh, J., and Yankner, B. A. 1995. β-amyloid fibrils induce tau phosphorylation and loss of microtubule binding. *Neuron* 14: 879–888.

Bush A. I., Pettingell W. H., Jr., Paradis M. D., & Tanzi R. E. 1994. Modulation of Aβ adhesiveness and secretase site cleavage by zinc. *J Biol Chem* 269(16): 12152–12158 (in eng).

Bush, A. I., Pettingell, W. H., Multhaup, G., D Paradis, M., Vonsattel, J. P., Gusella, J. F., Beyreuther, K., Masters, C. L., and Tanzi, R. E. 1994. Rapid induction of Alzheimer Aβ amyloid formation by zinc. *Science* 265: 1464–1467.

Busser, J., Geldmacher, D. S., and Herrup, K. 1998. Ectopic cell cycle proteins predict the sites of neuronal cell death in Alzheimer's disease brain. *J Neurosci* 18: 2801–2807.

Butterfield, D. A., Abdul, H. M., Opii, W., Newman, S. F., Joshi, G., Ansari, M. A., and Sultana, R. 2006. Pin1 in Alzheimer's disease. *J Neurochem* 98: 1697–1706.

Butterfield, D. A., and Boyd-Kimball, D. 2005. The critical role of methionine 35 in Alzheimer's amyloid β-peptide (1-42)-induced oxidative stress and neurotoxicity. *Biochim Biophys Acta* 1703: 149–156.

Butterfield, S. M., and Lashuel, H. A. 2010. Amyloidogenic protein-membrane interactions: Mechanistic insight from model systems. *Angew Chem Int Ed Engl* 49: 5628–5654.

Bystrom, R., Aisenbrey, C., Borowik, T., Bokvist, M., Lindstrom, F., Sani, M. A., Olofsson, A., and Grobner, G. 2008. Disordered proteins: Biological membranes as two-dimensional aggregation matrices. *Cell Biochem Biophys* 52: 175–189.

Cai, X. D., Golde, T. E., and Younkin, S. G. 1993. Release of excess amyloid β protein from a mutant amyloid β protein precursor. *Science* 259: 514–516.

Calloni, G., Zoffoli, S., Stefani, M., Dobson, C. M., and Chiti, F. 2005. Investigating the effects of mutations on protein aggregation in the cell. *J Biol Chem* 280: 10607–10613.

Cardoso, S. M., Santana, I., Swerdlow, R. H., and Oliveira, C. R. 2004. Mitochondria dysfunction of Alzheimer's disease cybrids enhances Aβ toxicity. *J Neurochem* 89: 1417–1426.

Carro, E., and Torres-Aleman, I. 2004. The role of insulin and insulin-like growth factor I in the molecular and cellular mechanisms underlying the pathology of Alzheimer's disease. *Eur J Pharmacol* 490: 127–133.

Caruso, A., Motolese, M., Iacovelli, L., Caraci, F., Copani, A., Nicoletti, F., Terstappen, G. C., Gaviraghi, G., and Caricasole, A. 2006. Inhibition of the canonical Wnt signaling pathway by apolipoprotein E4 in PC12 cells. *J Neurochem* 98: 364–371.

Caspersen, C., Wang, N., Yao, J., Sosunov, A., Chen, X., Lustbader, J. W., Xu, H. W., Stern, D., McKhann, G., and Yan, S. D. 2005. Mitochondrial Aβ: A potential focal point for neuronal metabolic dysfunction in Alzheimer's disease. *FASEB J* 19: 2040–2041.

Catalano, S. M., Dodson, E. C., Henze, D. A., Joyce, J. G., Krafft, G. A., and Kinney, G. G. 2006. The role of amyloid-β derived diffusible ligands (ADDLs) in Alzheimer's disease. *Curr Top Med Chem* 6: 597–608.

Caughey, B., and Lansbury, P. T. 2003. Protofibrils, pores, fibrils, and neurodegeneration: Separating the responsible protein aggregates from the innocent bystanders. *Annu Rev Neurosci* 26: 267–298.

Cedazo-Minguez, A., Popescu, B. O., Blanco-Millan, J. M., Akterin, S., Pei, J. J., Winblad, B., and Cowburn, R. F. 2003. Apolipoprotein E and β-amyloid (1-42) regulation of glycogen synthase kinase-3β. *J Neurochem* 87: 1152–1164.

Champagne, D., Pearson, D., Dea, D., Rochford, J., and Poirier, J. 2003. The cholesterol-lowering drug probucol increases apolipoprotein E production in the hippocampus of aged rats: Implications for Alzheimer's disease. *Neuroscience* 121: 99–110.

Chan, Y. H., and Boxer, S. G. 2007. Model membrane systems and their applications. *Curr Opin Chem Biol* 11: 581–587.

Chang, S., Ran Ma, T., Miranda, R. D., Balestra, M. E., Mahley, R. W., and Huang, Y. 2005. Lipid- and receptor-binding regions of apolipoprotein E4 fragments act in concert to cause mitochondrial dysfunction and neurotoxicity. *Proc Natl Acad Sci USA* 102: 18694–18699.

Chapman, P. F., Falinska, A. M., Knevett, S. G., and Ramsay, M. F. 2001. Genes, models and Alzheimer's disease. *Trends Genet* 17: 254–261.

Chapman, P. F., White, G. L., Jones, M. W., Cooper-Blacketer, D., Marshall, V. J., Irizarry, M., Younkin, L., Good, M. A., Bliss, T. V., Hyman, B. T., Younkin, S. G., and Hsiao, K. K. 1999. Impaired synaptic plasticity and learning in aged amyloid precursor protein transgenic mice. *Nat Neurosci* 2: 271–276.

Chasseigneaux, S., Dinc, L., Rose, C., Chabret, C., Coulpier, F., Topilko, P., Mauger, G., and Allinquant, B. 2011. Secreted amyloid precursor protein β and secreted amyloid precursor protein α induce axon outgrowth in vitro through Egr1 signaling pathway. *PLoS One* 6: e16301.

Chen, P. Y., Lin, C. C., Chang, Y. T., Lin, S. C., and Chan, S. I. 2002. One O-linked sugar can affect the Coil-to-β structural transition of the prion peptide. *Proc Natl Acad Sci USA* 99: 12633–12638.

Chen, S., Yadav, S. P., and Surewicz, W. K. 2010. Interaction between human prion protein and amyloid-β (Aβ) oligomers: Role of N-terminal residues. *J Biol Chem* 285: 26377–26383.

Chen, W., Mousseau, N., and Derreumaux, P. 2006. The conformations of the amyloid-β (21-30) fragment can be described by three families in solution. *J Chem Phys* 125: 084911.

Chen, W. T., Liao, Y. H., Yu, H. M., Cheng, I. H., and Chen, Y. R. 2011. Distinct effects of Zn2+, Cu2+, Fe3+, and Al3+ on amyloid-β stability, oligomerization, and aggregation: Amyloid-β destabilization promotes annular protofibril formation. *J Biol Chem* 286: 9646–9656.

Chen, Y., McPhie, D. L., Hirschberg, J., and Neve, R. L. 2000. The amyloid precursor protein-binding protein APP-BP1 drives the cell cycle through the S-M checkpoint and causes apoptosis in neurons. *J Biol Chem* 275: 8929–8935.

Cheng, I. H., Scearce-Levie, K., Legleiter, J., Palop, J. J., Gerstein, H., Bien-Ly, N., Puolivali, J., Lesne, S., Ashe, K. H., Muchowski, P. J., and Mucke, L. 2007. Accelerating amyloid-β fibrillization reduces oligomer levels and functional deficits in Alzheimer disease mouse models. *J Biol Chem* 282: 23818–23828.

Chi, E. Y., Ege, C., Winans, A., Majewski, J., Wu, G., Kjaer, K., and Lee, K. Y. 2008. Lipid membrane templates the ordering and induces the fibrillogenesis of Alzheimer's disease amyloid-β peptide. *Proteins* 72: 1–24.

Chi, E. Y., Frey, S. L., and Lee, K. Y. 2007. Ganglioside G(M1)-mediated amyloid-β fibrillogenesis and membrane disruption. *Biochemistry* 46: 1913–1924.

Chiti, F., Stefani, M., Taddei, N., Ramponi, G., and Dobson, C. M. 2003. Rationalization of the effects of mutations on peptide and protein aggregation rates. *Nature* 424: 805–808.

Cho, D. H., Nakamura, T., Fang, J., Cieplak, P., Godzik, A., Gu, Z., and Lipton, S. A. 2009. S-nitrosylation of Drp1 mediates β-amyloid-related mitochondrial fission and neuronal injury. *Science* 324: 102–105.

Cirrito, J. R., Yamada, K. A., Finn, M. B., Sloviter, R. S., Bales, K. R., May, P. C., Schoepp, D. D., Paul, S. M., Mennerick, S., and Holtzman, D. M. 2005. Synaptic activity regulates interstitial fluid amyloid-β levels in vivo. *Neuron* 48: 913–922.

Cisse, M., and Mucke, L. 2009. Alzheimer's disease: A prion protein connection. *Nature* 457: 1090–1091.

Clarke, A. R., Maandag, E. R., Van Roon, M., Van Der Lugt, N. M., Van Der Valk, M., Hooper, M. L., Berns, A., and Te Riele, H. 1992. Requirement for a functional Rb-1 gene in murine development. *Nature* 359: 328–330.

Cleary, J. P., Walsh, D. M., Hofmeister, J. J., Shankar, G. M., Kuskowski, M. A., Selkoe, D. J., and Ashe, K. H. 2005. Natural oligomers of the amyloid-β protein specifically disrupt cognitive function. *Nat Neurosci* 8: 79–84.

Clementi, M. E., Pezzotti, M., Orsini, F., Sampaolese, B., Mezzogori, D., Grassi, C., Giardina, B., and Misiti, F. 2006. Alzheimer's amyloid β-peptide (1-42) induces cell death in human neuroblastoma via bax/bcl-2 ratio increase: An intriguing role for methionine 35. *Biochem Biophys Res Commun* 342: 206–213.

Clements, A., Allsop, D., Walsh, D. M., and Williams, C. H. 1996. Aggregation and metal-binding properties of mutant forms of the amyloid Aβ peptide of Alzheimer's disease. *J Neurochem* 66: 740–747.

Clinton, L. K., Blurton-Jones, M., Myczek, K., Trojanowski, J. Q., and Laferla, F. M. 2010. Synergistic Interactions between Aβ, tau, and α-synuclein: Acceleration of neuropathology and cognitive decline. *J Neurosci* 30: 7281–7289.

Coles, M., Bicknell, W., Watson, A. A., Fairlie, D. P., and Craik, D. J. 1998. Solution structure of amyloid β-peptide(1-40) in a water-micelle environment. Is the membrane-spanning domain where we think it is? *Biochemistry* 37: 11064–11077.

Connell-Crowley, L., Le Gall, M., Vo, D. J., and Giniger, E. 2000. The cyclin-dependent kinase Cdk5 controls multiple aspects of axon patterning *in vivo*. *Curr Biol* 10: 599–602.

Cook, D. G., Forman, M. S., Sung, J. C., Leight, S., Kolson, D. L., Iwatsubo, T., Lee, V. M., and Doms, R. W. 1997. Alzheimer's Aβ(1-42) is generated in the endoplasmic reticulum/intermediate compartment of NT2N cells. *Nature Medicine* 3: 1021–1023.

Copani, A., Condorelli, F., Caruso, A., Vancheri, C., Sala, A., Giuffrida Stella, A. M., Canonico, P. L., Nicoletti, F., and Sortino, M. A. 1999. Mitotic signaling by beta-amyloid causes neuronal death. *FASEB J* 13: 2225–2234.

Copani, A., Uberti, D., Sortino, M. A., Bruno, V., Nicoletti, F., and Memo, M. 2001. Activation of cell-cycle-associated proteins in neuronal death: A mandatory or dispensable path? *Trends Neurosci* 24: 25–31.

Cope, G. A., and Deshaies, R. J. 2003. COP9 signalosome: A multifunctional regulator of SCF and other cullin-based ubiquitin ligases. *Cell* 114: 663–671.

Cordy, J. M., Hussain, I., Dingwall, C., Hooper, N. M., and Turner, A. J. 2003. Exclusively targeting beta-secretase to lipid rafts by GPI-anchor addition up-regulates β-site processing of the amyloid precursor protein. *Proc Natl Acad Sci USA* 100: 11735–11740.

Costello, D. A., O'Leary, D. M., and Herron, C. E. 2005. Agonists of peroxisome proliferator-activated receptor-γ attenuate the Aβ-mediated impairment of LTP in the hippocampus in vitro. *Neuropharmacology* 49: 359–366.

Crabbe, J. C., Wahlsten, D., and Dudek, B. C. 1999. Genetics of mouse behavior: interactions with laboratory environment. *Science* 284: 1670–1672.

Crescenzi, O., Tomaselli, S., Guerrini, R., Salvadori, S., D'Ursi, A. M., Temussi, P. A., and Picone, D. 2002. Solution structure of the Alzheimer amyloid β-peptide (1-42) in an apolar microenvironment. Similarity with a virus fusion domain. *Eur J Biochem* 269: 5642–5648.

Crook, R., Verkkoniemi, A., Perez-Tur, J., Mehta, N., Baker, M., Houlden, H., Farrer, M., Hutton, M., Lincoln, S., Hardy, J., Gwinn, K., Somer, M., Paetau, A., Kalimo, H., Ylikoski, R., Poyhonen, M., Kucera, S., and Haltia, M. 1998. A variant of Alzheimer's disease with spastic paraparesis and unusual plaques due to deletion of exon 9 of presenilin 1. *Nat Med* 4: 452–455.

Crouch, P. J., Barnham, K. J., Duce, J. A., Blake, R. E., Masters, C. L., and Trounce, I. A. 2006. Copper-dependent inhibition of cytochrome c oxidase by Aβ(1-42) requires reduced methionine at residue 35 of the Aβ peptide. *J Neurochem* 99: 226–236.

Crouch, P. J., Harding, S. M., White, A. R., Camakaris, J., Bush, A. I., and Masters, C. L. 2008. Mechanisms of Aβ mediated neurodegeneration in Alzheimer's disease. *Int J Biochem Cell Biol* 40: 181–198.

Cruz, L., Urbanc, B., Borreguero, J. M., Lazo, N. D., Teplow, D. B., and Stanley, H. E. 2005. Solvent and mutation effects on the nucleation of amyloid β-protein folding. *Proc Natl Acad Sci USA* 102: 18258–18263.

Cuajungco, M. P., Goldstein, L. E., Nunomura, A., Smith, M. A., Lim, J. T., Atwood, C. S., Huang, X., Farrag, Y. W., Perry, G., and Bush, A. I. 2000. Evidence that the β-amyloid plaques of Alzheimer's disease represent the redox-silencing and entombment of Aβ by zinc. *J Biol Chem* 275: 19439–19442.

Cummings, J. L., and Apostolova, L. G. 2007. The pathogenesis of Alzheimer's disease: General overview. In *Protein Misfolding, Aggregation, and Conformational Diseases*, ed. A. L. Fink and V. N. Uversky, 3–29. New York: Springer.

Curtain, C. C., Ali, F. E., Smith, D. G., Bush, A. I., Masters, C. L., and Barnham, K. J. 2003. Metal ions, pH, and cholesterol regulate the interactions of Alzheimer's disease amyloid-β peptide with membrane lipid. *J Biol Chem* 278: 2977–2982.

Curtain, C. C., Ali, F., Volitakis, I., Cherny, R. A., Norton, R. S., Beyreuther, K., Barrow, C. J., Masters, C. L., Bush, A. I., and Barnham, K. J. 2001. Alzheimer's disease amyloid-β binds copper and zinc to generate an allosterically ordered membrane-penetrating structure containing superoxide dismutase-like subunits. *J Biol Chem* 276: 20466–20473.

Dahlgren, K. N., Manelli, A. M., Stine, W. B., Jr., Baker, L. K., Krafft, G. A., and Ladu, M. J. 2002. Oligomeric and fibrillar species of amyloid-β peptides differentially affect neuronal viability. *J Biol Chem* 277: 32046–32053.

Danielsson, J., Pierattelli, R., Banci, L., and Graslund, A. 2007. High-resolution NMR studies of the zinc-binding site of the Alzheimer's amyloid β-peptide. *FEBS J* 274: 46–59.

Daugherty, B. L., and Green, S. A. 2001. Endosomal sorting of amyloid precursor protein-P-selectin chimeras influences secretase processing. *Traffic* 2: 908–916.

Davis, R. E., Miller, S., Herrnstadt, C., Ghosh, S. S., Fahy, E., Shinobu, L. A., Galasko, D., Thal, L. J., Beal, M. F., Howell, N., and Parker, W. D., Jr. 1997. Mutations in mitochondrial cytochrome c oxidase genes segregate with late-onset alzheimer disease. *Proc Natl Acad Sci USA* 94: 4526–4531.

De Ferrari, G. V., and Moon, R. T. 2006. The ups and downs of Wnt signaling in prevalent neurological disorders. *Oncogene* 25: 7545–7553.

De Ferrari, G. V., Papassotiropoulos, A., Biechele, T., Wavrant De-Vrieze, F., Avila, M. E., Major, M. B., Myers, A., Saez, K., Henriquez, J. P., Zhao, A., Wollmer, M. A., Nitsch, R. M., Hock, C., Morris, C. M., Hardy, J., and Moon, R. T. 2007. Common genetic variation within the low-density lipoprotein receptor-related protein 6 and late-onset alzheimer's disease. *Proc Natl Acad Sci USA* 104: 9434–9439.

De Strooper, B. 2007. Loss-of-function presenilin mutations in Alzheimer disease. Talking point on the role of presenilin mutations in Alzheimer disease. *EMBO Rep* 8: 141–146.

De Strooper, B., and Annaert, W. 2010. Novel research horizons for presenilins and γ-secretases in cell biology and disease. *Annu Rev Cell Dev Biol* 26: 235–260.

Debatin, L., Streffer, J., Geissen, M., Matschke, J., Aguzzi, A., and Glatzel, M. 2008. Association between deposition of beta-amyloid and pathological prion protein in sporadic Creutzfeldt-Jakob disease. *Neurodegener Dis* 5: 347–354.

Dekosky, S. T., and Scheff, S. W. 1990. Synapse loss in frontal cortex biopsies in Alzheimer's disease: Correlation with cognitive severity. *Ann Neurol* 27: 457–464.

Del Bo, R., Scarlato, M., Ghezzi, S., Martinelli-Boneschi, F., Fenoglio, C., Galimberti, G., Galbiati, S., Virgilio, R., Galimberti, D., Ferrarese, C., Scarpini, E., Bresolin, N., and Comi, G. P. 2006. Is M129V of PRNP gene associated with Alzheimer's disease? A case-control study and a meta-analysis. *Neurobiol Aging* 27: 770.e1–770.e5.

Demattos, R. B., Cirrito, J. R., Parsadanian, M., May, P. C., O'Dell, M. A., Taylor, J. W., Harmony, J. A., Aronow, B. J., Bales, K. R., Paul, S. M., and Holtzman, D. M. 2004. ApoE and clusterin cooperatively suppress Aβ levels and deposition: Evidence that ApoE regulates extracellular Aβ metabolism in vivo. *Neuron* 41: 193–202.

Dermaut, B., Croes, E. A., Rademakers, R., Van Den Broeck, M., Cruts, M., Hofman, A., Van Duijn, C. M., and Van Broeckhoven. 2003. C. PRNP Val129 homozygosity increases risk for early-onset alzheimer's disease. *Ann Neurol* 53: 409–412.

Deshaies, R. J. 1999. SCF and Cullin/Ring H2-based ubiquitin ligases. *Annu Rev Cell Dev Biol* 15: 435–467.

Deshpande, A., Mina, E., Glabe, C., and Busciglio, J. 2006. Different conformations of amyloid beta induce neurotoxicity by distinct mechanisms in human cortical neurons. *J Neurosci* 26: 6011–6018.

Devi, L., Prabhu, B. M., Galati, D. F., Avadhani, N. G., and Anandatheerthavarada, H. K. 2006. Accumulation of amyloid precursor protein in the mitochondrial import channels of human Alzheimer's disease brain is associated with mitochondrial dysfunction. *J Neurosci* 26: 9057–9068.

Dhavan, R., and Tsai, L. H. 2001. A decade of CDK5. *Nat Rev Mol Cell Biol* 2: 749–759.

Di Paolo, G., and Kim, T. W. 2011. Linking lipids to Alzheimer's disease: cholesterol and beyond. *Nat Rev Neurosci* 12: 284–296.

Dickey, C. A., Yue, M., Lin, W. L., Dickson, D. W., Dunmore, J. H., Lee, W. C., Zehr, C., West, G., Cao, S., Clark, A. M., Caldwell, G. A., Caldwell, K. A., Eckman, C., Patterson, C., Hutton, M., and Petrucelli, L. 2006. Deletion of the ubiquitin ligase CHIP leads to the accumulation, but not the aggregation, of both endogenous phospho- and caspase-3-cleaved tau species. *J Neurosci* 26: 6985–6996.

Dickinson, A. G., Meikle, V. M., and Fraser, H. 1968. Identification of a gene which controls the incubation period of some strains of scrapie agent in mice. *J Comp Pathol* 78: 293–299.

Dodart, J. C., Marr, R. A., Koistinaho, M., Gregersen, B. M., Malkani, S., Verma, I. M., and Paul, S. M. 2005. Gene delivery of human apolipoprotein E alters brain Aβ burden in a mouse model of Alzheimer's disease. *Proc Natl Acad Sci USA* 102: 1211–1216.

Dong, J., Atwood, C. S., Anderson, V. E., Siedlak, S. L., Smith, M. A., Perry, G., and Carey, P. R. 2003. Metal binding and oxidation of amyloid-β within isolated senile plaque cores: Raman microscopic evidence. *Biochemistry* 42: 2768–2773.

Drew, S. C., Noble, C. J., Masters, C. L., Hanson, G. R., and Barnham, K. J. 2009. Pleomorphic copper coordination by Alzheimer's disease amyloid-β peptide. *J Am Chem Soc* 131: 1195–1207.

Du, H., Guo, L., Fang, F., Chen, D., Sosunov, A. A., McKhann, G. M., Yan, Y., Wang, C., Zhang, H., Molkentin, J. D., Gunn-Moore, F. J., Vonsattel, J. P., Arancio, O., Chen, J. X., and Yan, S. D. 2008. Cyclophilin D deficiency attenuates mitochondrial and neuronal perturbation and ameliorates learning and memory in Alzheimer's disease. *Nat Med* 14: 1097–1105.

Dumanis, S. B., Tesoriero, J. A., Babus, L. W., Nguyen, M. T., Trotter, J. H., Ladu, M. J., Weeber, E. J., Turner, R. S., Xu, B., Rebeck, G. W., and Hoe, H. S. 2009. ApoE4 decreases spine density and dendritic complexity in cortical neurons in vivo. *J Neurosci* 29: 15317–15322.

Duyckaerts, C., and Dickson, D. W. 2003. *Neuropathology of Alzheimer's disease*. Basel: ISN Neuropath Press.

Dzwolak, W., Grudzielanek, S., Smirnovas, V., Ravindra, R., Nicolini, C., Jansen, R., Loksztejn, A., Porowski, S., and Winter, R. 2005. Ethanol-perturbed amyloidogenic self-assembly of insulin: Looking for origins of amyloid strains. *Biochemistry* 44: 8948–8958.

Ehehalt, R., Keller, P., Haass, C., Thiele, C., and Simons, K. 2003. Amyloidogenic processing of the Alzheimer β-amyloid precursor protein depends on lipid rafts. *J Cell Biol* 160: 113–123.

Endoh, R., Ogawara, M., Iwatsubo, T., Nakano, I., and Mori, H. 1993. Lack of the carboxyl terminal sequence of tau in ghost tangles of Alzheimer's disease. *Brain Res* 601: 164–172.

Esler, W. P., Stimson, E. R., Jennings, J. M., Ghilardi, J. R., Mantyh, P. W., and Maggio, J. E. 1996. Zinc-induced aggregation of human and rat β-amyloid peptides in vitro. *J Neurochem* 66: 723–732.

Evans, K. C., Berger, E. P., Cho, C. G., Weisgraber, K. H., and Lansbury, P. T., Jr. 1995. Apolipoprotein E is a kinetic but not a thermodynamic inhibitor of amyloid formation: Implications for the pathogenesis and treatment of Alzheimer disease. *Proc Natl Acad Sci USA* 92: 763–767.

Faller, P. 2009. Copper and zinc binding to amyloid-beta: Coordination, dynamics, aggregation, reactivity and metal-ion transfer. *Chembiochem* 10: 2837–2845.

Faller, P., and Hureau, C. 2009. Bioinorganic chemistry of copper and zinc ions coordinated to amyloid-β peptide. *Dalton Trans* 1080–1094.

Fändrich, M. 2007. On the structural definition of amyloid fibrils and other polypeptide aggregates. *Cell Mol Life Sci* 64: 2066–2078.

Fändrich, M., Schmidt, M., and Grigorieff, N. 2011. Recent progress in understanding Alzheimer's β-amyloid structures. *Trends Biochem Sci* 36: 338–345.

Fang, C. L., Wu, W. H., Liu, Q., Sun, X., Ma, Y., Zhao, Y. F., and Li, Y. M. 2010. Dual functions of β-amyloid oligomer and fibril in Cu(II)-induced H2O2 production. *Regul Pept* 163: 1–6.

Farris, W., Mansourian, S., Leissring, M. A., Eckman, E. A., Bertram, L., Eckman, C. B., Tanzi, R. E., and Selkoe, D. J. 2004. Partial loss-of-function mutations in insulin-degrading enzyme that induce diabetes also impair degradation of amyloid β-protein. *Am J Pathol* 164: 1425–1434.

Fassbender, K., Simons, M., Bergmann, C., Stroick, M., Lutjohann, D., Keller, P., Runz, H., Kuhl, S., Bertsch, T., Von Bergmann, K., Hennerici, M., Beyreuther, K., and Hartmann, T. 2001. Simvastatin strongly reduces levels of Alzheimer's disease β-amyloid peptides Aβ 42 and Aβ 40 *in vitro* and *in vivo*. *Proc Natl Acad Sci USA* 98: 5856–5861.

Favit, A., Grimaldi, M., and Alkon, D. L. 2000. Prevention of β-amyloid neurotoxicity by blockade of the ubiquitin-proteasome proteolytic pathway. *J Neurochem* 75: 1258–1263.

Fawzi, N. L., Phillips, A. H., Ruscio, J. Z., Doucleff, M., Wemmer, D. E., and Head-Gordon, T. 2008. Structure and dynamics of the Aβ(21-30) peptide from the interplay of NMR experiments and molecular simulations. *J Am Chem Soc* 130: 6145–6158.

Feany, M. B., and Dickson, D. W. 1996. Neurodegenerative disorders with extensive tau pathology: A comparative study and review. *Ann Neurol* 40: 139–148.

Feddersen, R. M., Ehlenfeldt, R., Yunis, W. S., Clark, H. B., and Orr, H. T. 1992. Disrupted cerebellar cortical development and progressive degeneration of Purkinje cells in SV40 T antigen transgenic mice. *Neuron* 9: 955–966.

Ferreiro, E., Oliveira, C. R., and Pereira, C. M. 2008. The release of calcium from the endoplasmic reticulum induced by amyloid-beta and prion peptides activates the mitochondrial apoptotic pathway. *Neurobiol Dis* 30: 331–342.

Fiala, M., Cribbs, D. H., Rosenthal, M., and Bernard, G. 2007. Phagocytosis of amyloid-β and inflammation: Two faces of innate immunity in Alzheimer's disease. *J Alzheimer's Dis* 11: 457–463.

Fiala, M., Lin, J., Ringman, J., Kermani-Arab, V., Tsao, G., Patel, A., Lossinsky, A. S., Graves, M. C., Gustavson, A., Sayre, J., Sofroni, E., Suarez, T., Chiappelli, F., and Bernard, G. 2005. Ineffective phagocytosis of amyloid-beta by macrophages of Alzheimer's disease patients. *J Alzheimer's Dis* 7: 221–232; discussion 255–262.

Floyd, S. R., Porro, E. B., Slepnev, V. I., Ochoa, G. C., Tsai, L. H., and De Camilli, P. 2001. Amphiphysin 1 binds the cyclin-dependent kinase (cdk) 5 regulatory subunit p35 and is phosphorylated by cdk5 and cdc2. *J Biol Chem* 276: 8104–8110.

Foley, P. 2010. Lipids in Alzheimer's disease: A century-old story. *Biochim Biophys Acta* 1801: 750–753.

Fratta, P., Engel, W. K., McFerrin, J., Davies, K. J., Lin, S. W., and Askanas, V. 2005. Proteasome inhibition and aggresome formation in sporadic inclusion-body myositis and in amyloid-beta precursor protein-overexpressing cultured human muscle fibers. *Am J Pathol* 167: 517–526.

Freed, E., Lacey, K. R., Huie, P., Lyapina, S. A., Deshaies, R. J., Stearns, T., and Jackson, P. K. 1999. Components of an SCF ubiquitin ligase localize to the centrosome and regulate the centrosome duplication cycle. *Genes Dev* 13: 2242–2257.

Friedhoff, P., Von Bergen, M., Mandelkow, E. M., Davies, P., and Mandelkow, E. 1998. A nucleated assembly mechanism of Alzheimer paired helical filaments. *Proc Natl Acad Sci USA* 95: 15712–15717.

Frolich, L., Blum-Degen, D., Bernstein, H. G., Engelsberger, S., Humrich, J., Laufer, S., Muschner, D., Thalheimer, A., Turk, A., Hoyer, S., Zochling, R., Boissl, K. W., Jellinger, K., and Riederer, P. 1998. Brain insulin and insulin receptors in aging and sporadic Alzheimer's disease. *J Neural Transm* 105: 423–438.

Fu, A. K., Fu, W. Y., Cheung, J., Tsim, K. W., Ip, F. C., Wang, J. H., and Ip, N. Y. 2001. Cdk5 is involved in neuregulin-induced AChR expression at the neuromuscular junction. *Nat Neurosci* 4: 374–381.

Gabbita, S. P., Aksenov, M. Y., Lovell, M. A., and Markesbery, W. R. 1999. Decrease in peptide methionine sulfoxide reductase in Alzheimer's disease brain. *J Neurochem* 73: 1660–1666.

Gao, C. Y., Zakeri, Z., Zhu, Y., He, H., and Zelenka, P. S. 1997. Expression of Cdk5, p35, and Cdk5-associated kinase activity in the developing rat lens. *Dev Genet* 20: 267–275.

Garzon-Rodriguez, W., Yatsimirsky, A. K., and Glabe, C. G. 1999. Binding of Zn(II), Cu(II), and Fe(II) ions to Alzheimer's A beta peptide studied by fluorescence. *Bioorg Med Chem Lett* 9: 2243–2248.

Gehman, J. D., O'Brien, C. C., Shabanpoor, F., Wade, J. D., and Separovic, F. 2008. Metal effects on the membrane interactions of amyloid-β peptides. *Eur Biophys J* 37: 333–344.

Giaccone, G., Mangieri, M., Capobianco, R., Limido, L., Hauw, J. J., Haik, S., Fociani, P., Bugiani, O., and Tagliavini, F. 2008. Tauopathy in human and experimental variant Creutzfeldt-Jakob disease. *Neurobiol Aging* 29: 1864–1873.

Giasson, B. I., Lee, V. M., and Trojanowski, J. Q. 2003. Interactions of amyloidogenic proteins. *Neuromolecular Med* 4: 49–58.

Gibb, G. M., Pearce, J., Betts, J. C., Lovestone, S., Hoffmann, M. M., Maerz, W., Blackstock, W. P., and Anderton, B. H. 2000. Differential effects of apolipoprotein E isoforms on phosphorylation at specific sites on tau by glycogen synthase kinase-3β identified by nano-electrospray mass spectrometry. *FEBS Lett* 485: 99–103.

Gilmore, E. C., Ohshima, T., Goffinet, A. M., Kulkarni, A. B., and Herrup, K. 1998. Cyclin-dependent kinase 5-deficient mice demonstrate novel developmental arrest in cerebral cortex. *J Neurosci* 18: 6370–6377.

Gimbel, D. A., Nygaard, H. B., Coffey, E. E., Gunther, E. C., Lauren, J., Gimbel, Z. A., and Strittmatter, S. M. 2010. Memory impairment in transgenic Alzheimer mice requires cellular prion protein. *J Neurosci* 30: 6367–6374.

Glabe, C. G. 2008. Structural classification of toxic amyloid oligomers. *J Biolog Chem* 283: 29639–29643.

Glenner, G. G., and Wong, C. W. 1984a. Alzheimer's disease and Down's syndrome: Sharing of a unique cerebrovascular amyloid fibril protein. *Biochem Biophys Res Commun* 122: 1131–1135.

Glenner, G. G., and Wong, C. W. 1984b. Alzheimer's disease: Initial report of the purification and characterization of a novel cerebrovascular amyloid protein. *Biochem Biophys Res Commun* 120: 885–890.

Glodzik-Sobanska, L., Pirraglia, E., Brys, M., De Santi, S., Mosconi, L., Rich, K. E., Switalski, R., Saint Louis, L., Sadowski, M. J., Martiniuk, F., Mehta, P., Pratico, D., Zinkowski, R. P., Blennow, K., and De Leon, M. J. 2009. The effects of normal aging and ApoE genotype on the levels of CSF biomarkers for Alzheimer's disease. *Neurobiol Aging* 30: 672–681.

Goedert, M. 2003. *Introduction to the Tauopathies.* Basel: ISN Neuropath Press.

Goldgaber, D., Lerman, M. I., McBride, O. W., Saffiotti, U., and Gajdusek, D. C. 1987. Characterization and chromosomal localization of a cDNA encoding brain amyloid of Alzheimer's disease. *Science* 235: 877–880.

Gotz, J., Chen, F., Van Dorpe, J., and Nitsch, R. M. 2001. Formation of neurofibrillary tangles in P301l tau transgenic mice induced by Aβ 42 fibrils. *Science* 293: 1491–1495.

Gotz, J., Ittner, L. M., and Lim, Y. A. 2009. Common features between diabetes mellitus and Alzheimer's disease. *Cell Mol Life Sci* 66: 1321–1325.

Grant, M. A., Lazo, N. D., Lomakin, A., Condron, M. M., Arai, H., Yamin, G., Rigby, A. C., and Teplow, D. B. 2007. Familial Alzheimer's disease mutations alter the stability of the amyloid β-protein monomer folding nucleus. *Proc Natl Acad Sci USA* 104: 16522–16527.

Greengard, P., Benfenati, F., and Valtorta, F. 1994. Synapsin I, an actin-binding protein regulating synaptic vesicle traffic in the nerve terminal. *Adv Second Messenger Phosphoprotein Res* 29: 31–45.

Gregori, L., Fuchs, C., Figueiredo-Pereira, M. E., Van Nostrand, W. E., and Goldgaber, D. 1995. Amyloid β-protein inhibits ubiquitin-dependent protein degradation *in vitro*. *J Biol Chem* 270: 19702–19708.

Gregori, L., Hainfeld, J. F., Simon, M. N., and Goldgaber, D. 1997. Binding of amyloid β protein to the 20 S proteasome. *J Biol Chem* 272: 58–62.

Grziwa, B., Grimm, M. O., Masters, C. L., Beyreuther, K., Hartmann, T., and Lichtenthaler, S. F. 2003. The transmembrane domain of the amyloid precursor protein in microsomal membranes is on both sides shorter than predicted. *J Biol Chem* 278: 6803–6808.

Guilloreau, L. et al. 2006. Structural and thermodynamical properties of CuII amyloid-β16/28 complexes associated with Alzheimer's disease. *J Biol Inorg Chem* 11(8): 1024–1038.

Gunther, E. C., and Strittmatter, S. M. 2010. β-amyloid oligomers and cellular prion protein in Alzheimer's disease. *J Mol Med* 88: 331–338.

Guo, M., Gorman, P. M., Rico, M., Chakrabartty, A., and Laurents, D. V. 2005. Charge substitution shows that repulsive electrostatic interactions impede the oligomerization of Alzheimer amyloid peptides. *FEBS Lett* 579: 3574–3578.

Gustafson, D. R., Skoog, I., Rosengren, L., Zetterberg, H., and Blennow, K. 2007. Cerebrospinal fluid β-amyloid 1-42 concentration may predict cognitive decline in older women. *J Neurol, Neurosurg, and Psych* 78: 461–464.

Haass, C., Koo, E. H., Mellon, A., Hung, A. Y., and Selkoe, D. J. 1992. Targeting of cell-surface β-amyloid precursor protein to lysosomes: Alternative processing into amyloid-bearing fragments. *Nature* 357: 500–503.

Haass, C., and Selkoe, D. J. 1993. Cellular processing of β-amyloid precursor protein and the genesis of amyloid β-peptide. *Cell* 75: 1039–1042.

Haass, C., and Selkoe, D. J. 2007. Soluble protein oligomers in neurodegeneration: Lessons from the Alzheimer's amyloid β-peptide. *Nat Rev Mol Cell Biol* 8: 101–112.

Hajieva, P., Kuhlmann, C., Luhmann, H. J., and Behl, C. 2009. Impaired calcium homeostasis in aged hippocampal neurons. *Neurosci Lett* 451: 119–123.

Halleskog, C., Mulder, J., Dahlstrom, J., Mackie, K., Hortobagyi, T., Tanila, H., Kumar Puli, L., Farber, K., Harkany, T., and Schulte, G. 2011. WNT signaling in activated microglia is proinflammatory. *Glia* 59: 119–131.

Hamdane, M., Smet, C., Sambo, A. V., Leroy, A., Wieruszeski, J. M., Delobel, P., Maurage, C. A., Ghestem, A., Wintjens, R., Begard, S., Sergeant, N., Delacourte, A., Horvath, D., Landrieu, I., Lippens, G., and Buee, L. 2002. Pin1: A therapeutic target in Alzheimer neurodegeneration. *J Mol Neurosci* 19: 275–287.

Hamid, R., Kilger, E., Willem, M., Vassallo, N., Kostka, M., Bornhovd, C., Reichert, A. S., Kretzschmar, H. A., Haass, C., and Herms, J. 2007. Amyloid precursor protein intracellular domain modulates cellular calcium homeostasis and ATP content. *J Neurochem* 102: 1264–1275.

Hansson, C. A., Frykman, S., Farmery, M. R., Tjernberg, L. O., Nilsberth, C., Pursglove, S. E., Ito, A., Winblad, B., Cowburn, R. F., Thyberg, J., and Ankarcrona, M. 2004. Nicastrin, presenilin, APH-1, and PEN-2 form active γ-secretase complexes in mitochondria. *J Biol Chem* 279: 51654–51660.

Hansson Petersen, C. A., Alikhani, N., Behbahani, H., Wiehager, B., Pavlov, P. F., Alafuzoff, I., Leinonen, V., Ito, A., Winblad, B., Glaser, E., and Ankarcrona, M. 2008. The amyloid β-peptide is imported into mitochondria via the TOM import machinery and localized to mitochondrial cristae. *Proc Natl Acad Sci USA* 105: 13145–13150.

Hardy, J. A., and Higgins, G. A. 1992. Alzheimer's disease: The amyloid cascade hypothesis. *Science* 256: 184–185.

Harper, J. D., and Lansbury, P. T., Jr. 1997a. Models of amyloid seeding in Alzheimer's disease and scrapie: mechanistic truths and physiological consequences of the time-dependent solubility of amyloid proteins. *Annu Rev Biochem* 66: 385–407.

Harper, J. D., Wong, S. S., Lieber, C. M., and Lansbury, P. T. 1997b. Observation of metastable Aβ amyloid protofibrils by atomic force microscopy. *Chem Biol* 4: 119–125.

Harper, J. D., Wong, S. S., Lieber, C. M., and Lansbury, P. T., Jr. 1999. Assembly of Aβ amyloid protofibrils: An in vitro model for a possible early event in Alzheimer's disease. *Biochemistry* 38: 8972–8980.

Harris, F. M., Brecht, W. J., Xu, Q., Tesseur, I., Kekonius, L., Wyss-Coray, T., Fish, J. D., Masliah, E., Hopkins, P. C., Scearce-Levie, K., Weisgraber, K. H., Mucke, L., Mahley, R. W., and Huang, Y. 2003. Carboxyl-terminal-truncated apolipoprotein E4 causes Alzheimer's disease-like neurodegeneration and behavioral deficits in transgenic mice. *Proc Natl Acad Sci USA* 100: 10966–10971.

Hartley, D. M., Walsh, D. M., Ye, C. P., Diehl, T., Vasquez, S., Vassilev, P. M., Teplow, D. B., and Selkoe, D. J. 1999. Protofibrillar intermediates of amyloid β-protein induce acute electrophysiological changes and progressive neurotoxicity in cortical neurons. *J Neurosci* 19: 8876–8884.

Hartman, R. E., Wozniak, D. F., Nardi, A., Olney, J. W., Sartorius, L., and Holtzman, D. M. 2001. Behavioral phenotyping of GFAP-apoE3 and -apoE4 transgenic mice: Apoe4 mice show profound working memory impairments in the absence of Alzheimer's-like neuropathology. *Exp Neurol* 170: 326–344.

Hartmann, T., Bieger, S. C., Bruhl, B., Tienari, P. J., Ida, N., Allsop, D., Roberts, G. W., Masters, C. L., Dotti, C. G., Unsicker, K., and Beyreuther, K. 1997. Distinct sites of intracellular production for Alzheimer's disease Aβ40/42 amyloid peptides. *Nature Medicine* 3: 1016–1020.

Hartmann, T., Kuchenbecker, J., and Grimm, M. O. 2007. Alzheimer's disease: The lipid connection. *J Neurochem* 103 Suppl 1: 159–170.

Hatcher, L. Q., Hong, L., Bush, W. D., Carducci, T., and Simon, J. D. 2008. Quantification of the binding constant of copper(II) to the amyloid-β peptide. *J Phys Chem B* 112: 8160–8164.

Hegde, A. N. 2010. The ubiquitin-proteasome pathway and synaptic plasticity. *Learn Mem* 17: 314–327.

Heneka, M. T., and O'Banion, M. K. 2007. Inflammatory processes in Alzheimer's disease. *J Neuroimmunol* 184: 69–91.

Hensley, K., Hall, N., Subramaniam, R., Cole, P., Harris, M., Aksenov, M., Aksenova, M., Gabbita, S. P., Wu, J. F., Carney, J. M., et al. 1995. Brain regional correspondence between Alzheimer's disease histopathology and biomarkers of protein oxidation. *J Neurochem* 65: 2146–2156.

Hernandez-Ortega, K., Ferrera, P., and Arias, C. 2007. Sequential expression of cell-cycle regulators and Alzheimer's disease-related proteins in entorhinal cortex after hippocampal excitotoxic damage. *J Neurosci Res* 85: 1744–1751.

Herreman, A., Hartmann, D., Annaert, W., Saftig, P., Craessaerts, K., Serneels, L., Umans, L., Schrijvers, V., Checler, F., Vanderstichele, H., Baekelandt, V., Dressel, R., Cupers, P., Huylebroeck, D., Zwijsen, A., Van Leuven, F., and De Strooper, B. 1999. Presenilin 2 deficiency causes a mild pulmonary phenotype and no changes in amyloid precursor protein processing but enhances the embryonic lethal phenotype of presenilin 1 deficiency. *Proc Natl Acad Sci USA* 96: 11872–11877.

Herrup, K., and Arendt, T. 2002. Re-expression of cell cycle proteins induces neuronal cell death during Alzheimer's disease. *J Alzheimer's Dis* 4: 243–247.

Herrup, K., and Busser, J. C. 1995. The induction of multiple cell cycle events precedes target-related neuronal death. *Development* 121: 2385–2395.

Herrup, K., Neve, R., Ackerman, S. L., and Copani, A. 2004. Divide and die: Cell cycle events as triggers of nerve cell death. *J Neurosci* 24: 9232–9239.

Ho, L., Qin, W., Pompl, P. N., Xiang, Z., Wang, J., Zhao, Z., Peng, Y., Cambareri, G., Rocher, A., Mobbs, C. V., Hof, P. R., and Pasinetti, G. M. 2004. Diet-induced insulin resistance promotes amyloidosis in a transgenic mouse model of Alzheimer's disease. *FASEB J* 18: 902–904.

Hoe, H. S., Freeman, J., and Rebeck, G. W. 2006. Apolipoprotein E decreases tau kinases and phospho-tau levels in primary neurons. *Mol Neurodegener* 1: 18.

Hof, P. R. 1997. Morphology and neurochemical characteristics of the vulnerable neurons in brain aging and Alzheimer's disease. *Eur Neurol* 37: 71–81.

Hoglinger, G. U., Breunig, J. J., Depboylu, C., Rouaux, C., Michel, P. P., Alvarez-Fischer, D., Boutillier, A. L., Degregori, J., Oertel, W. H., Rakic, P., Hirsch, E. C., and Hunot, S. 2007. The pRb/E2F cell-cycle pathway mediates cell death in Parkinson's disease. *Proc Natl Acad Sci USA* 104: 3585–3590.

Hollingworth, P., Harold, D., Sims, R., Gerrish, A., Lambert, J. C., Carrasquillo, M. M., Abraham, R. et al. 2010. Common variants at ABCA7, MS4A6A/MS4A4E, EPHA1, CD33 and CD2AP are associated with Alzheimer's disease. *Nat Genet* 43: 429–435.

Holtzman, D. M., Bales, K. R., Tenkova, T., Fagan, A. M., Parsadanian, M., Sartorius, L. J., Mackey, B., Olney, J., McKeel, D., Wozniak, D., and Paul, S. M. 2000. Apolipoprotein E isoform-dependent amyloid deposition and neuritic degeneration in a mouse model of Alzheimer's disease. *Proc Natl Acad Sci USA* 97: 2892–2897.

Holtzman, D. M., Pitas, R. E., Kilbridge, J., Nathan, B., Mahley, R. W., Bu, G., and Schwartz, A. L. 1995. Low density lipoprotein receptor-related protein mediates apolipoprotein E-dependent neurite outgrowth in a central nervous system-derived neuronal cell line. *Proc Natl Acad Sci USA* 92: 9480–9484.

Holzer, M., Gartner, U., Stobe, A., Hartig, W., Gruschka, H., Bruckner, M. K., and Arendt, T. 2002. Inverse association of Pin1 and tau accumulation in Alzheimer's disease hippocampus. *Acta Neuropathol* 104: 471–481.

Hortschansky, P., Schroeckh, V., Christopeit, T., Zandomeneghi, G., and Fandrich, M. 2005. The aggregation kinetics of Alzheimer's β-amyloid peptide is controlled by stochastic nucleation. *Protein Sci* 14: 1753–1759.

Hoshi, M., Sato, M., Matsumoto, S., Noguchi, A., Yasutake, K., Yoshida, N., and Sato, K. 2003. Spherical aggregates of β-amyloid (amylospheroid) show high neurotoxicity and activate tau protein kinase I/glycogen synthase kinase-3β. *Proc Natl Acad Sci USA* 100: 6370–6375.

Hou, L., Shao, H., Zhang, Y., Li, H., Menon, N. K., Neuhaus, E. B., Brewer, J. M., Byeon, I. J., Ray, D. G., Vitek, M. P., Iwashita, T., Makula, R. A., Przybyla, A. B., and Zagorski, M. G. 2004. Solution NMR studies of the Aβ(1-40) and Aβ(1-42) peptides establish that the Met35 oxidation state affects the mechanism of amyloid formation. *J Am Chem Soc* 126: 1992–2005.

Hou, L., and Zagorski, M. G. 2006. NMR reveals anomalous copper(II) binding to the amyloid Aβ peptide of Alzheimer's disease. *J Am Chem Soc* 128: 9260–9261.

House, E., Collingwood, J., Khan, A., Korchazkina, O., Berthon, G., and Exley, C. 2004. Aluminium, iron, zinc and copper influence the in vitro formation of amyloid fibrils of Aβ42 in a manner which may have consequences for metal chelation therapy in Alzheimer's disease. *J Alzheimer's Dis* 6: 291–301.

Hsia, A. Y., Masliah, E., McConlogue, L., Yu, G. Q., Tatsuno, G., Hu, K., Kholodenko, D., Malenka, R. C., Nicoll, R. A., and Mucke, L. 1999. Plaque-independent disruption of neural circuits in Alzheimer's disease mouse models. *Proc Natl Acad Sci USA* 96: 3228–3233.

Hsiao, K., Baker, H. F., Crow, T. J., Poulter, M., Owen, F., Terwilliger, J. D., Westaway, D., Ott, J., and Prusiner, S. B. 1989. Linkage of a prion protein missense variant to Gerstmann-Straussler syndrome. *Nature* 338: 342–345.

Hsieh, H., Boehm, J., Sato, C., Iwatsubo, T., Tomita, T., Sisodia, S., and Malinow, R. 2006. AMPA-R removal underlies Aβ-induced synaptic depression and dendritic spine loss. *Neuron* 52: 831–843.

Hu, J., and Van Eldik, L. J. 1999. Glial-derived proteins activate cultured astrocytes and enhance beta amyloid-induced glial activation. *Brain Res* 842: 46–54.

Hu, X., Crick, S. L., Bu, G., Frieden, C., Pappu, R. V., and Lee, J. M. 2009. Amyloid seeds formed by cellular uptake, concentration, and aggregation of the amyloid-beta peptide. *Proc Natl Acad Sci USA* 106: 20324–20329.

Huang, D. Y., Weisgraber, K. H., Goedert, M., Saunders, A. M., Roses, A. D., and Strittmatter, W. J. 1995. ApoE3 binding to tau tandem repeat I is abolished by tau serine(262) phosphorylation. *Neurosci Lett* 192: 209–212.

Huang, X., Atwood, C. S., Hartshorn, M. A., Multhaup, G., Goldstein, L. E., Scarpa, R. C., Cuajungco, M. P., Gray, D. N., Lim, J., Moir, R. D., Tanzi, R. E., and Bush, A. 1999a. I. The Aβ peptide of Alzheimer's disease directly produces hydrogen peroxide through metal ion reduction. *Biochemistry* 38: 7609–7616.

Huang, X., Atwood, C. S., Moir, R. D., Hartshorn, M. A., Tanzi, R. E., and Bush, A. I. 2004. Trace metal contamination initiates the apparent auto-aggregation, amyloidosis, and oligomerization of Alzheimer's Aβ peptides. *J Biol Inorg Chem* 9: 954–960.

Huang, X., Cuajungco, M. P., Atwood, C. S., Hartshorn, M. A., Tyndall, J. D., Hanson, G. R., Stokes, K. C., Leopold, M., Multhaup, G., Goldstein, L. E., Scarpa, R. C., Saunders, A. J., Lim, J., Moir, R. D., Glabe, C., Bowden, E. F., Masters, C. L., Fairlie, D. P., Tanzi, R. E., and Bush, A. I. 1999b. Cu(II) potentiation of alzheimer Aβ neurotoxicity. Correlation with cell-free hydrogen peroxide production and metal reduction. *J Biol Chem* 274: 37111–37116.

Huang, Y. 2010. Aβ-independent roles of apolipoprotein E4 in the pathogenesis of Alzheimer's disease. *Trends Mol Med* 16: 287–294.

Huang, Y., Liu, X. Q., Wyss-Coray, T., Brecht, W. J., Sanan, D. A., and Mahley, R. W. 2001. Apolipoprotein E fragments present in Alzheimer's disease brains induce neurofibrillary tangle-like intracellular inclusions in neurons. *Proc Natl Acad Sci USA* 98: 8838–8843.

Humbert, S., Lanier, L. M., and Tsai, L. H. 2000. Synaptic localization of p39, a neuronal activator of cdk5. *Neuroreport* 11: 2213–2216.

Huse, J. T., Pijak, D. S., Leslie, G. J., Lee, V. M., and Doms, R. W. 2000. Maturation and endosomal targeting of β-site amyloid precursor protein-cleaving enzyme. The Alzheimer's disease β-secretase. *J Biol Chem* 275: 33729–33737.

Ignatius, M. J., Shooter, E. M., Pitas, R. E., and Mahley, R. W. 1987. Lipoprotein uptake by neuronal growth cones in vitro. *Science* 236: 959–962.

Iijima, K., Ando, K., Takeda, S., Satoh, Y., Seki, T., Itohara, S., Greengard, P., Kirino, Y., Nairn, A. C., and Suzuki, T. 2000. Neuron-specific phosphorylation of Alzheimer's β-amyloid precursor protein by cyclin-dependent kinase 5. *J Neurochem* 75: 1085–1091.

Ikeda, S. I., Yanagisawa, N., Allsop, D., and Glenner, G. G. 1994. Gerstmann-Straussler-Scheinker disease showing β-protein type cerebellar and cerebral amyloid angiopathy. *Acta Neuropathol* 88: 262–266.

Inayathullah, M., and Teplow, D. B. 2011. Structural dynamics of the ΔE22 (Osaka) familial Alzheimer's disease-linked amyloid β-protein. *Amyloid: Int J Prot Folding Dis* 18: 98–107.

Ittner, L. M., Ke, Y. D., Delerue, F., Bi, M., Gladbach, A., Van Eersel, J., Wolfing, H., Chieng, B. C., Christie, M. J., Napier, I. A., Eckert, A., Staufenbiel, M., Hardeman, E., and Gotz, J. 2010. Dendritic function of tau mediates amyloid-β toxicity in Alzheimer's disease mouse models. *Cell* 142: 387–397.

Jacks, T., Fazeli, A., Schmitt, E. M., Bronson, R. T., Goodell, M. A., and Weinberg, R. A. 1992. Effects of an Rb mutation in the mouse. *Nature* 359: 295–300.

Jan, A., Adolfsson, O., Allaman, I., Buccarello, A. L., Magistretti, P. J., Pfeifer, A., Muhs, A., and Lashuel, H. A. 2011. Aβ42 neurotoxicity is mediated by ongoing nucleated polymerization process rather than by discrete Aβ42 species. *J Biol Chem* 286: 8585–8596.

Jang, H., Arce, F. T., Ramachandran, S., Capone, R., Azimova, R., Kagan, B. L., Nussinov, R., and Lal, R. 2010. Truncated β-amyloid peptide channels provide an alternative mechanism for Alzheimer's Disease and Down syndrome. *Proc Natl Acad Sci USA* 107: 6538–6543.

Jarrett, J. T., Berger, E. P., and Lansbury, P. T., Jr. 1993a. The carboxy terminus of the β amyloid protein is critical for the seeding of amyloid formation: Implications for the pathogenesis of Alzheimer's disease. *Biochemistry* 32: 4693–4697.

Jarrett, J. T., and Lansbury, P. T., Jr. 1993b. Seeding "one-dimensional crystallization" of amyloid: A pathogenic mechanism in Alzheimer's disease and scrapie? *Cell* 73: 1055–1058.

Jeffrey, P. D., Russo, A. A., Polyak, K., Gibbs, E., Hurwitz, J., Massague, J., and Pavletich, N. P. 1995. Mechanism of CDK activation revealed by the structure of a cyclinA-CDK2 complex. *Nature* 376: 313–320.

Jellinger, K. A., and Attems, J. 2007. Neurofibrillary tangle-predominant dementia: comparison with classical Alzheimer disease. *Acta Neuropathol* 113: 107–117.

Ji, Y., Gong, Y., Gan, W., Beach, T., Holtzman, D. M., and Wisniewski, T. 2003. Apolipoprotein E isoform-specific regulation of dendritic spine morphology in apolipoprotein E transgenic mice and Alzheimer's disease patients. *Neuroscience* 122: 305–315.

Jordan-Sciutto, K. L., Dorsey, R., Chalovich, E. M., Hammond, R. R., and Achim, C. L. 2003. Expression patterns of retinoblastoma protein in Parkinson disease. *J Neuropathol Exp Neurol* 62: 68–74.

Jordan-Sciutto, K. L., Wang, G., Murphy-Corb, M., and Wiley, C. A. 2000. Induction of cell-cycle regulators in simian immunodeficiency virus encephalitis. *Am J Pathol* 157: 497–507.

Jordan-Sciutto, K. L., Wang, G., Murphey-Corb, M., and Wiley, C. A. 2002. Cell cycle proteins exhibit altered expression patterns in lentiviral-associated encephalitis. *J Neurosci* 22: 2185–2195.

Kagan, B. L., Azimov, R., and Azimova, R. 2004. Amyloid peptide channels. *J Membr Biol* 202: 1–10.

Kagan, B. L., Hirakura, Y., Azimov, R., Azimova, R., and Lin, M. C. 2002. The channel hypothesis of Alzheimer's disease: Current status. *Peptides* 23: 1311–1315.

Kamal, A., Almenar-Queralt, A., Leblanc, J. F., Roberts, E. A., and Goldstein, L. S. 2001. Kinesin-mediated axonal transport of a membrane compartment containing β-secretase and presenilin-1 requires APP. *Nature* 414: 643–648.

Kamenetz, F., Tomita, T., Hsieh, H., Seabrook, G., Borchelt, D., Iwatsubo, T., Sisodia, S., and Malinow, R. 2003. APP processing and synaptic function. *Neuron* 37: 925–937.

Kamino, K., Orr, H. T., Payami, H., Wijsman, E. M., Alonso, M. E., Pulst, S. M., Anderson, L., O'Dahl, S., Nemens, E., White, J. A., et al. 1992. Linkage and mutational analysis of familial Alzheimer disease kindreds for the APP gene region. *Am J Hum Genet* 51: 998–1014.

Kang, J., Lemaire, H. G., Unterbeck, A., Salbaum, J. M., Masters, C. L., Grzeschik, K. H., Multhaup, G., Beyreuther, K., and Muller-Hill, B. 1987. The precursor of Alzheimer's disease amyloid A4 protein resembles a cell-surface receptor. *Nature* 325: 733–736.

Karr, J. W., Akintoye, H., Kaupp L. J., & Szalai, V. A. 2005. N-Terminal deletions modify the Cu2+ binding site in amyloid-β. *Biochemistry* 44(14): 5478–5487.

Karr, J. W., and Szalai, V. A. 2008. Cu(II) binding to monomeric, oligomeric, and fibrillar forms of the Alzheimer's disease amyloid-β peptide. *Biochemistry* 47: 5006–5016.

Kato, G., and Maeda, S. 1999. Neuron-specific Cdk5 kinase is responsible for mitosis-independent phosphorylation of c-Src at Ser75 in human Y79 retinoblastoma cells. *J Biochem* 126: 957–961.

Kawahara, M., Arispe, N., Kuroda, Y., and Rojas, E. 1997. Alzheimer's disease amyloid β-protein forms Zn(2+)-sensitive, cation-selective channels across excised membrane patches from hypothalamic neurons. *Biophys J* 73: 67–75.

Kawarabayashi, T., Shoji, M., Younkin, L. H., Wen-Lang, L., Dickson, D. W., Murakami, T., Matsubara, E., Abe, K., Ashe, K. H., and Younkin, S. G. 2004. Dimeric amyloid β protein rapidly accumulates in lipid rafts followed by apolipoprotein E and phosphorylated tau accumulation in the Tg2576 mouse model of Alzheimer's disease. *J Neurosci* 24: 3801–3809.

Kayed, R., Head, E., Thompson, J. L., McIntire, T. M., Milton, S. C., Cotman, C. W., and Glabe, C. G. 2003. Common structure of soluble amyloid oligomers implies common mechanism of pathogenesis. *Science* 300: 486–489.

Kayed, R., Pensalfini, A., Margol, L., Sokolov, Y., Sarsoza, F., Head, E., Hall, J., and Glabe, C. 2009. Annular protofibrils are a structurally and functionally distinct type of amyloid oligomer. *J Biol Chem* 284: 4230–4237.

Kayed, R., Sokolov, Y., Edmonds, B., McIntire, T. M., Milton, S. C., Hall, J. E., and Glabe, C. G. 2004. Permeabilization of lipid bilayers is a common conformation-dependent activity of soluble amyloid oligomers in protein misfolding diseases. *J Biol Chem* 279: 46363–46366.

Keil, U., Bonert, A., Marques, C. A., Scherping, I., Weyermann, J., Strosznajder, J. B., Muller-Spahn, F., Haass, C., Czech, C., Pradier, L., Muller, W. E., and Eckert, A. 2004. Amyloid β-induced changes in nitric oxide production and mitochondrial activity lead to apoptosis. *J Biol Chem* 279: 50310–50320.

Kellett, K. A., and Hooper, N. M. 2009. Prion protein and Alzheimer disease. *Prion* 3: 190–194.

Kessels, H. W., Nguyen, L. N., Nabavi, S., and Malinow, R. 2010. The prion protein as a receptor for amyloid-β. *Nature* 466: E3–4; discussion E4–5.

Kheterpal, I., Chen, M., Cook, K. D., and Wetzel, R. 2006. Structural differences in Aβ amyloid protofibrils and fibrils mapped by hydrogen exchange: Mass spectrometry with on-line proteolytic fragmentation. *J Mol Biol* 361: 785–795.

Kim, S. I., Yi, J. S., and Ko, Y. G. 2006. Amyloid β oligomerization is induced by brain lipid rafts. *Journal of Cellular Biochemistry* 99: 878–889.

Kinoshita, A., Fukumoto, H., Shah, T., Whelan, C. M., Irizarry, M. C., and Hyman, B. T. 2003. Demonstration by FRET of BACE interaction with the amyloid precursor protein at the cell surface and in early endosomes. *J Cell Sci* 116: 3339–3346.

Kipreos, E. T., Lander, L. E., Wing, J. P., He, W. W., and Hedgecock, E. M. 1996. cul-1 is required for cell cycle exit in *C. elegans* and identifies a novel gene family. *Cell* 85: 829–839.

Kirkitadze, M. D., Bitan, G., and Teplow, D. B. 2002. Paradigm shifts in Alzheimer's disease and other neurodegenerative disorders: The emerging role of oligomeric assemblies. *J Neurosci Res* 69: 567–577.

Klein, W. L. 2002. Aβ toxicity in Alzheimer's disease: Globular oligomers (ADDLs) as new vaccine and drug targets. *Neurochem Int* 41: 345–352.

Klyubin, I., Walsh, D. M., Lemere, C. A., Cullen, W. K., Shankar, G. M., Betts, V., Spooner, E. T., Jiang, L., Anwyl, R., Selkoe, D. J., and Rowan, M. J. 2005. Amyloid β protein immunotherapy neutralizes Aβ oligomers that disrupt synaptic plasticity *in vivo*. *Nat Med* 11: 556–561.

Kobayashi, S., Ishiguro, K., Omori, A., Takamatsu, M., Arioka, M., Imahori, K., and Uchida, T. 1993. A cdc2-related kinase PSSALRE/cdk5 is homologous with the 30 kDa subunit of tau protein kinase II, a proline-directed protein kinase associated with microtubule. *FEBS Lett* 335: 171–175.

Kokubo, H., Kayed, R., Glabe, C. G., Staufenbiel, M., Saido, T. C., Iwata, N., and Yamaguchi, H. 2009. Amyloid Beta annular protofibrils in cell processes and synapses accumulate with aging and Alzheimer-associated genetic modification. *Int J Alzheimer's Dis*, doi:10.4061/2009/689285.

Koo, E. H., and Squazzo, S. L. 1994. Evidence that production and release of amyloid β-protein involves the endocytic pathway. *J Biol Chem* 269: 17386–17389.

Koppal, T., Subramaniam, R., Drake, J., Prasad, M. R., Dhillon, H., and Butterfield, D. A. 1998. Vitamin E protects against Alzheimer's amyloid peptide (25-35)-induced changes in neocortical synaptosomal membrane lipid structure and composition. *Brain Res* 786: 270–273.

Kovacs, D. M., Fausett, H. J., Page, K. J., Kim, T. W., Moir, R. D., Merriam, D. E., Hollister, R. D., Hallmark, O. G., Mancini, R., Felsenstein, K. M., Hyman, B. T., Tanzi, R. E., and Wasco, W. 1996. Alzheimer-associated presenilins 1 and 2: Neuronal expression in brain and localization to intracellular membranes in mammalian cells. *Nat Med* 2: 224–229.

Kovacs, D. M., Gersbacher, M. T., and Kim, D. Y. 2010. Alzheimer's secretases regulate voltage-gated sodium channels. *Neurosci Lett* 486: 68–72.

Kowalik-Jankowska, T., Ruta, M., Wisniewska, K., and Lankiewicz, L. 2003. Coordination abilities of the 1-16 and 1-28 fragments of beta-amyloid peptide towards copper(II) ions: A combined potentiometric and spectroscopic study. *J Inorg Biochem* 95: 270–282.

Kraepelin, Emil. 2007. *Clinical psychiatry: A textbook for students and physicians* (reprint). Translated by A. Ross Diefendorf. Whitefish, MT: Kessinger Publishing.

Krone, M. G., Baumketner, A., Bernstein, S. L., Wyttenbach, T., Lazo, N. D., Teplow, D. B., Bowers, M. T., and Shea, J. E. 2008. Effects of familial Alzheimer's disease mutations on the folding nucleation of the amyloid β-protein. *J Mol Biol* 381: 221–228.

Kuan, C. Y., Schloemer, A. J., Lu, A., Burns, K. A., Weng, W. L., Williams, M. T., Strauss, K. I., Vorhees, C. V., Flavell, R. A., Davis, R. J., Sharp, F. R., and Rakic, P. 2004. Hypoxia-ischemia induces DNA synthesis without cell proliferation in dying neurons in adult rodent brain. *J Neurosci* 24: 10763–10772.

Kuhn, T. S. 1962. *The structure of scientific revolutions.* Chicago: University of Chicago Press.

Kumar, S., Yoshida, Y., and Noda, M. 1993. Cloning of a cDNA which encodes a novel ubiquitin-like protein. *Biochem Biophys Res Commun* 195: 393–399.

Kusakawa, G., Saito, T., Onuki, R., Ishiguro, K., Kishimoto, T., and Hisanaga, S. 2000. Calpain-dependent proteolytic cleavage of the p35 cyclin-dependent kinase 5 activator to p25. *J Biol Chem* 275: 17166–17172.

Ladu, M. J., Pederson, T. M., Frail, D. E., Reardon, C. A., Getz, G. S., and Falduto, M. T. 1995. Purification of apolipoprotein E attenuates isoform-specific binding to β-amyloid. *J Biol Chem* 270: 9039–9042.

Laferla, F. M. 2010. Pathways linking Aβ and tau pathologies. *Biochem Soc Trans* 38: 993–995.

Laferla, F. M., Green, K. N., and Oddo, S. 2007. Intracellular amyloid-β in Alzheimer's disease. *Nat Rev Neurosci* 8: 499–509.

Lam, A. R., Teplow, D. B., Stanley, H. E., and Urbanc, B. 2008. Effects of the Arctic (E22->G) mutation on amyloid β-protein folding: Discrete molecular dynamics study. *J Am Chem Soc* 130: 17413–17422.

Lambert, M. P., Barlow, A. K., Chromy, B. A., Edwards, C., Freed, R., Liosatos, M., Morgan, T. E., Rozovsky, I., Trommer, B., Viola, K. L., Wals, P., Zhang, C., Finch, C. E., Krafft, G. A., and Klein, W. L. 1998. Diffusible, nonfibrillar ligands derived from Aβ1-42 are potent central nervous system neurotoxins. *Proc Natl Acad Sci USA* 95: 6448–6453.

Langui, D., Girardot, N., El Hachimi, K. H., Allinquant, B., Blanchard, V., Pradier, L., and Duyckaerts, C. 2004. Subcellular topography of neuronal Aβ peptide in APPxPS1 transgenic mice. *American J of Path* 165: 1465–1477.

Lashuel, H. A., Hartley, D., Petre, B. M., Walz, T., and Lansbury, P. T., Jr. 2002. Neurodegenerative disease: Amyloid pores from pathogenic mutations. *Nature* 418: 291.

Lashuel, H. A., and Lansbury, P. T., Jr. 2006. Are amyloid diseases caused by protein aggregates that mimic bacterial pore-forming toxins? *Q Rev Biophys* 39: 167–201.

Lauren, J., Gimbel, D. A., Nygaard, H. B., Gilbert, J. W., and Strittmatter, S. M. 2009. Cellular prion protein mediates impairment of synaptic plasticity by amyloid-β oligomers. *Nature* 457: 1128–1132.

Lawson, V. A., Collins, S. J., Masters, C. L., and Hill, A. F. 2005. Prion protein glycosylation. *J Neurochem* 93: 793–801.

Lazaro, J. B., Kitzmann, M., Poul, M. A., Vandromme, M., Lamb, N. J., and Fernandez, A. 1997. Cyclin dependent kinase 5, cdk5, is a positive regulator of myogenesis in mouse C2 cells. *J Cell Sci* 110 (Pt 10): 1251–1260.

Lazo, N. D., Grant, M. A., Condron, M. C., Rigby, A. C., and Teplow, D. B. 2005. On the nucleation of amyloid β-protein monomer folding. *Protein Sci* 14: 1581–1596.

Leduc, V., Jasmin-Belanger, S., and Poirier, J. 2010. APOE and cholesterol homeostasis in Alzheimer's disease. *Trends Mol Med* 16: 469–477.

Lee, E. Y., Chang, C. Y., Hu, N., Wang, Y. C., Lai, C. C., Herrup, K., Lee, W. H., and Bradley, A. 1992. Mice deficient for Rb are nonviable and show defects in neurogenesis and haematopoiesis. *Nature* 359: 288–294.

Lee, E. Y., Hu, N., Yuan, S. S., Cox, L. A., Bradley, A., Lee, W. H., and Herrup, K. 1994. Dual roles of the retinoblastoma protein in cell cycle regulation and neuron differentiation. *Genes Dev* 8: 2008–2021.

Lee, H. G., Casadesus, G., Zhu, X., Castellani, R. J., McShea, A., Perry, G., Petersen, R. B., Bajic, V., and Smith, M. A. 2009. Cell cycle re-entry mediated neurodegeneration and its treatment role in the pathogenesis of Alzheimer's disease. *Neurochem Int* 54: 84–88.

Lee, H. G., Castellani, R. J., Zhu, X., Perry, G., and Smith, M. A. 2005. Amyloid-β in Alzheimer's disease: The horse or the cart? Pathogenic or protective? *Int J Exp Pathol* 86: 133–138.

Lee, M. S., Kwon, Y. T., Li, M., Peng, J., Friedlander, R. M., and Tsai, L. H. 2000. Neurotoxicity induces cleavage of p35 to p25 by calpain. *Nature* 405: 360–364.

Lee, S. J. 1998. Endoplasmic reticulum retention and degradation of T cell antigen receptor β chain. *Exp Mol Med* 30: 159–164.

Lee, V. M., Balin, B. J., Otvos, L., Jr., and Trojanowski, J. Q. 1991. A68: A major subunit of paired helical filaments and derivatized forms of normal Tau. *Science* 251: 675–678.

Lesne, S., Koh, M. T., Kotilinek, L., Kayed, R., Glabe, C. G., Yang, A., Gallagher, M., and Ashe, K. H. 2006. A specific amyloid-β protein assembly in the brain impairs memory. *Nature* 440: 352–357.

Levitan, D., and Greenwald, I. 1995. Facilitation of lin-12-mediated signalling by sel-12, a *Caenorhabditis elegans* S182 Alzheimer's disease gene. *Nature* 377: 351–354.

Levy-Lahad, E., Wasco, W., Poorkaj, P., Romano, D. M., Oshima, J., Pettingell, W. H., Yu, C. E., Jondro, P. D., Schmidt, S. D., Wang, K., et al. 1995. Candidate gene for the chromosome 1 familial Alzheimer's disease locus. *Science* 269: 973–977.

Lewis, J., Dickson, D. W., Lin, W. L., Chisholm, L., Corral, A., Jones, G., Yen, S. H., Sahara, N., Skipper, L., Yager, D., Eckman, C., Hardy, J., Hutton, M., and McGowan, E. 2001. Enhanced neurofibrillary degeneration in transgenic mice expressing mutant tau and APP. *Science* 293: 1487–1491.

Li, J., Xu, M., Zhou, H., Ma, J., and Potter, H. 1997. Alzheimer presenilins in the nuclear membrane, interphase kinetochores, and centrosomes suggest a role in chromosome segregation. *Cell* 90: 917–927.

Liakopoulos, D., Busgen, T., Brychzy, A., Jentsch, S., and Pause, A. 1999. Conjugation of the ubiquitin-like protein NEDD8 to cullin-2 is linked to von Hippel-Lindau tumor suppressor function. *Proc Natl Acad Sci USA* 96: 5510–5515.

Liang, W. S., Dunckley, T., Beach, T. G., Grover, A., Mastroeni, D., Walker, D. G., Caselli, R. J., Kukull, W. A., McKeel, D., Morris, J. C., Hulette, C., Schmechel, D., Alexander, G. E., Reiman, E. M., Rogers, J., and Stephan, D. A. 2007. Gene expression profiles in anatomically and functionally distinct regions of the normal aged human brain. *Physiol Genomics* 28: 311–322.

Liochev, S. I. 1999. The mechanism of "Fenton-like" reactions and their importance for biological systems. A biologist's view. *Met Ions Biol Syst* 36: 1–39.

Liou, Y. C., Sun, A., Ryo, A., Zhou, X. Z., Yu, Z. X., Huang, H. K., Uchida, T., Bronson, R., Bing, G., Li, X., Hunter, T., and Lu, K. P. 2003. Role of the prolyl isomerase Pin1 in protecting against age-dependent neurodegeneration. *Nature* 424: 556–561.

Liu, R. Q., Zhou, Q. H., Ji, S. R., Zhou, Q., Feng, D., Wu, Y., and Sui, S. F. 2010. Membrane localization of β-amyloid 1-42 in lysosomes: A possible mechanism for lysosome labilization. *J Biol Chem* 285: 19986–19996.

Liu, S. T., Howlett, G., and Barrow, C. J. 1999. Histidine-13 is a crucial residue in the zinc ion-induced aggregation of the Aβ peptide of Alzheimer's disease. *Biochemistry* 38: 9373–9378.

Lomakin, A., Teplow, D. B., Kirschner, D. A., and Benedek, G. B. 1997. Kinetic theory of fibrillogenesis of amyloid β-protein. *Proc Natl Acad Sci USA* 94: 7942–7947.

Lomakina, N. F., and Rybakov, S. S. 1996. Nucleotide sequence of the RNA polymerase gene attenuated by a variant of foot-and-mouth disease virus and its comparison with the virulence of related variants of subtype A22. *Mol Gen Mikrobiol Virusol* 35–40.

Lopes, J. P., Oliveira, C. R., and Agostinho, P. 2009. Cdk5 acts as a mediator of neuronal cell cycle re-entry triggered by amyloid-β and prion peptides. *Cell Cycle* 8: 97–104.

Lord, A., Englund, H., Soderberg, L., Tucker, S., Clausen, F., Hillered, L., Gordon, M., Morgan, D., Lannfelt, L., Pettersson, F. E., and Nilsson, L. N. 2009. Amyloid-β protofibril levels correlate with spatial learning in Arctic Alzheimer's disease transgenic mice. *FEBS J* 276: 995–1006.

Love, S. 2003. Neuronal expression of cell cycle-related proteins after brain ischaemia in man. *Neurosci Lett* 353: 29–32.

Lovell, M. A., Robertson, J. D., Teesdale, W. J., Campbell, J. L., and Markesbery, W. R. 1998. Copper, iron and zinc in Alzheimer's disease senile plaques. *J Neurol Sci* 158: 47–52.

Lovell, M. A., Xie, C., Gabbita, S. P., and Markesbery, W. R. 2000. Decreased thioredoxin and increased thioredoxin reductase levels in Alzheimer's disease brain. *Free Radic Biol Med* 28: 418–427.

Lovell, M. A., Xie, C., Xiong, S., and Markesbery, W. R. 2003. Protection against amyloid beta peptide and iron/hydrogen peroxide toxicity by alpha lipoic acid. *J Alzheimer's Dis* 5: 229–239.

Lu, K. P., Hanes, S. D., and Hunter, T. 1996. A human peptidyl-prolyl isomerase essential for regulation of mitosis. *Nature* 380: 544–547.

Lührs, T., Ritter, C., Adrian, M., Riek-Loher, D., Bohrmann, B., DöBeli, H., Schubert, D., and Riek, R. 2005. 3D structure of Alzheimer's amyloid-β(1–42) fibrils. *Proc Natl Acad Sci USA* 102: 17342–17347.

Luo, L. 2000. Rho GTPases in neuronal morphogenesis. *Nat Rev Neurosci* 1: 173–180.

Lustbader, J. W., Cirilli, M., Lin, C., Xu, H. W., Takuma, K., Wang, N., Caspersen, C., Chen, X., Pollak, S., Chaney, M., Trinchese, F., Liu, S., Gunn-Moore, F., Lue, L. F., Walker, D. G., Kuppusamy, P., Zewier, Z. L., Arancio, O., Stern, D., Yan, S. S., and Wu, H. 2004. ABAD directly links Aβ to mitochondrial toxicity in Alzheimer's disease. *Science* 304: 448–452.

Lyras, L., Cairns, N. J., Jenner, A., Jenner, P., and Halliwell, B. 1997. An assessment of oxidative damage to proteins, lipids, and DNA in brain from patients with Alzheimer's disease. *J Neurochem* 68: 2061–2069.

Ma, Q. F., et al. 2006. Characterization of copper binding to the peptide amyloid-β(1-16) associated with Alzheimer's disease. *Biopolymers* 83(1): 20–31.

Mahley, R. W. 1988. Apolipoprotein E: Cholesterol transport protein with expanding role in cell biology. *Science* 240: 622–630.

Makin, O. S., and Serpell, L. C. 2005. Structures for amyloid fibrils. *FEBS Journal* 272: 5950–5961.

Maler, L., and Graslund, A. 2009. Artificial membrane models for the study of macromolecular delivery. *Methods Mol Biol* 480: 129–139.

Mancuso, M., Orsucci, D., Siciliano, G., and Murri, L. 2008. Mitochondria, mitochondrial DNA and Alzheimer's disease. What comes first? *Curr Alzheimer Res* 5: 457–468.

Manczak, M., Anekonda, T. S., Henson, E., Park, B. S., Quinn, J., and Reddy, P. H. 2006. Mitochondria are a direct site of Aβ accumulation in Alzheimer's disease neurons: Implications for free radical generation and oxidative damage in disease progression. *Hum Mol Genet* 15: 1437–1449.

Mantyh, P. W., Ghilardi, J. R., Rogers, S., Demaster, E., Allen, C. J., Stimson, E. R., and Maggio, J. E. 1993. Aluminum, iron, and zinc ions promote aggregation of physiological concentrations of β-amyloid peptide. *J Neurochem* 61: 1171–1174.

Mark, R. J., Pang, Z., Geddes, J. W., Uchida, K., and Mattson, M. P. 1997. Amyloid β-peptide impairs glucose transport in hippocampal and cortical neurons: Involvement of membrane lipid peroxidation. *J Neurosci* 17: 1046–1054.

Markesbery, W. R. 1997. Oxidative stress hypothesis in Alzheimer's disease. *Free Radic Biol Med* 23: 134–147.

Markesbery, W. R., and Lovell, M. A. 1998. Four-hydroxynonenal, a product of lipid peroxidation, is increased in the brain in Alzheimer's disease. *Neurobiol Aging* 19: 33–36.

Marquer, C., Devauges, V., Cossec, J. C., Liot, G., Lecart, S., Saudou, F., Duyckaerts, C., Leveque-Fort, S., and Potier, M. C. 2011. Local cholesterol increase triggers amyloid precursor protein-Bace1 clustering in lipid rafts and rapid endocytosis. *FASEB J* 25: 1295–1305.

Martins, I. C., Kuperstein, I., Wilkinson, H., Maes, E., Vanbrabant, M., Jonckheere, W., Van Gelder, P., Hartmann, D., D'Hooge, R., De Strooper, B., Schymkowitz, J., and Rousseau, F. 2008. Lipids revert inert Aβ amyloid fibrils to neurotoxic protofibrils that affect learning in mice. *Embo J* 27: 224–233.

Martins, I. J., Hone, E., Foster, J. K., Sunram-Lea, S. I., Gnjec, A., Fuller, S. J., Nolan, D., Gandy, S. E., and Martins, R. N. 2006. Apolipoprotein E, cholesterol metabolism, diabetes, and the convergence of risk factors for Alzheimer's disease and cardiovascular disease. *Mol Psychiatry* 11: 721–736.

Martins, R. N., Harper, C. G., Stokes, G. B., and Masters, C. L. 1986. Increased cerebral glucose-6-phosphate dehydrogenase activity in Alzheimer's disease may reflect oxidative stress. *J Neurochem* 46: 1042–1045.

Marzolo, M. P., and Bu, G. 2009. Lipoprotein receptors and cholesterol in APP trafficking and proteolytic processing, implications for Alzheimer's disease. *Semin Cell Dev Biol* 20: 191–200.

Masoumi, A., Goldenson, B., Ghirmai, S., Avagyan, H., Zaghi, J., Abel, K., Zheng, X., Espinosa-Jeffrey, A., Mahanian, M., Liu, P. T., Hewison, M., Mizwickie, M., Cashman, J., and Fiala, M. 2009. 1α,25-dihydroxyvitamin D3 interacts with curcuminoids to stimulate amyloid-β clearance by macrophages of Alzheimer's disease patients. *J Alzheimer's Dis* 17: 703–717.

Masters, C. L., Gajdusek, D. C., and Gibbs, C. J., Jr. 1981. Creutzfeldt-Jakob disease virus isolations from the Gerstmann-Straussler syndrome with an analysis of the various forms of amyloid plaque deposition in the virus-induced spongiform encephalopathies. *Brain* 104: 559–588.

Masters, C. L., Harris, J. O., Gajdusek, D. C., Gibbs, C. J., Jr., Bernoulli, C., and Asher, D. M. 1979. Creutzfeldt-Jakob disease: Patterns of worldwide occurrence and the significance of familial and sporadic clustering. *Ann Neurol* 5: 177–188.

Masters, C. L., Multhaup, G., Simms, G., Pottgiesser, J., Martins, R. N., and Beyreuther, K. 1985. Neuronal origin of a cerebral amyloid: neurofibrillary tangles of Alzheimer's disease contain the same protein as the amyloid of plaque cores and blood vessels. *Embo J* 4: 2757–2763.

Matsumura, S., Shinoda, K., Yamada, M., Yokojima, S., Inoue, M., Ohnishi, T., Shimada, T., Kikuchi, K., Masui, D., Hashimoto, S., Sato, M., Ito, A., Akioka, M., Takagi, S., Nakamura, Y., Nemoto, K., Hasegawa, Y., Takamoto, H., Inoue, H., Nakamura, S., Nabeshima, Y., Teplow, D. B., Kinjo, M., and Hoshi, M. 2011. Two distinct amyloid β-protein (Aβ) assembly pathways leading to oligomers and fibrils identified by combined fluorescence correlation spectroscopy, morphology, and toxicity analyses. *J Bio Chem* 286: 11555–11562.

Mattson, M. P. 1997. Cellular actions of β-amyloid precursor protein and its soluble and fibrillogenic derivatives. *Physiol Rev* 77: 1081–1132.

Mattson, M. P. 2002. Brain evolution and lifespan regulation: Conservation of signal transduction pathways that regulate energy metabolism. *Mech Ageing Dev* 123: 947–953.

Mattson, M. P., and Chan, S. L. 2001. Dysregulation of cellular calcium homeostasis in Alzheimer's disease: Bad genes and bad habits. *J Mol Neurosci* 17: 205–224.

Mattson, M. P., and Chan, S. L. 2003. Neuronal and glial calcium signaling in Alzheimer's disease. *Cell Calcium* 34: 385–397.

McAlpine, F. E., Lee, J. K., Harms, A. S., Ruhn, K. A., Blurton-Jones, M., Hong, J., Das, P., Golde, T. E., Laferla, F. M., Oddo, S., Blesch, A., and Tansey, M. G. 2009. Inhibition of soluble TNF signaling in a mouse model of Alzheimer's disease prevents pre-plaque amyloid-associated neuropathology. *Neurobiol Dis* 34: 163–177.

McDonald, D. R., Bamberger, M. E., Combs, C. K., and Landreth, G. E. 1998. β-amyloid fibrils activate parallel mitogen-activated protein kinase pathways in microglia and THP1 monocytes. *J Neurosci* 18: 4451–4460.

McGeer, E. G., and McGeer, P. L. 2003. Inflammatory processes in Alzheimer's disease. *Prog Neuropsy Biol Psy* 27: 741–749.

McGeer, P. L., and McGeer, E. G. 1996. Anti-inflammatory drugs in the fight against Alzheimer's disease. *Ann N Y Acad Sci* 777: 213–220.

McLaurin, J., and Chakrabartty, A. 1996. Membrane disruption by Alzheimer β-amyloid peptides mediated through specific binding to either phospholipids or gangliosides: Implications for neurotoxicity. *J Biol Chem* 271: 26482–26489.

McShea, A., Harris, P. L., Webster, K. R., Wahl, A. F., and Smith, M. A. 1997. Abnormal expression of the cell cycle regulators P16 and CDK4 in Alzheimer's disease. *Am J Pathol* 150: 1933–1939.

Meinhardt, J., Sachse, C., Hortschansky, P., Grigorieff, N., and Fändrich, M. 2009. Aβ(1-40) fibril polymorphism implies diverse interaction patterns in amyloid fibrils. *J of Mol Biol* 386: 869–877.

Melo, M. N., Ferre, R., and Castanho, M. A. 2009. Antimicrobial peptides: Linking partition, activity and high membrane-bound concentrations. *Nat Rev Microbiol* 7: 245–250.

Meloni, G., Sonois, V., Delaine, T., Guilloreau, L., Gillet, A., Teissie, J., Faller, P., and Vasak, M. 2008. Metal swap between Zn7-metallothionein-3 and amyloid-β-Cu protects against amyloid-β toxicity. *Nat Chem Biol* 4: 366–372.

Meyer-Luehmann, M., Coomaraswamy, J., Bolmont, T., Kaeser, S., Schaefer, C., Kilger, E., Neuenschwander, A., Abramowski, D., Frey, P., Jaton, A. L., Vigouret, J. M., Paganetti, P., Walsh, D. M., Mathews, P. M., Ghiso, J., Staufenbiel, M., Walker, L. C., and Jucker, M. 2006. Exogenous induction of cerebral β-amyloidogenesis is governed by agent and host. *Science* 313: 1781–1784.

Mi, W., Pawlik, M., Sastre, M., Jung, S. S., Radvinsky, D. S., Klein, A. M., Sommer, J., Schmidt, S. D., Nixon, R. A., Mathews, P. M., and Levy, E. 2007. Cystatin C inhibits amyloid-β deposition in Alzheimer's disease mouse models. *Nat Genet* 39: 1440–1442.

Miller, L. M., Wang, Q., Telivala, T. P., Smith, R. J., Lanzirotti, A., and Miklossy, J. 2006. Synchrotron-based infrared and X-ray imaging shows focalized accumulation of Cu and Zn co-localized with β-amyloid deposits in Alzheimer's disease. *J Struct Biol* 155: 30–37.

Milward, E. A., Papadopoulos, R., Fuller, S. J., Moir, R. D., Small, D., Beyreuther, K., and Masters, C. L. 1992. The amyloid protein precursor of Alzheimer's disease is a mediator of the effects of nerve growth factor on neurite outgrowth. *Neuron* 9: 129–137.

Minogue, A. M., Schmid, A. W., Fogarty, M. P., Moore, A. C., Campbell, V. A., Herron, C. E., and Lynch, M. A. 2003. Activation of the c-Jun N-terminal kinase signaling cascade mediates the effect of amyloid-β on long-term potentiation and cell death in hippocampus: A role for interleukin-1β? *J Biol Chem* 278: 27971–27980.

Misumi, Y., Ando, Y., Ueda, M., Obayashi, K., Jono, H., Su, Y., Yamashita, T., and Uchino, M. 2009. Chain reaction of amyloid fibril formation with induction of basement membrane in familial amyloidotic polyneuropathy. *J Pathol* 219: 481–490.

Miyazono, M., Kitamoto, T., Iwaki, T., and Tateishi, J. 1992. Colocalization of prion protein and β protein in the same amyloid plaques in patients with Gerstmann-Straussler syndrome. *Acta Neuropathol* 83: 333–339.

Mohamed, A., and Posse De Chaves, E. 2011. Aβ internalization by neurons and glia. *Int J Alzheimer's Disease*, doi: 10.4061/2011/127984.

Mohorko, N., Repovs, G., Popovic, M., Kovacs, G. G., and Bresjanac, M. 2010. Curcumin labeling of neuronal fibrillar tau inclusions in human brain samples. *J Neuropathol Exp Neurol* 69: 405–414.

Moloney, A. M., Griffin, R. J., Timmons, S., O'Connor, R., Ravid, R., and O'Neill, C. 2010. Defects in IGF-1 receptor, insulin receptor and IRS-1/2 in Alzheimer's disease indicate possible resistance to IGF-1 and insulin signalling. *Neurobiol Aging* 31: 224–243.

Monaco, E. A., III, and Vallano, M. L. 2005. Role of protein kinases in neurodegenerative disease: Cyclin-dependent kinases in Alzheimer's disease. *Front Biosci* 10: 143–159.

Moreira, P. I., Santos, M. S., Moreno, A., Rego, A. C., and Oliveira, C. 2002. Effect of amyloid β-peptide on permeability transition pore: A comparative study. *J Neurosci Res* 69: 257–267.

Moskovitz, J., Berlett, B. S., Poston, J. M., and Stadtman, E. R. 1999. Methionine sulfoxide reductase in antioxidant defense. *Methods Enzymol* 300: 239–244.

Mueller-Steiner, S., Zhou, Y., Arai, H., Roberson, E. D., Sun, B., Chen, J., Wang, X., Yu, G., Esposito, L., Mucke, L., and Gan, L. 2006. Antiamyloidogenic and neuroprotective functions of cathepsin B: Implications for Alzheimer's disease. *Neuron* 51: 703–714.

Muller, T., Loosse, C., Schrotter, A., Schnabel, A., Helling, S., Egensperger, R., and Marcus, K. 2011. The AICD interacting protein DAB1 is up-regulated in Alzheimer frontal cortex brain samples and causes deregulation of proteins involved in gene expression changes. *Curr Alzheimer Res* 8: 573–582.

Mura, E., Lanni, C., Preda, S., Pistoia, F., Sara, M., Racchi, M., Schettini, G., Marchi, M., and Govoni, S. 2010. β-amyloid: A disease target or a synaptic regulator affecting age-related neurotransmitter changes? *Curr Pharm Des* 16: 672–683.

Murakami, K., Hara, H., Masuda, Y., Ohigashi, H., and Irie, K. 2007. Distance measurement between Tyr10 and Met35 in amyloid β by site-directed spin-labeling ESR spectroscopy: Implications for the stronger neurotoxicity of Aβ42 than Aβ40. *Chembiochem* 8: 2308–2314.

Murakami, K., Irie, K., Ohigashi, H., Hara, H., Nagao, M., Shimizu, T., and Shirasawa, T. 2005. Formation and stabilization model of the 42-mer Aβ radical: Implications for the long-lasting oxidative stress in Alzheimer's disease. *J Am Chem Soc* 127: 15168–15174.

Murakami, Y., Ohsawa, I., Kasahara, T., and Ohta, S. 2009. Cytoprotective role of mitochondrial amyloid β peptide-binding alcohol dehydrogenase against a cytotoxic aldehyde. *Neurobiol Aging* 30: 325–329.

Murray, I. V., Liu, L., Komatsu, H., Uryu, K., Xiao, G., Lawson, J. A., and Axelsen, P. H. 2007. Membrane-mediated amyloidogenesis and the promotion of oxidative lipid damage by amyloid β proteins. *J Biol Chem* 282: 9335–9345.

Murray, I. V., Sindoni, M. E., and Axelsen, P. H. 2005. Promotion of oxidative lipid membrane damage by amyloid β proteins. *Biochemistry* 44: 12606–12613.

Murray, M. M., Krone, M. G., Bernstein, S. L., Baumketner, A., Condron, M. M., Lazo, N. D., Teplow, D. B., Wyttenbach, T., Shea, J. E., and Bowers, M. T. 2009. Amyloid β-protein: Experiment and theory on the 21-30 fragment. *J Phys Chem B* 113: 6041–6046.

Nagy, Z., Esiri, M. M., Cato, A. M., and Smith, A. D. 1997a. Cell cycle markers in the hippocampus in Alzheimer's disease. *Acta Neuropathol* 94: 6–15.

Nagy, Z., Esiri, M. M., and Smith, A. D. 1997b. Expression of cell division markers in the hippocampus in Alzheimer's disease and other neurodegenerative conditions. *Acta Neuropathol* 93: 294–300.

Naj, A. C., Jun, G., Beecham, G. W., Wang, L. S., Vardarajan, B. N., Buros, J., Gallins, P. J., et al. 2010. Common variants at MS4A4/MS4A6E, CD2AP, CD33 and EPHA1 are associated with late-onset alzheimer's disease. *Nat Genet* 43: 436–441.

Nath, R., Davis, M., Probert, A. W., Kupina, N. C., Ren, X., Schielke, G. P., and Wang, K. K. 2000. Processing of Cdk5 activator p35 to its truncated form (p25) by calpain in acutely injured neuronal cells. *Biochem Biophys Res Commun* 274: 16–21.

Nathan, B. P., Chang, K. C., Bellosta, S., Brisch, E., Ge, N., Mahley, R. W., and Pitas, R. E. 1995. The inhibitory effect of apolipoprotein E4 on neurite outgrowth is associated with microtubule depolymerization. *J Biol Chem* 270: 19791–19799.

Nelson, O., Tu, H., Lei, T., Bentahir, M., De Strooper, B., and Bezprozvanny, I. 2007. Familial Alzheimer disease-linked mutations specifically disrupt Ca2+ leak function of presenilin 1. *J Clin Invest* 117: 1230–1239.

Nelson, R., Sawaya, M. R., Balbirnie, M., Madsen, A. O., Riekel, C., Grothe, R., and Eisenberg, D. 2005. Structure of the cross-β spine of amyloid-like fibrils. *Nature* 435: 773–778.

Neve, R. L., and McPhie, D. L. 2006. The cell cycle as a therapeutic target for Alzheimer's disease. *Pharmacol Ther* 111: 99–113.

Nico, P. B., De-Paris, F., Vinade, E. R., Amaral, O. B., Rockenbach, I., Soares, B. L., Guarnieri, R., Wichert-Ana, L., Calvo, F., Walz, R., Izquierdo, I., Sakamoto, A. C., Brentani, R., Martins, V. R., and Bianchin, M. M. 2005. Altered behavioural response to acute stress in mice lacking cellular prion protein. *Behav Brain Res* 162: 173–181.

Nikolic, M., Chou, M. M., Lu, W., Mayer, B. J., and Tsai, L. H. 1998. The p35/Cdk5 kinase is a neuron-specific Rac effector that inhibits Pak1 activity. *Nature* 395: 194–198.

Nilsberth, C., Westlind-Danielsson, A., Eckman, C. B., Condron, M. M., Axelman, K., Forsell, C., Stenh, C., Luthman, J., Teplow, D. B., Younkin, S. G., Naslund, J., and Lannfelt, L. 2001. The "Arctic" APP mutation (E693G) causes Alzheimer's disease by enhanced Aβ protofibril formation. *Nat Neurosci* 4: 887–893.

Nitsch, R. M., Blusztajn, J. K., Pittas, A. G., Slack, B. E., Growdon, J. H., and Wurtman, R. J. 1992. Evidence for a membrane defect in Alzheimer disease brain. *Proc Natl Acad Sci USA* 89: 1671–1675.

Noguchi, A., Matsumura, S., Dezawa, M., Tada, M., Yanazawa, M., Ito, A., Akioka, M., Kikuchi, S., Sato, M., Ideno, S., Noda, M., Fukunari, A., Muramatsu, S., Itokazu, Y., Sato, K., Takahashi, H., Teplow, D. B., Nabeshima, Y., Kakita, A., Imahori, K., and Hoshi, M. 2009. Isolation and characterization of patient-derived, toxic, high mass amyloid β-protein (Aβs) assembly from Alzheimer disease brains. *J Bio Chem* 284: 32895–32905.

Nunomura, A., Hofer, T., Moreira, P. I., Castellani, R. J., Smith, M. A., and Perry, G. 2009. RNA oxidation in Alzheimer disease and related neurodegenerative disorders. *Acta Neuropathol* 118: 151–166.

Nygaard, H. B., and Strittmatter, S. M. 2009. Cellular prion protein mediates the toxicity of β-amyloid oligomers: Implications for Alzheimer disease. *Arch Neurol* 66: 1325–1328.

O'Nuallain, B., Shivaprasad, S., Kheterpal, I., and Wetzel, R. 2005. Thermodynamics of Aβ(1- 40) amyloid fibril elongation. *Biochemistry* 44: 12709–12718.

Oakley, H., Cole, S. L., Logan, S., Maus, E., Shao, P., Craft, J., Guillozet-Bongaarts, A., Ohno, M., Disterhoft, J., Van Eldik, L., Berry, R., and Vassar, R. 2006. Intraneuronal β-amyloid aggregates, neurodegeneration, and neuron loss in transgenic mice with five familial Alzheimer's disease mutations: potential factors in amyloid plaque formation. *J Neurosci* 26: 10129–10140.

Obin, M., Mesco, E., Gong, X., Haas, A. L., Joseph, J., and Taylor, A. 1999. Neurite outgrowth in PC12 cells. Distinguishing the roles of ubiquitylation and ubiquitin-dependent proteolysis. *J Biol Chem* 274: 11789–11795.

Oddo, S., Billings, L., Kesslak, J. P., Cribbs, D. H., and Laferla, F. M. 2004. Aβ immunotherapy leads to clearance of early, but not late, hyperphosphorylated tau aggregates via the proteasome. *Neuron* 43: 321–332.

Oddo, S., Caccamo, A., Cheng, D., Jouleh, B., Torp, R., and Laferla, F. M. 2007. Genetically augmenting tau levels does not modulate the onset or progression of Aβ pathology in transgenic mice. *J Neurochem* 102: 1053–1063.

Oddo, S., Caccamo, A., Tran, L., Lambert, M. P., Glabe, C. G., Klein, W. L., and Laferla, F. M. 2006. Temporal profile of amyloid-β (Aβ) oligomerization in an in vivo model of Alzheimer disease: A link between Aβ and tau pathology. *J Biol Chem* 281: 1599–1604.

Oddo, S., Caccamo, A., Tseng, B., Cheng, D., Vasilevko, V., Cribbs, D. H., and Laferla, F. M. 2008. Blocking Aβ42 accumulation delays the onset and progression of tau pathology via the C terminus of heat shock protein70-interacting protein: A mechanistic link between Abeta and tau pathology. *J Neurosci* 28: 12163–12175.

Oesch, B., Westaway, D., Walchli, M., McKinley, M. P., Kent, S. B., Aebersold, R., Barry, R. A., Tempst, P., Teplow, D. B., Hood, L. E., et al. 1985. A cellular gene encodes scrapie PrP 27-30 protein. *Cell* 40: 735–746.

Ogawa, O., Zhu, X., Lee, H. G., Raina, A., Obrenovich, M. E., Bowser, R., Ghanbari, H. A., Castellani, R. J., Perry, G., and Smith, M. A. 2003. Ectopic localization of phosphorylated histone H3 in Alzheimer's disease: A mitotic catastrophe? *Acta Neuropathol* 105: 524–528.

Oh, S., Hong, H. S., Hwang, E., Sim, H. J., Lee, W., Shin, S. J., and Mook-Jung, I. 2005. Amyloid peptide attenuates the proteasome activity in neuronal cells. *Mech Ageing Dev* 126: 1292–1299.

Ohkubo, N., Lee, Y. D., Morishima, A., Terashima, T., Kikkawa, S., Tohyama, M., Sakanaka, M., Tanaka, J., Maeda, N., Vitek, M. P., and Mitsuda, N. 2003. Apolipoprotein E and Reelin ligands modulate tau phosphorylation through an apolipoprotein E receptor/disabled-1/glycogen synthase kinase-3β cascade. *Faseb J* 17: 295–297.

Ohshima, T., Gilmore, E. C., Longenecker, G., Jacobowitz, D. M., Brady, R. O., Herrup, K., and Kulkarni, A. B. 1999. Migration defects of cdk5(-/-) neurons in the developing cerebellum is cell autonomous. *J Neurosci* 19: 6017–6026.

Ohshima, T., Ward, J. M., Huh, C. G., Longenecker, G., Veeranna, Pant, H. C., Brady, R. O., Martin, L. J., and Kulkarni, A. B. 1996. Targeted disruption of the cyclin-dependent kinase 5 gene results in abnormal corticogenesis, neuronal pathology and perinatal death. *Proc Natl Acad Sci USA* 93: 11173–11178.

Ohta, S., and Ohsawa, I. 2006. Dysfunction of mitochondria and oxidative stress in the pathogenesis of Alzheimer's disease: On defects in the cytochrome c oxidase complex and aldehyde detoxification. *J Alzheimer's Dis* 9: 155–166.

Okada, T., Wakabayashi, M., Ikeda, K., and Matsuzaki, K. 2007. Formation of toxic fibrils of Alzheimer's amyloid β-protein-(1-40) by monosialoganglioside GM1, a neuronal membrane component. *J Mol Biol* 371: 481–489.

Ono, K., Condron, M. M., and Teplow, D. B. 2009. Structure-neurotoxicity relationships of amyloid β-protein oligomers. *Proc Natl Acad Sci USA* 106: 14745–14750.

Opazo, C., Huang, X., Cherny, R. A., Moir, R. D., Roher, A. E., White, A. R., Cappai, R., Masters, C. L., Tanzi, R. E., Inestrosa, N. C., and Bush, A. I. 2002. Metalloenzyme-like activity of Alzheimer's disease β-amyloid. Cu-dependent catalytic conversion of dopamine, cholesterol, and biological reducing agents to neurotoxic H(2)O(2). *J Biol Chem* 277: 40302–40308.

Osenkowski, P., Ye, W., Wang, R., Wolfe, M. S., and Selkoe, D. J. 2008. Direct and potent regulation of γ-secretase by its lipid microenvironment. *J Biol Chem* 283: 22529–22540.

Overmyer, M., Helisalmi, S., Soininen, H., Laakso, M., Riekkinen, P., Sr., and Alafuzoff, I. 1999. Reactive microglia in aging and dementia: An immunohistochemical study of postmortem human brain tissue. *Acta Neuropathol* 97: 383–392.

Paglini, G., Pigino, G., Kunda, P., Morfini, G., Maccioni, R., Quiroga, S., Ferreira, A., and Caceres, A. 1998. Evidence for the participation of the neuron-specific CDK5 activator P35 during laminin-enhanced axonal growth. *J Neurosci* 18: 9858–9869.

Paivio, A., Jarvet, J., Graslund, A., Lannfelt, L., and Westlind-Danielsson, A. 2004. Unique physicochemical profile of β-amyloid peptide variant Abeta1-40E22G protofibrils: Conceivable neuropathogen in arctic mutant carriers. *J Mol Biol* 339: 145–159.

Palop, J. J., and Mucke, L. 2010. Amyloid-β-induced neuronal dysfunction in Alzheimer's disease: From synapses toward neural networks. *Nat Neurosci* 13: 812–818.

Pamplona, R., Dalfo, E., Ayala, V., Bellmunt, M. J., Prat, J., Ferrer, I., and Portero-Otin, M. 2005. Proteins in human brain cortex are modified by oxidation, glycoxidation, and lipoxidation: Effects of Alzheimer disease and identification of lipoxidation targets. *J Biol Chem* 280: 21522–21530.

Pan, K. M., Baldwin, M., Nguyen, J., Gasset, M., Serban, A., Groth, D., Mehlhorn, I., Huang, Z., Fletterick, R. J., Cohen, F. E., et al. 1993. Conversion of α-helices into β-sheets features in the formation of the scrapie prion proteins. *Proc Natl Acad Sci USA* 90: 10962–10966.

Parameshwaran, K., Dhanasekaran, M., and Suppiramaniam, V. 2008. Amyloid beta peptides and glutamatergic synaptic dysregulation. *Exp Neurol* 210: 7–13.

Park, D. S., Farinelli, S. E., and Greene, L. A. 1996. Inhibitors of cyclin-dependent kinases promote survival of post-mitotic neuronally differentiated PC12 cells and sympathetic neurons. *J Biol Chem* 271: 8161–8169.

Park, D. S., Levine, B., Ferrari, G., and Greene, L. A. 1997. Cyclin dependent kinase inhibitors and dominant negative cyclin dependent kinase 4 and 6 promote survival of NGF-deprived sympathetic neurons. *J Neurosci* 17: 8975–8983.

Parkin, E. T., Watt, N. T., Hussain, I., Eckman, E. A., Eckman, C. B., Manson, J. C., Baybutt, H. N., Turner, A. J., and Hooper, N. M. 2007. Cellular prion protein regulates β-secretase cleavage of the Alzheimer's amyloid precursor protein. *Proc Natl Acad Sci USA* 104: 11062–11067.

Parvathy, S., Hussain, I., Karran, E. H., Turner, A. J., and Hooper, N. M. 1999. Cleavage of Alzheimer's amyloid precursor protein by α-secretase occurs at the surface of neuronal cells. *Biochemistry* 38: 9728–9734.

Patrick, G. N., Zukerberg, L., Nikolic, M., De La Monte, S., Dikkes, P., and Tsai, L. H. 1999. Conversion of p35 to p25 deregulates Cdk5 activity and promotes neurodegeneration. *Nature* 402: 615–622.

Paudel, H. K., Lew, J., Ali, Z., and Wang, J. H. 1993. Brain proline-directed protein kinase phosphorylates tau on sites that are abnormally phosphorylated in tau associated with Alzheimer's paired helical filaments. *J Biol Chem* 268: 23512–23518.

Pei, J. J., Grundke-Iqbal, I., Iqbal, K., Bogdanovic, N., Winblad, B., and Cowburn, R. F. 1998. Accumulation of cyclin-dependent kinase 5 (cdk5) in neurons with early stages of Alzheimer's disease neurofibrillary degeneration. *Brain Res* 797: 267–277.

Pena, F., Ordaz, B., Balleza-Tapia, H., Bernal-Pedraza, R., Marquez-Ramos, A., Carmona-Aparicio, L., and Giordano, M. 2010. β-amyloid protein (25-35) disrupts hippocampal network activity: Role of Fyn-kinase. *Hippocampus* 20: 78–96.

Perez, R. G., Soriano, S., Hayes, J. D., Ostaszewski, B., Xia, W., Selkoe, D. J., Chen, X., Stokin, G. B., and Koo, E. H. 1999. Mutagenesis identifies new signals for β-amyloid precursor protein endocytosis, turnover, and the generation of secreted fragments, including Aβ42. *J Biol Chem* 274: 18851–18856.

Peters, J. M., Franke, W. W., and Kleinschmidt, J. A. 1994. Distinct 19 S and 20 S subcomplexes of the 26 S proteasome and their distribution in the nucleus and the cytoplasm. *J Biol Chem* 269: 7709–7718.

Petkova, A. T., Ishii, Y., Balbach, J. J., Antzutkin, O. N., Leapman, R. D., Delaglio, F., and Tycko, R. 2002. A structural model for Alzheimer's β-amyloid fibrils based on experimental constraints from solid state NMR. *Proc Natl Acad Sci* 99: 16742–16747.

Petrucelli, L., Dickson, D., Kehoe, K., Taylor, J., Snyder, H., Grover, A., De Lucia, M., McGowan, E., Lewis, J., Prihar, G., Kim, J., Dillmann, W. H., Browne, S. E., Hall, A., Voellmy, R., Tsuboi, Y., Dawson, T. M., Wolozin, B., Hardy, J., and Hutton, M. 2004. CHIP and Hsp70 regulate tau ubiquitination, degradation and aggregation. *Hum Mol Genet* 13: 703–714.

Phinney, A. L., Horne, P., Yang, J., Janus, C., Bergeron, C., and Westaway, D. 2003. Mouse models of Alzheimer's disease: The long and filamentous road. *Neurol Res* 25: 590–600.

Pigino, G., Paglini, G., Ulloa, L., Avila, J., and Caceres, A. 1997. Analysis of the expression, distribution and function of cyclin dependent kinase 5 (cdk5) in developing cerebellar macroneurons. *J Cell Sci* 110 (Pt 2): 257–270.

Pines, J. 1993. Cyclins and cyclin-dependent kinases: Take your partners. *Trends Biochem Sci* 18: 195–197.

Podust, V. N., Brownell, J. E., Gladysheva, T. B., Luo, R. S., Wang, C., Coggins, M. B., Pierce, J. W., Lightcap, E. S., and Chau, V. 2000. A Nedd8 conjugation pathway is essential for proteolytic targeting of p27Kip1 by ubiquitination. *Proc Natl Acad Sci USA* 97: 4579–4584.

Poirier, J. 2003. Apolipoprotein E and cholesterol metabolism in the pathogenesis and treatment of Alzheimer's disease. *Trends Mol Med* 9: 94–101.

Poirier, J. 2008. Apolipoprotein E represents a potent gene-based therapeutic target for the treatment of sporadic Alzheimer's disease. *Alzheimer's Dement* 4: S91–97.

Poirier, J., Hess, M., May, P. C., and Finch, C. E. 1991. Cloning of hippocampal poly(A) RNA sequences that increase after entorhinal cortex lesion in adult rat. *Brain Res Mol Brain Res* 9: 191–195.

Pralle, A., Keller, P., Florin, E. L., Simons, K., and Horber, J. K. 2000. Sphingolipid-cholesterol rafts diffuse as small entities in the plasma membrane of mammalian cells. *J Cell Biol* 148: 997–1008.

Price, D. L., and Sisodia, S. S. 1994. Cellular and molecular biology of Alzheimer's disease and animal models. *Annu Rev Med* 45: 435–446.

Probst, A., Taylor, K. I., and Tolnay, M. 2007. Hippocampal sclerosis dementia: A reappraisal. *Acta Neuropathol* 114: 335–345.

Prusiner, S. B. 1991. Molecular biology of prion diseases. *Science* 252: 1515–1522.

Prusiner, S. B. 2001. Shattuck lecture: Neurodegenerative diseases and prions. *N Engl J Med* 344: 1516–1526.

Puglielli, L., Ellis, B. C., Saunders, A. J., and Kovacs, D. M. 2003. Ceramide stabilizes β-site amyloid precursor protein-cleaving enzyme 1 and promotes amyloid β-peptide biogenesis. *J Biol Chem* 278: 19777–19783.

Pyo, H., Jou, I., Jung, S., Hong, S., and Joe, E. H. 1998. Mitogen-activated protein kinases activated by lipopolysaccharide and β-amyloid in cultured rat microglia. *Neuroreport* 9: 871–874.

Qi, Z., Huang, Q. Q., Lee, K. Y., Lew, J., and Wang, J. H. 1995. Reconstitution of neuronal Cdc2-like kinase from bacteria-expressed Cdk5 and an active fragment of the brain-specific activator: Kinase activation in the absence of Cdk5 phosphorylation. *J Biol Chem* 270: 10847–10854.

Quist, A., Doudevski, I., Lin, H., Azimova, R., Ng, D., Frangione, B., Kagan, B., Ghiso, J., and Lal, R. 2005. Amyloid ion channels: A common structural link for protein-misfolding disease. *Proc Natl Acad Sci USA* 102: 10427–10432.

Radde, R., Duma, C., Goedert, M., and Jucker, M. 2008. The value of incomplete mouse models of Alzheimer's disease. *Eur J Nucl Med Mol Imaging* 35 Suppl 1: S70–74.

Ramakrishnan, P., Dickson, D. W., and Davies, P. 2003. Pin1 colocalization with phosphorylated tau in Alzheimer's disease and other tauopathies. *Neurobiol Dis* 14: 251–264.

Raman, B., et al. 2005. Metal ion-dependent effects of clioquinol on the fibril growth of an amyloid β peptide. *J Biol Chem* 280(16): 16157–16162.

Ranganathan, S., and Bowser, R. 2003. Alterations in G(1) to S phase cell-cycle regulators during amyotrophic lateral sclerosis. *Am J Pathol* 162: 823–835.

Rangel, A., Burgaya, F., Gavin, R., Soriano, E., Aguzzi, A., and Del Rio, J. A. 2007. Enhanced susceptibility of Prnp-deficient mice to kainate-induced seizures, neuronal apoptosis, and death: Role of AMPA/kainate receptors. *J Neurosci Res* 85: 2741–2755.

Read, M. A., Brownell, J. E., Gladysheva, T. B., Hottelet, M., Parent, L. A., Coggins, M. B., Pierce, J. W., Podust, V. N., Luo, R. S., Chau, V., and Palombella, V. J. 2000. Nedd8 modification of Cul-1 activates SCF(β(TrCP))-dependent ubiquitination of IkappaBalpha. *Mol Cell Biol* 20: 2326–2333.

Refolo, L. M., Pappolla, M. A., Lafrancois, J., Malester, B., Schmidt, S. D., Thomas-Bryant, T., Tint, G. S., Wang, R., Mercken, M., Petanceska, S. S., and Duff, K. E. 2001. A cholesterol-lowering drug reduces β-amyloid pathology in a transgenic mouse model of Alzheimer's disease. *Neurobiol Dis* 8: 890–899.

Relini, A., Cavalleri, O., Rolandi, R., and Gliozzi, A. 2009. The two-fold aspect of the interplay of amyloidogenic proteins with lipid membranes. *Chem Phys Lipids* 158: 1–9.

Revesz, T., and Holton, J. L. 2003. Anatamopathological spectrum of tauopathies. 2003. *Mov Disord* 18 Suppl 6: S13–20.

Rhein, V., Baysang, G., Rao, S., Meier, F., Bonert, A., Muller-Spahn, F., and Eckert, A. 2009a. Amyloid-beta leads to impaired cellular respiration, energy production and mito-chondrial electron chain complex activities in human neuroblastoma cells. *Cell Mol Neurobiol* 29: 1063–1071.

Rhein, V., Song, X., Wiesner, A., Ittner, L. M., Baysang, G., Meier, F., Ozmen, L., Bluethmann, H., Drose, S., Brandt, U., Savaskan, E., Czech, C., Gotz, J., and Eckert, A. 2009b. Amyloid-β and tau synergistically impair the oxidative phosphorylation system in triple transgenic Alzheimer's disease mice. *Proc Natl Acad Sci USA* 106: 20057–20062.

Ricchelli, F., Drago, D., Filippi, B., Tognon, G., and Zatta, P. 2005. Aluminum-triggered structural modifications and aggregation of β-amyloids. *Cell Mol Life Sci* 62: 1724–1733.

Richter, R. P., Berat, R., and Brisson, A. R. 2006. Formation of solid-supported lipid bilayers: An integrated view. *Langmuir* 22: 3497–3505.

Riddell, D. R., Christie, G., Hussain, I., and Dingwall, C. 2001. Compartmentalization of β-secretase (Asp2) into low-buoyant density, noncaveolar lipid rafts. *Curr Biol* 11: 1288–1293.

Riek, R., Guntert, P., Dobeli, H., Wipf, B., and Wuthrich, K. 2001. NMR studies in aqueous solution fail to identify significant conformational differences between the monomeric forms of two Alzheimer peptides with widely different plaque-competence, Aβ(1-40) (ox) and Aβ(1-42)(ox). *Eur J Biochem* 268: 5930–5936.

Riek, R., Hornemann, S., Wider, G., Billeter, M., Glockshuber, R., and Wuthrich, K. 1996. NMR structure of the mouse prion protein domain PrP(121-321). *Nature* 382: 180–182.

Riemenschneider, M., Klopp, N., Xiang, W., Wagenpfeil, S., Vollmert, C., Muller, U., Forstl, H., Illig, T., Kretzschmar, H., and Kurz, A. 2004. Prion protein codon 129 polymor-phism and risk of Alzheimer disease. *Neurology* 63: 364–366.

Rival, T., Page, R. M., Chandraratna, D. S., Sendall, T. J., Ryder, E., Liu, B., Lewis, H., Rosahl, T., Hider, R., Camargo, L. M., Shearman, M. S., Crowther, D. C., and Lomas, D. A. 2009. Fenton chemistry and oxidative stress mediate the toxicity of the β-amyloid peptide in a *Drosophila* model of Alzheimer's disease. *Eur J Neurosci* 29: 1335–1347.

Robakis, N. K., Ramakrishna, N., Wolfe, G., and Wisniewski, H. M. 1987. Molecular cloning and characterization of a cDNA encoding the cerebrovascular and the neuritic plaque amyloid peptides. *Proc Natl Acad Sci USA* 84: 4190–4194.

Roberson, E. D., Halabisky, B., Yoo, J. W., Yao, J., Chin, J., Yan, F., Wu, T., Hamto, P., Devidze, N., Yu, G. Q., Palop, J. J., Noebels, J. L., and Mucke, L. 2011. Amyloid-β/Fyn-induced synaptic, network, and cognitive impairments depend on tau levels in multiple mouse models of Alzheimer's disease. *J Neurosci* 31: 700–711.

Roberson, E. D., Scearce-Levie, K., Palop, J. J., Yan, F., Cheng, I. H., Wu, T., Gerstein, H., Yu, G. Q., and Mucke, L. 2007. Reducing endogenous tau ameliorates amyloid β-induced deficits in an Alzheimer's disease mouse model. *Science* 316: 750–754.

Roberson, E. D., et al. 2006. 100 Years and counting: Prospects for defeating Alzheimer's disease. *Science* 314: 781–784.

Rogaev, E. I., Sherrington, R., Rogaeva, E. A., Levesque, G., Ikeda, M., Liang, Y., Chi, H., Lin, C., Holman, K., Tsuda, T., et al. 1995. Familial Alzheimer's disease in kindreds with missense mutations in a gene on chromosome 1 related to the Alzheimer's disease type 3 gene. *Nature* 376: 775–778.

Rogaeva, E., Meng, Y., Lee, J. H., Gu, Y., Kawarai, T., Zou, F., Katayama, T., Baldwin, C. T., Cheng, R., Hasegawa, H., Chen, F., Shibata, N., Lunetta, K. L., Pardossi-Piquard, R., Bohm, C., Wakutani, Y., Cupples, L. A., Cuenco, K. T., Green, R. C., Pinessi, L., Rainero, I., Sorbi, S., Bruni, A., Duara, R., Friedland, R. P., Inzelberg, R., Hampe, W., Bujo, H., Song, Y. Q., Andersen, O. M., Willnow, T. E., Graff-Radford, N., Petersen, R. C., Dickson, D., Der, S. D., Fraser, P. E., Schmitt-Ulms, G., Younkin, S., Mayeux, R., Farrer, L. A., and St. George-Hyslop, P. 2007. The neuronal sortilin-related receptor SORL1 is genetically associated with Alzheimer disease. *Nature Genetics* 39: 168–177.

Rojo, L. E., Fernandez, J. A., Maccioni, A. A., Jimenez, J. M., and Maccioni, R. B. 2008. Neuroinflammation: Implications for the pathogenesis and molecular diagnosis of Alzheimer's disease. *Arch Med Res* 39: 1–16.

Rosales, J. L., Nodwell, M. J., Johnston, R. N., and Lee, K. Y. 2000. Cdk5/p25(nck5a) interaction with synaptic proteins in bovine brain. *J Cell Biochem* 78: 151–159.

Roses, A. D., Saunders, A. M., Alberts, M. A., Strittmatter, W. J., Schmechel, D., Gorder, E., and Pericak-Vance, M. A. 1995. 2007. Apolipoprotein E E4 allele and risk of dementia. *JAMA* 273: 374–375; author reply 375–376.

Rossi, C., and Chopineau, J. 2007. Biomimetic tethered lipid membranes designed for membrane-protein interaction studies. *Eur Biophys J* 36: 955–965.

Rovelet-Lecrux, A., Hannequin, D., Raux, G., Le Meur, N., Laquerriere, A., Vital, A., Dumanchin, C., Feuillette, S., Brice, A., Vercelletto, M., Dubas, F., Frebourg, T., and Campion, D. 2006. APP locus duplication causes autosomal dominant early-onset alzheimer disease with cerebral amyloid angiopathy. *Nat Genet* 38: 24–26.

Rowan, M. J., Klyubin, I., Wang, Q., and Anwyl, R. 2005. Synaptic plasticity disruption by amyloid β protein: Modulation by potential Alzheimer's disease modifying therapies. *Biochem Soc Trans* 33: 563–567.

Roychaudhuri, R., Yang, M., Hoshi, M. M., and Teplow, D. B. 2009. Amyloid β-protein assembly and Alzheimer disease. *J Biol Chem* 284: 4749–4753.

Rozga, M., Protas, A. M., Jablonowska, A., Dadlez, M., and Bal, W. 2009. The Cu(II) complex of Aβ40 peptide in ammonium acetate solutions. Evidence for ternary species formation. *Chem Commun* (Camb): 1374–1376.

Rubenstein, R., Kascsak, R. J., Merz, P. A., Wisniewski, H. M., Carp, R. I., and Iqbal, K. 1986. Paired helical filaments associated with Alzheimer disease are readily soluble structures. *Brain Res* 372: 80–88.

Sachse, C., Xu, C., Wieligmann, K., Diekmann, S., Grigorieff, N., and Fändrich, M. 2006. Quaternary structure of a mature amyloid fibril from Alzheimer's Aβ(1-40) peptide. *J Mol Biol* 362: 347–354.

Sandberg, A., Luheshi, L. M., Sollvander, S., Pereira De Barros, T., Macao, B., Knowles, T. P., Biverstal, H., Lendel, C., Ekholm-Petterson, F., Dubnovitsky, A., Lannfelt, L., Dobson, C. M., and Hard, T. 2010. Stabilization of neurotoxic Alzheimer amyloid-β oligomers by protein engineering. *Proc Natl Acad Sci USA* 107: 15595–15600.

Sarell, C. J., Wilkinson, S. R., and Viles, J. H. 2010. Substoichiometric levels of Cu2+ ions accelerate the kinetics of fiber formation and promote cell toxicity of amyloid-β from Alzheimer disease. *J Biol Chem* 285: 41533–41540.

Sastre, M., Dewachter, I., Landreth, G. E., Willson, T. M., Klockgether, T., Van Leuven, F., and Heneka, M. T. 2003. Nonsteroidal anti-inflammatory drugs and peroxisome proliferator-activated receptor-γ agonists modulate immunostimulated processing of amyloid precursor protein through regulation of β-secretase. *J Neurosci* 23: 9796–9804.

Saunders, A. M., Schmader, K., Breitner, J. C., Benson, M. D., Brown, W. T., Goldfarb, L., Goldgaber, D., Manwaring, M. G., Szymanski, M. H., McCown, N., et al. 1993a. Apolipoprotein E ε4 allele distributions in late-onset alzheimer's disease and in other amyloid-forming diseases. *Lancet* 342: 710–711.

Saunders, A. M., Strittmatter, W. J., Schmechel, D., George-Hyslop, P. H., Pericak-Vance, M. A., Joo, S. H., Rosi, B. L., Gusella, J. F., Crapper-Maclachlan, D. R., Alberts, M. J., et al. 1993b. Association of apolipoprotein E allele ε4 with late-onset familial and sporadic Alzheimer's disease. *Neurology* 43: 1467–1472.

Sawaya, M. R., Sambashivan, S., Nelson, R., Ivanova, M. I., Sievers, S. A., Apostol, M. I., Thompson, M. J., Balbirnie, M., Wiltzius, J. J. W., McFarlane, H. T., Madsen, A. O., Riekel, C., and Eisenberg, D. 2007. Atomic structures of amyloid cross-β spines reveal varied steric zippers. *Nature* 447: 453–457.

Sayre, L. M., Zelasko, D. A., Harris, P. L., Perry, G., Salomon, R. G., and Smith, M. A. 1997. 4-Hydroxynonenal-derived advanced lipid peroxidation end products are increased in Alzheimer's disease. *J Neurochem* 68: 2092–2097.

Scarmeas, N., Stern, Y., Tang, M. X., Mayeux, R., and Luchsinger, J. A. 2006. Mediterranean diet and risk for Alzheimer's disease. *Ann Neurol* 59: 912–921.

Scheidt, H. A., Morgado, I., Rothemund, S., Huster, D., and Fandrich, M. 2011. Solid-state NMR spectroscopic investigation of Aβ protofibrils: Implication of Aβ-sheet remodeling upon maturation into terminal amyloid fibrils. *Angew Chem Int Ed Engl* 50: 2837–2840.

Schipper, H. M. 2004. Heme oxygenase expression in human central nervous system disorders. *Free Radic Biol Med* 37: 1995–2011.

Schmidt, A. M., Yan, S. D., Yan, S. F., and Stern, D. M. 2001. The multiligand receptor RAGE as a progression factor amplifying immune and inflammatory responses. *J Clin Invest* 108: 949–955.

Schmidt, C., Lepsverdize, E., Chi, S. L., Das, A. M., Pizzo, S. V., Dityatev, A., and Schachner, M. 2008. Amyloid precursor protein and amyloid β-peptide bind to ATP synthase and regulate its activity at the surface of neural cells. *Mol Psychiatry* 13: 953–969.

Schubert, D., and Chevion, M. 1995. The role of iron in beta amyloid toxicity. *Biochem Biophys Res Commun* 216: 702–707.

Schubert, D., Cole, G., Saitoh, T., and Oltersdorf, T. 1989. Amyloid beta protein precursor is a mitogen. *Biochem Biophys Res Commun* 162: 83–88.

Selkoe, D. J. 2008. Soluble oligomers of the amyloid β-protein impair synaptic plasticity and behavior. *Behav Brain Res* 192: 106–113.

Selkoe, D. J., Yamazaki, T., Citron, M., Podlisny, M. B., Koo, E. H., Teplow, D. B., and Haass, C. 1996. The role of APP processing and trafficking pathways in the formation of amyloid β-protein. *Ann N Y Acad Sci* 777: 57–64.

Sengupta, P., Garai, K., Sahoo, B., Shi, Y., Callaway, D. J., and Maiti, S. 2003. The amyloid β peptide (Aβ(1-40)) is thermodynamically soluble at physiological concentrations. *Biochemistry* 42: 10506–10513.

Serneels, L., Van Biervliet, J., Craessaerts, K., Dejaegere, T., Horre, K., Van Houtvin, T., Esselmann, H., Paul, S., Schafer, M. K., Berezovska, O., Hyman, B. T., Sprangers, B., Sciot, R., Moons, L., Jucker, M., Yang, Z., May, P. C., Karran, E., Wiltfang, J., D'Hooge, R., and De Strooper, B. 2009. γ-Secretase heterogeneity in the Aph1 subunit: Relevance for Alzheimer's disease. *Science* 324: 639–642.

Seubert, P., Vigo-Pelfrey, C., Esch, F., Lee, M., Dovey, H., Davis, D., Sinha, S., Schlossmacher, M., Whaley, J., Swindlehurst, C., et al. 1992. Isolation and quantification of soluble Alzheimer's β-peptide from biological fluids. *Nature* 359: 325–327.

Shankar, G. M., Bloodgood, B. L., Townsend, M., Walsh, D. M., Selkoe, D. J., and Sabatini, B. L. 2007. Natural oligomers of the Alzheimer amyloid-β protein induce reversible synapse loss by modulating an NMDA-type glutamate receptor-dependent signaling pathway. *J Neurosci* 27: 2866–2875.

Shankar, G. M., Li, S., Mehta, T. H., Garcia-Munoz, A., Shepardson, N. E., Smith, I., Brett, F. M., Farrell, M. A., Rowan, M. J., Lemere, C. A., Regan, C. M., Walsh, D. M., Sabatini, B. L., and Selkoe, D. J. 2008. Amyloid-β protein dimers isolated directly from Alzheimer's brains impair synaptic plasticity and memory. *Nat Med* 14: 837–842.

Sheffield, L. G., Marquis, J. G., and Berman, N. E. 2000. Regional distribution of cortical microglia parallels that of neurofibrillary tangles in Alzheimer's disease. *Neurosci Lett* 285: 165–168.

Shen, J., and Kelleher, R. J., III. 2007. The presenilin hypothesis of Alzheimer's disease: Evidence for a loss-of-function pathogenic mechanism. *Proc Natl Acad Sci USA* 104: 403–409.

Shen, M., Stukenberg, P. T., Kirschner, M. W., and Lu, K. P. 1998. The essential mitotic peptidyl-prolyl isomerase Pin1 binds and regulates mitosis-specific phosphoproteins. *Genes Dev* 12: 706–720.

Sheng, J. G., Zhu, S. G., Jones, R. A., Griffin, W. S., and Mrak, R. E. 2000. Interleukin-1 promotes expression and phosphorylation of neurofilament and tau proteins in vivo. *Exp Neurol* 163: 388–391.

Sherrington, R., Froelich, S., Sorbi, S., Campion, D., Chi, H., Rogaeva, E. A., Levesque, G., Rogaev, E. I., Lin, C., Liang, Y., Ikeda, M., Mar, L., Brice, A., Agid, Y., Percy, M. E., Clerget-Darpoux, F., Piacentini, S., Marcon, G., Nacmias, B., Amaducci, L., Frebourg, T., Lannfelt, L., Rommens, J. M., and St, George-Hyslop, P. H. 1996. Alzheimer's disease associated with mutations in presenilin 2 is rare and variably penetrant. *Hum Mol Genet* 5: 985–988.

Sherrington, R., Rogaev, E. I., Liang, Y., Rogaeva, E. A., Levesque, G., Ikeda, M., Chi, H., Lin, C., Li, G., Holman, K., Tsuda, T., Mar, L., Foncin, J. F., Bruni, A. C., Montesi, M. P., Sorbi, S., Rainero, I., Pinessi, L., Nee, L., Chumakov, I., Pollen, D., Brookes, A., Sanseau, P., Polinsky, R. J., Wasco, W., Da Silva, H. A., Haines, J. L., Perkicak-Vance, M. A., Tanzi, R. E., Roses, A. D., Fraser, P. E., Rommens, J. M., and St. George-Hyslop, P. H. 1995. Cloning of a gene bearing missense mutations in early-onset familial Alzheimer's disease. *Nature* 375: 754–760.

Shipton, O. A., Leitz, J. R., Dworzak, J., Acton, C. E., Tunbridge, E. M., Denk, F., Dawson, H. N., Vitek, M. P., Wade-Martins, R., Paulsen, O., and Vargas-Caballero, M. 2011. Tau protein is required for amyloid β-induced impairment of hippocampal long-term potentiation. *J Neurosci* 31: 1688–1692.

Siegel, S. J., Bieschke, J., Powers, E. T., and Kelly, J. W. 2007. The oxidative stress metabolite 4-hydroxynonenal promotes Alzheimer protofibril formation. *Biochemistry* 46: 1503–1510.

Simons, K., and Toomre, D. 2000. Lipid rafts and signal transduction. *Nat Rev Mol Cell Biol* 1: 31–39.

Simons, M., Keller, P., De Strooper, B., Beyreuther, K., Dotti, C. G., and Simons, K. 1998. Cholesterol depletion inhibits the generation of β-amyloid in hippocampal neurons. *Proc Natl Acad Sci USA* 95: 6460–6464.

Sjogren, M., Mielke, M., Gustafson, D., Zandi, P., and Skoog, I. 2006. Cholesterol and Alzheimer's disease: Is there a relation? *Mech Ageing Dev* 127: 138–147.

Skovronsky, D. M., Doms, R. W., and Lee, V. M. 1998. Detection of a novel intraneuronal pool of insoluble amyloid β protein that accumulates with time in culture. *J Cell Biol* 141: 1031–1039.

Small, S. A., and Duff, K. 2008. Linking Aβ and tau in late-onset alzheimer's disease: A dual pathway hypothesis. *Neuron* 60: 534–542.

Smith, D. G., Cappai, R., and Barnham, K. J. 2007. The redox chemistry of the Alzheimer's disease amyloid β peptide. *Biochim Biophys Acta* 1768: 1976–1990.

Smith, I. F., Green, K. N., and Laferla, F. M. 2005. Calcium dysregulation in Alzheimer's disease: Recent advances gained from genetically modified animals. *Cell Calcium* 38: 427–437.

Smith, M. A., Harris, P. L., Sayre, L. M., and Perry, G. 1997. Iron accumulation in Alzheimer disease is a source of redox-generated free radicals. *Proc Natl Acad Sci USA* 94: 9866–9868.

Smith, T. W., and Lippa, C. F. 1995. Ki-67 immunoreactivity in Alzheimer's disease and other neurodegenerative disorders. *J Neuropathol Exp Neurol* 54: 297–303.

Sokolov, Y., Kozak, J. A., Kayed, R., Chanturiya, A., Glabe, C., and Hall, J. E. 2006. Soluble amyloid oligomers increase bilayer conductance by altering dielectric structure. *J Gen Physiol* 128: 637–647.

Sokolowska, M., and Bal, W. 2005. Cu(II) complexation by "non-coordinating" N-2-hydroxyethylpiperazine-N'-2-ethanesulfonic acid (HEPES buffer). *J Inorg Biochem* 99: 1653–1660.

Sparks, D. L., Kuo, Y. M., Roher, A., Martin, T., and Lukas, R. J. 2000. Alterations of Alzheimer's disease in the cholesterol-fed rabbit, including vascular inflammation. Preliminary observations. *Ann N Y Acad Sci* 903: 335–344.

Sparks, D. L., Liu, H., Gross, D. R., and Scheff, S. W. 1995. Increased density of cortical apolipoprotein E immunoreactive neurons in rabbit brain after dietary administration of cholesterol. *Neurosci Lett* 187: 142–144.

Sparr, E., Engel, M. F., Sakharov, D. V., Sprong, M., Jacobs, J., De Kruijff, B., Hoppener, J. W., and Killian, J. A. 2004. Islet amyloid polypeptide-induced membrane leakage involves uptake of lipids by forming amyloid fibers. *FEBS Lett* 577: 117–120.

Spasic, D., and Annaert, W. 2008. Building γ-secretase: The bits and pieces. *J Cell Sci* 121: 413–420.

St. George-Hyslop, P. H., and Petit, A. Molecular biology and genetics of Alzheimer's disease. 2005. *C R Biol* 328: 119–130.

Stahl, N., Borchelt, D. R., Hsiao, K., and Prusiner, S. B. 1987. Scrapie prion protein contains a phosphatidylinositol glycolipid. *Cell* 51: 229–240.

Stewart, W. F., Kawas, C., Corrada, M., and Metter, E. J. 1997. Risk of Alzheimer's disease and duration of NSAID use. *Neurology* 48: 626–632.

Sticht, H., Bayer, P., Willbold, D., Dames, S., Hilbich, C., Beyreuther, K., Frank, R. W., and Rosch, P. 1995. Structure of amyloid A4-(1-40)-peptide of Alzheimer's disease. *Eur J Biochem* 233: 293–298.

Strittmatter, W. J., and Roses, A. D. 1995. Apolipoprotein E and Alzheimer disease. *Proc Natl Acad Sci USA* 92: 4725–4727.

Strittmatter, W. J., Weisgraber, K. H., Huang, D. Y., Dong, L. M., Salvesen, G. S., Pericak-Vance, M., Schmechel, D., Saunders, A. M., Goldgaber, D., and Roses, A. D. 1993. Binding of human apolipoprotein E to synthetic amyloid beta peptide: Isoform-specific effects and implications for late-onset alzheimer disease. *Proc Natl Acad Sci USA* 90: 8098–8102.

Strozyk, D., Blennow, K., White, L. R., and Launer, L. J. 2003. CSF Aβ 42 levels correlate with amyloid-neuropathology in a population-based autopsy study. *Neurology* 60: 652–656.

Stukenberg, P. T., and Kirschner, M. W. 2001. Pin1 acts catalytically to promote a conformational change in Cdc25. *Mol Cell* 7: 1071–1083.

Sultana, R., Boyd-Kimball, D., Poon, H. F., Cai, J., Pierce, W. M., Klein, J. B., Markesbery, W. R., Zhou, X. Z., Lu, K. P., and Butterfield, D. A. 2006a. Oxidative modification and down-regulation of Pin1 in Alzheimer's disease hippocampus: A redox proteomics analysis. *Neurobiol Aging* 27: 918–925.

Sultana, R., Boyd-Kimball, D., Poon, H. F., Cai, J., Pierce, W. M., Klein, J. B., Merchant, M., Markesbery, W. R., and Butterfield, D. A. 2006b. Redox proteomics identification of oxidized proteins in Alzheimer's disease hippocampus and cerebellum: An approach to understand pathological and biochemical alterations in AD. *Neurobiol Aging* 27: 1564–1576.

Supnet, C., and Bezprozvanny, I. 2010. Neuronal calcium signaling, mitochondrial dysfunction, and Alzheimer's disease. *J Alzheimer's Dis* 20 Suppl 2: S487–498.

Syme, C. D., Nadal, R. C., Rigby, S. E., and Viles, J. H. 2004. Copper binding to the amyloid-β (Aβ) peptide associated with Alzheimer's disease: Folding, coordination geometry, pH dependence, stoichiometry, and affinity of Aβ-(1-28): Insights from a range of complementary spectroscopic techniques. *J Biol Chem* 279: 18169–18177.

Takahashi, R. H., Milner, T. A., Li, F., Nam, E. E., Edgar, M. A., Yamaguchi, H., Beal, M. F., Xu, H., Greengard, P., and Gouras, G. K. 2002. Intraneuronal Alzheimer Aβ42 accumulates in multivesicular bodies and is associated with synaptic pathology. *American J Path* 161: 1869–1879.

Takeda, S., Sato, N., Rakugi, H., and Morishita, R. 2011. Molecular mechanisms linking diabetes mellitus and Alzheimer disease: Beta-amyloid peptide, insulin signaling, and neuronal function. *Mol Biosyst* 7: 1822–1827.

Talmard, C., Bouzan, A., & Faller, P. 2007. Zinc binding to amyloid-β: isothermal titration calorimetry and Zn competition experiments with Zn sensors. *Biochemistry* 46(47): 13658–13666.

Talmard, C., Guilloreau, L., Coppel, Y., Mazarguil, H., and Faller, P. 2007. Amyloid-β peptide forms monomeric complexes with Cu(II) and Zn(II) prior to aggregation. *Chembiochem* 8: 163–165.

Talmard, C., Leuma Yona, R., and Faller, P. 2009. Mechanism of zinc(II)-promoted amyloid formation: Zinc(II) binding facilitates the transition from the partially α-helical conformer to aggregates of amyloid β protein(1-28). *J Biol Inorg Chem* 14: 449–455.

Tannoch, V. J., Hinds, P. W., and Tsai, L. H. 2000. Cell cycle control. *Adv Exp Med Biol* 465: 127–140.

Tanzi, R. E., and Bertram, L. 2001. New frontiers in Alzheimer's disease genetics. *Neuron* 32: 181–184.

Tanzi, R. E., Bird, E. D., Latt, S. A., and Neve, R. L. 1987. The amyloid beta protein gene is not duplicated in brains from patients with Alzheimer's disease. *Science* 238: 666–669.

Tarus, B., Straub, J. E., and Thirumalai, D. 2008. Structures and free-energy landscapes of the wild type and mutants of the Abeta(21-30) peptide are determined by an interplay between intrapeptide electrostatic and hydrophobic interactions. *J Mol Biol* 379: 815–829.

Tateishi, K., Omata, M., Tanaka, K., and Chiba, T. 2001. The NEDD8 system is essential for cell cycle progression and morphogenetic pathway in mice. *J Cell Biol* 155: 571–579.

Teplow, D. B. 2006. Preparation of amyloid β-protein for structural and functional studies. *Methods Enzymol* 413: 20–33.

Terry, R. D., Masliah, E., Salmon, D. P., Butters, N., Deteresa, R., Hill, R., Hansen, L. A., and Katzman, R. 1991. Physical basis of cognitive alterations in Alzheimer's disease: Synapse loss is the major correlate of cognitive impairment. *Ann Neurol* 30: 572–580.

Terwel, D., Muyllaert, D., Dewachter, I., Borghgraef, P., Croes, S., Devijver, H., and Van Leuven, F. 2008. Amyloid activates GSK-3β to aggravate neuronal tauopathy in bigenic mice. *Am J Pathol* 172: 786–798.

Teter, B., Xu, P. T., Gilbert, J. R., Roses, A. D., Galasko, D., and Cole, G. M. 2002. Defective neuronal sprouting by human apolipoprotein E4 is a gain-of-negative function. *J Neurosci Res* 68: 331–336.

Tillement, L., Lecanu, L., and Papadopoulos, V. 2011. Alzheimer's disease: Effects of β-amyloid on mitochondria. *Mitochondrion* 11: 13–21.

Tillement, L., Lecanu, L., Yao, W., Greeson, J., and Papadopoulos, V. 2006. The spirostenol (22R, 25R)-20α-spirost-5-en-3β-yl hexanoate blocks mitochondrial uptake of Aβ in neuronal cells and prevents Aβ-induced impairment of mitochondrial function. *Steroids* 71: 725–735.

Tiraboschi, P., Hansen, L. A., Masliah, E., Alford, M., Thal, L. J., and Corey-Bloom, J. 2004. Impact of APOE genotype on neuropathologic and neurochemical markers of Alzheimer disease. *Neurology* 62: 1977–1983.

Tomaselli, S., Esposito, V., Vangone, P., Van Nuland, N. A., Bonvin, A. M., Guerrini, R., Tancredi, T., Temussi, P. A., and Picone, D. 2006. The α-to-β conformational transition of Alzheimer's Aβ-(1-42) peptide in aqueous media is reversible: A step by step conformational analysis suggests the location of β conformation seeding. *Chembiochem* 7: 257–267.

Tougu, V., Karafin, A., & Palumaa, P. 2008. Binding of zinc(II) and copper(II) to the full-length Alzheimer's amyloid-β peptide. *J Neurochem* 104(5): 1249–1259.

Townsend, M., Shankar, G. M., Mehta, T., Walsh, D. M., and Selkoe, D. J. 2006. Effects of secreted oligomers of amyloid β-protein on hippocampal synaptic plasticity: a potent role for trimers. *J Physiol* 572: 477–492.

Tseng, B. P., Green, K. N., Chan, J. L., Blurton-Jones, M., and Laferla, F. M. 2008. Aβ inhibits the proteasome and enhances amyloid and tau accumulation. *Neurobiol Aging* 29: 1607–1618.

Tseng, H. C., Zhou, Y., Shen, Y., and Tsai, L. H. 2002. A survey of Cdk5 activator p35 and p25 levels in Alzheimer's disease brains. *FEBS Lett* 523: 58–62.

Turk, E., Teplow, D. B., Hood, L. E., and Prusiner, S. B. 1988. Purification and properties of the cellular and scrapie hamster prion proteins. *Eur J Biochem* 176: 21–30.

Turnbull, S., Tabner, B. J., El-Agnaf, O. M., Twyman, L. J., and Allsop, D. 2001. New evidence that the Alzheimer β-amyloid peptide does not spontaneously form free radicals: An ESR study using a series of spin-traps. *Free Radic Biol Med* 30: 1154–1162.

Turrens, J. F. 2003. Mitochondrial formation of reactive oxygen species. *J Physiol* 552: 335–344.

Tycko, R. 2004. Progress towards a molecular-level structural understanding of amyloid fibrils. *Curr Opin in Struc Biol* 14: 96–103.

Tycko, R., Savtchenko, R., Ostapchenko, V. G., Makarava, N., and Baskakov, I. V. 2010. The α-helical C-terminal domain of full-length recombinant PrP converts to an in-register parallel β-sheet structure in PrP fibrils: Evidence from solid state nuclear magnetic resonance. *Biochemistry* 49: 9488–9497.

Ueberham, U., and Arendt, T. 2005. The expression of cell cycle proteins in neurons and its relevance for Alzheimer's disease. *Curr Drug Targets CNS Neurol Disord* 4: 293–306.

Ueda, K., Fukui, Y., and Kageyama, H. 1994. Amyloid β protein-induced neuronal cell death: Neurotoxic properties of aggregated amyloid beta protein. *Brain Res* 639: 240–244.

Urbanc, B., Betnel, M., Cruz, L., Bitan, G., and Teplow, D. B. 2010. Elucidation of amyloid β-protein oligomerization mechanisms: Discrete molecular dynamics study. *J American Chem Soc* 132: 4266–4280.

Urbanc, B., Cruz, L., Yun, S., Buldyrev, S. V., Bitan, G., Teplow, D. B., and Stanley, H. E. 2004. In silico study of amyloid β-protein folding and oligomerization. *Proc Natl Acad Sci USA* 101: 17345–17350.

Van Den Haute, C., Spittaels, K., Van Dorpe, J., Lasrado, R., Vandezande, K., Laenen, I., Geerts, H., and Van Leuven, F. 2001. Coexpression of human cdk5 and its activator p35 with human protein tau in neurons in brain of triple transgenic mice. *Neurobiol Dis* 8: 32–44.

Van Den Heuvel, S., and Harlow, E. 1993. Distinct roles for cyclin-dependent kinases in cell cycle control. *Science* 262: 2050–2054.

Van Hoesen, G. W., Augustinack, J. C., Dierking, J., Redman, S. J., and Thangavel, R. 2000. The parahippocampal gyrus in Alzheimer's disease. Clinical and preclinical neuroanatomical correlates. *Ann N Y Acad Sci* 911: 254–274.

Vassar, R. 2001. The β-secretase, BACE: A prime drug target for Alzheimer's disease. *J Mol Neurosci* 17: 157–170.

Vestergaard, M., Hamada, T., and Takagi, M. 2008. Using model membranes for the study of amyloid beta:lipid interactions and neurotoxicity. *Biotechnol Bioeng* 99: 753–763.

Vetrivel, K. S., Cheng, H., Kim, S. H., Chen, Y., Barnes, N. Y., Parent, A. T., Sisodia, S. S., and Thinakaran, G. 2005. Spatial segregation of γ-secretase and substrates in distinct membrane domains. *J Biol Chem* 280: 25892–25900.

Vetrivel, K. S., Cheng, H., Lin, W., Sakurai, T., Li, T., Nukina, N., Wong, P. C., Xu, H., and Thinakaran, G. 2004. Association of γ-secretase with lipid rafts in post-Golgi and endosome membranes. *J Biol Chem* 279: 44945–44954.

Vetrivel, K. S., and Thinakaran, G. 2010. Membrane rafts in Alzheimer's disease beta-amyloid production. *Biochim Biophys Acta* 1801: 860–867.

Vincent, I., Jicha, G., Rosado, M., and Dickson, D. W. 1997. Aberrant expression of mitotic cdc2/cyclin B1 kinase in degenerating neurons of Alzheimer's disease brain. *J Neurosci* 17: 3588–3598.

Vincent, I., Pae, C. I., and Hallows, J. L. 2003. The cell cycle and human neurodegenerative disease. *Prog Cell Cycle Res* 5: 31–41.

Vincent, I., Zheng, J. H., Dickson, D. W., Kress, Y., and Davies, P. 1998. Mitotic phospho-epitopes precede paired helical filaments in Alzheimer's disease. *Neurobiol Aging* 19: 287–296.

Vito, P., Lacana, E., and D'Adamio, L. 1996. Interfering with apoptosis: Ca(2+)-binding protein ALG-2 and Alzheimer's disease gene ALG-3. *Science* 271: 521–525.

Volicer, L., and Crino, P. B. 1990. Involvement of free radicals in dementia of the Alzheimer type: A hypothesis. *Neurobiol Aging* 11: 567–571.

Wahlsten, D., Metten, P., Phillips, T. J., Boehm, S. L., II, Burkhart-Kasch, S., Dorow, J., Doerksen, S., Downing, C., Fogarty, J., Rodd-Henricks, K., Hen, R., McKinnon, C. S., Merrill, C. M., Nolte, C., Schalomon, M., Schlumbohm, J. P., Sibert, J. R., Wenger, C. D., Dudek, B. C., and Crabbe, J. C. 2003. Different data from different labs: Lessons from studies of gene-environment interaction. *J Neurobiol* 54: 283–311.

Wakabayashi, T., and De Strooper, B. 2008. Presenilins: Members of the gamma-secretase quartets, but part-time soloists too. *Physiology* (Bethesda) 23: 194–204.

Walsh, D. M., Hartley, D. M., Kusumoto, Y., Fezoui, Y., Condron, M. M., Lomakin, A., Benedek, G. B., Selkoe, D. J., and Teplow, D. B. 1999. Amyloid beta-protein fibrillogenesis. Structure and biological activity of protofibrillar intermediates. *J Biol Chem* 274: 25945–25952.

Walsh, D. M., Klyubin, I., Fadeeva, J. V., Cullen, W. K., Anwyl, R., Wolfe, M. S., Rowan, M. J., and Selkoe, D. J. 2002. Naturally secreted oligomers of amyloid beta protein potently inhibit hippocampal long-term potentiation in vivo. *Nature* 416: 535–539.

Walsh, D. M., Lomakin, A., Benedek, G. B., Condron, M. M., and Teplow, D. B. 1997. Amyloid beta-protein fibrillogenesis. Detection of a protofibrillar intermediate. *J Biol Chem* 272: 22364–22372.

Wang, X., Su, B., Lee, H. G., Li, X., Perry, G., Smith, M. A., and Zhu, X. 2009. Impaired balance of mitochondrial fission and fusion in Alzheimer's disease. *J Neurosci* 29: 9090–9103.

Wang, X., Su, B., Perry, G., Smith, M. A., and Zhu, X. 2007. Insights into amyloid-β-induced mitochondrial dysfunction in Alzheimer disease. *Free Radic Biol Med* 43: 1569–1573.

Wang, X., Su, B., Siedlak, S. L., Moreira, P. I., Fujioka, H., Wang, Y., Casadesus, G., and Zhu, X. 2008. Amyloid-β overproduction causes abnormal mitochondrial dynamics via differential modulation of mitochondrial fission/fusion proteins. *Proc Natl Acad Sci USA* 105: 19318–19323.

Ward, R. V., Jennings, K. H., Jepras, R., Neville, W., Owen, D. E., Hawkins, J., Christie, G., Davis, J. B., George, A., Karran, E. H., and Howlett, D. R. 2000. Fractionation and characterization of oligomeric, protofibrillar and fibrillar forms of β-amyloid peptide. *Biochem J* 348 Pt 1: 137–144.

Weggen, S., Eriksen, J. L., Das, P., Sagi, S. A., Wang, R., Pietrzik, C. U., Findlay, K. A., Smith, T. E., Murphy, M. P., Bulter, T., Kang, D. E., Marquez-Sterling, N., Golde, T. E., and Koo, E. H. 2001. A subset of NSAIDs lower amyloidogenic Aβ42 independently of cyclooxygenase activity. *Nature* 414: 212–216.

Weggen, S., Eriksen, J. L., Sagi, S. A., Pietrzik, C. U., Ozols, V., Fauq, A., Golde, T. E., and Koo, E. H. 2003. Evidence that nonsteroidal anti-inflammatory drugs decrease amyloid β 42 production by direct modulation of γ-secretase activity. *J Biol Chem* 278: 31831–31837.

Weinberg, R. A. 1995. The retinoblastoma protein and cell cycle control. *Cell* 81: 323–330.

Weisgraber, K. H. 1994. Apolipoprotein E: structure-function relationships. *Adv Protein Chem* 45: 249–302.

Weisgraber, K. H., and Mahley, R. W. 1996. Human apolipoprotein E: The Alzheimer's disease connection. *FASEB J* 10: 1485–1494.

Westlind-Danielsson, A., and Arnerup, G. 2001. Spontaneous in vitro formation of supramolecular β-amyloid structures, "βamy balls", by β-amyloid 1-40 peptide. *Biochemistry* 40: 14736–14743.

Wetzel, M. K., Naska, S., Laliberte, C. L., Rymar, V. V., Fujitani, M., Biernaskie, J. A., Cole, C. J., Lerch, J. P., Spring, S., Wang, S. H., Frankland, P. W., Henkelman, R. M., Josselyn, S. A., Sadikot, A. F., Miller, F. D., and Kaplan, D. R. 2008. p73 regulates neurodegeneration and phospho-tau accumulation during aging and Alzheimer's disease. *Neuron* 59: 708–721.

Whalen, B. M., Selkoe, D. J., and Hartley, D. M. 2005. Small non-fibrillar assemblies of amyloid β-protein bearing the Arctic mutation induce rapid neuritic degeneration. *Neurobiol Dis* 20: 254–266.

Whitson, J. S., Glabe, C. G., Shintani, E., Abcar, A., and Cotman, C. W. 1990. β-Amyloid protein promotes neuritic branching in hippocampal cultures. *Neurosci Lett* 110: 319–324.

Whitson, J. S., Selkoe, D. J., and Cotman, C. W. 1989. Amyloid beta protein enhances the survival of hippocampal neurons in vitro. *Science* 243: 1488–1490.

Wiesehan, K., Funke, S. A., Fries, M., and Willbold, D. 2007. Purification of recombinantly expressed and cytotoxic human amyloid-beta peptide 1-42. *J Chromatogr B Analyt Technol Biomed Life Sci* 856: 229–233.

Wilcock, D. M., Gharkholonarehe, N., Van Nostrand, W. E., Davis, J., Vitek, M. P., and Colton, C. A. 2009. Amyloid reduction by amyloid-β vaccination also reduces mouse tau pathology and protects from neuron loss in two mouse models of Alzheimer's disease. *J Neurosci* 29: 7957–7965.

Wild-Bode, C., Yamazaki, T., Capell, A., Leimer, U., Steiner, H., Ihara, Y., and Haass, C. 1997. Intracellular generation and accumulation of amyloid β-peptide terminating at amino acid 42. *J Biol Chem* 272: 16085–16088.

Williams, A. D., Sega, M., Chen, M., Kheterpal, I., Geva, M., Berthelier, V., Kaleta, D. T., Cook, K. D., and Wetzel, R. 2005. Structural properties of Aβ protofibrils stabilized by a small molecule. *Proc Natl Acad Sci USA* 102: 7115–7120.

Williams, T. I., Lynn, B. C., Markesbery, W. R., and Lovell, M. A. 2006. Increased levels of 4-hydroxynonenal and acrolein, neurotoxic markers of lipid peroxidation, in the brain in Mild Cognitive Impairment and early Alzheimer's disease. *Neurobiol Aging* 27: 1094–1099.

Wisniewski, T., Aucouturier, P., Soto, C., and Frangione, B. 1998. The prionoses and other conformational disorders. *Amyloid* 5: 212–224.

Wolfe, M. S. 2009. Tau mutations in neurodegenerative diseases. *J Biol Chem* 284: 6021–6025.

Wolfe, M. S. 2010. Structure, mechanism and inhibition of gamma-secretase and presenilin-like proteases. *Biol Chem* 391: 839–847.

Wolfe, M. S., and Kopan, R. 2004. Intramembrane proteolysis: Theme and variations. *Science* 305: 1119–1123.

Wolfer, D. P., Stagljar-Bozicevic, M., Errington, M. L., and Lipp, H. P. 1998. Spatial memory and learning in transgenic mice: Fact or artifact? *News Physiol Sci* 13: 118–123.

Wolozin, B., Iwasaki, K., Vito, P., Ganjei, J. K., Lacana, E., Sunderland, T., Zhao, B., Kusiak, J. W., Wasco, W., and D'Adamio, L. 1996. Participation of presenilin 2 in apoptosis: Enhanced basal activity conferred by an Alzheimer mutation. *Science* 274: 1710–1713.

Wong, P. T., Schauerte, J. A., Wisser, K. C., Ding, H., Lee, E. L., Steel, D. G., and Gafni, A. 2009. Amyloid-β membrane binding and permeabilization are distinct processes influenced separately by membrane charge and fluidity. *J Mol Biol* 386: 81–96.

Wood, S. J., Maleeff, B., Hart, T., and Wetzel, R. 1996. Physical, morphological and functional differences between ph 5.8 and 7.4 aggregates of the Alzheimer's amyloid peptide Aβ. *J Mol Biol* 256: 870–877.

Wu, K., Chen, A., and Pan, Z. Q. 2000. Conjugation of Nedd8 to CUL1 enhances the ability of the ROC1-CUL1 complex to promote ubiquitin polymerization. *J Biol Chem* 275: 32317–32324.

Xie, C. W. 2004. Calcium-regulated signaling pathways: Role in amyloid β-induced synaptic dysfunction. *Neuromolecular Med* 6: 53–64.

Xiong, H., Callaghan, D., Jones, A., Walker, D. G., Lue, L. F., Beach, T. G., Sue, L. I., Woulfe, J., Xu, H., Stanimirovic, D. B., and Zhang, W. 2008. Cholesterol retention in Alzheimer's brain is responsible for high β- and γ-secretase activities and Aβ production. *Neurobiol Dis* 29: 422–437.

Yan, Y., and Wang, C. 2006. Abeta42 is more rigid than Abeta40 at the C terminus: Implications for Abeta aggregation and toxicity. *J Mol Biol* 364: 853–862.

Yang, M., and Teplow, D. B. 2008. Amyloid β-protein monomer folding: Free-energy surfaces reveal alloform-specific differences. *J Mol Biol* 384: 450–464.

Yang, Y., Geldmacher, D. S., and Herrup, K. 2001. DNA replication precedes neuronal cell death in Alzheimer's disease. *J Neurosci* 21: 2661–2668.

Yang, Y., and Herrup, K. 2005. Loss of neuronal cell cycle control in ataxia-telangiectasia: A unified disease mechanism. *J Neurosci* 25: 2522–2529.

Yankner, B. A., Duffy, L. K., and Kirschner, D. A. 1990. Neurotrophic and neurotoxic effects of amyloid beta protein: Reversal by tachykinin neuropeptides. *Science* 250: 279–282.

Ye, C. P., Selkoe, D. J., and Hartley, D. M. 2003. Protofibrils of amyloid β-protein inhibit specific K+ currents in neocortical cultures. *Neurobiol Dis* 13: 177–190.

Yong, W., Lomakin, A., Kirkitadze, M. D., Teplow, D. B., Chen, S. H., and Benedek, G. B. 2002. Structure determination of micelle-like intermediates in amyloid β-protein fibril assembly by using small angle neutron scattering. *Proc Natl Acad Sci USA* 99: 150–154.

Zaghi, J., Goldenson, B., Inayathullah, M., Lossinsky, A. S., Masoumi, A., Avagyan, H., Mahanian, M., Bernas, M., Weinand, M., Rosenthal, M. J., Espinosa-Jeffrey, A., De Vellis, J., Teplow, D. B., and Fiala, M. 2009. Alzheimer disease macrophages shuttle amyloid-beta from neurons to vessels, contributing to amyloid angiopathy. *Acta Neuropathol* 117: 111–124.

Zandi, P. P., Anthony, J. C., Khachaturian, A. S., Stone, S. V., Gustafson, D., Tschanz, J. T., Norton, M. C., Welsh-Bohmer, K. A., and Breitner, J. C. 2004. Reduced risk of Alzheimer disease in users of antioxidant vitamin supplements: The Cache County study. *Arch Neurol* 61: 82–88.

Zerbinatti, C. V., Wozniak, D. F., Cirrito, J., Cam, J. A., Osaka, H., Bales, K. R., Zhuo, M., Paul, S. M., Holtzman, D. M., and Bu, G. 2004. Increased soluble amyloid-β peptide and memory deficits in amyloid model mice overexpressing the low-density lipoprotein receptor-related protein. *Proc Natl Acad Sci USA* 101: 1075–1080.

Zhang, S., Iwata, K., Lachenmann, M. J., Peng, J. W., Li, S., Stimson, E. R., Lu, Y., Felix, A. M., Maggio, J. E., and Lee, J. P. 2000. The Alzheimer's peptide Aβ adopts a collapsed coil structure in water. *J Struct Biol* 130: 130–141.

Zhao, X., and Yang, J. 2010. Amyloid-β peptide is a substrate of the human 20S proteasome. *ACS Chem Neurosci* 1: 655–660.

Zhou, X. Z., Kops, O., Werner, A., Lu, P. J., Shen, M., Stoller, G., Kullertz, G., Stark, M., Fischer, G., and Lu, K. P. 2000. Pin1-dependent prolyl isomerization regulates dephosphorylation of Cdc25C and tau proteins. *Mol Cell* 6: 873–883.

Zhu, X., Lee, H. G., Perry, G., and Smith, M. A. 2007. Alzheimer disease, the two-hit hypothesis: An update. *Biochim Biophys Acta* 1772: 494–502.

Zhu, X., Raina, A. K., Perry, G., and Smith, M. A. 2004. Alzheimer's disease: The two-hit hypothesis. *Lancet Neurol* 3: 219–226.

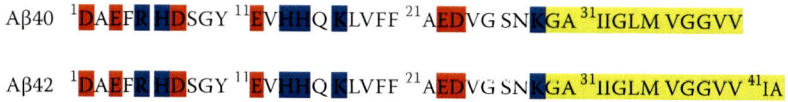

Aβ40 ^{1}DAEFR HDSGY ^{11}EVHHQ KLVFF ^{21}AEDVG SNKGA ^{31}IIGLM VGGVV

Aβ42 ^{1}DAEFR HDSGY ^{11}EVHHQ KLVFF ^{21}AEDVG SNKGA ^{31}IIGLM VGGVV ^{41}IA

FIGURE 1.1   The primary structures of Aβ40 and Aβ42 are presented. Acidic residues are shaded red, basic residues are shaded blue, and the putative intramembrane peptide segments are shaded yellow.

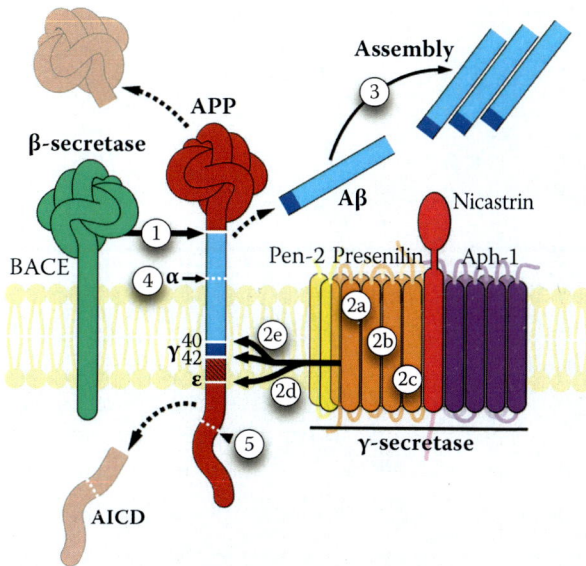

FIGURE 1.2   (1) β-secretase (BACE) cleavage of APP and (2) (a–e) by a multisubunit γ-secretase complex (Nicastrin, Aph-1, Presenilin and Pen-2) to generate Aβ. 2a–2c refer to the active site, docking site and ATP binding site of γ-secretase. 2e refers to the predilection of γ-secretase for γ or ε(2d) cleavage generating Aβ40 or Aβ42. (3) Production and self-assembly of Aβ to toxic species. (4) APP cleavage by α-secretases (ADAM family of proteins) precludes the production of Aβ. (5) Caspase cleavage of Aβ intracellular domain (AICD) generates a C31 fragment that may affect toxicity by Aβ or an independent mechanism. (From E. D. Roberson et al., 2006. "100 Years and Counting: Prospects for Defeating Alzheimer's Disease." *Science* 314 (5800): 781–784.)

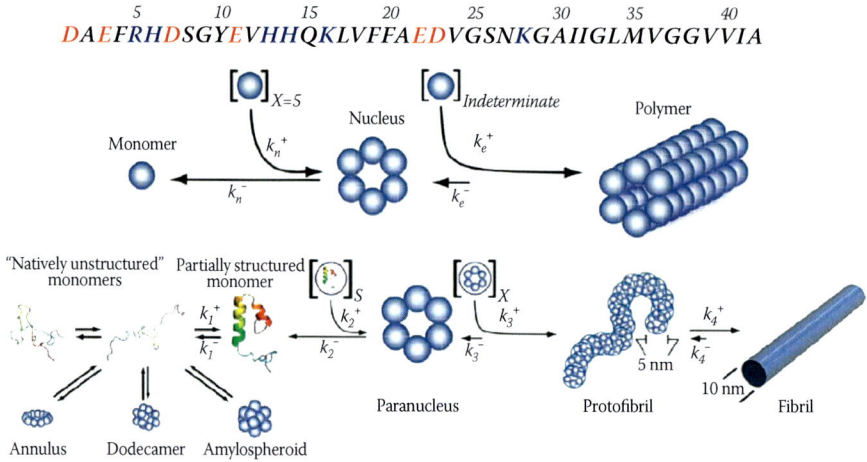

$$\overset{5}{D A} \overset{10}{E F R H D} \overset{15}{S G Y E} \overset{20}{V H H Q K L V F F A} \overset{25}{E D} \overset{30}{V G S N K G A} \overset{35}{I I G L M} \overset{40}{V G G V V I A}$$

FIGURE 1.3 Pathways of Aβ assembly. (From R. Roychaudhuri, M. Yang, M. M. Hoshi, and D. B. Teplow. "Amyloid β-Protein Assembly and Alzheimer Disease." 2009. *Journal of Biological Chemistry* 284: 4749–4753. With permission.)

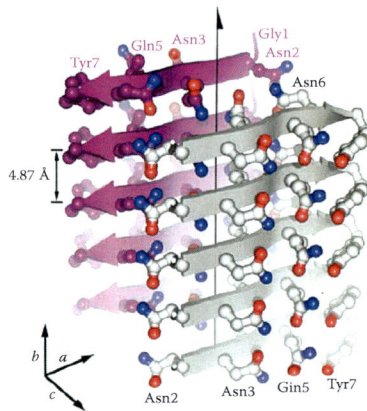

FIGURE 1.4 "The pair-of-sheets structure, showing the backbone of each β-strand as an arrow, with side chains protruding. The dry interface is between the two sheets, with the wet interfaces on the outside surfaces. Side chains Asn 2, Gln 4 and Asn 6 point inwards, forming the dry interface. The 21 screw axis of the crystal is shown as the vertical line. It rotates one of the strands of the near sheet 1808 about the axis and moves it up 4.87A°/2 so that it is superimposed on one of the strands of the far sheet." (From R. Nelson, M. R. Sawaya, M. Balbirnie, A. O. Madsen, C. Riekel, R. Grothe, and D. Eisenberg. "Structure of the Cross-β Spine of Amyloid-like Fibrils." 2005. *Nature* 435: 773–778. With permission.)

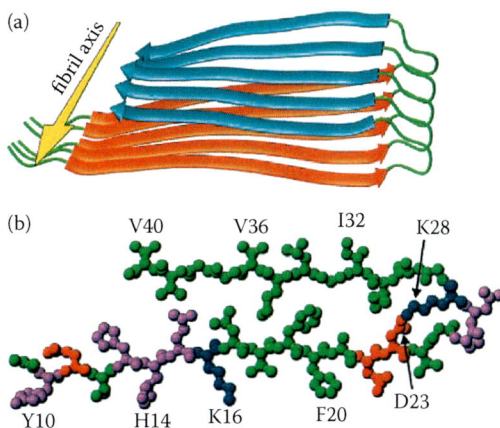

FIGURE 1.5   Structural model of Aβ40 fibrils.

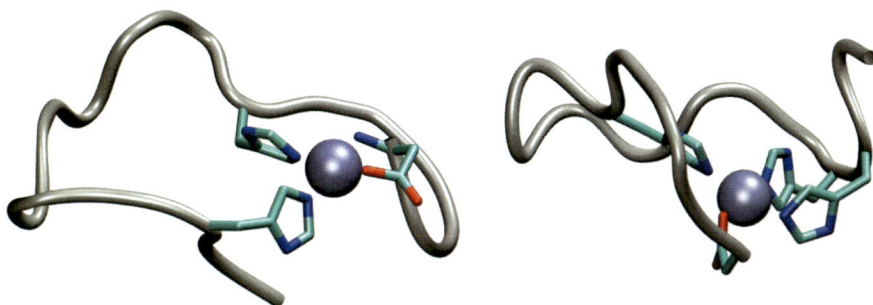

FIGURE 1.7A   Models of Cu(II) binding to Aβ: (N-term, His6, His13 or His14, Asp1-COO-) (left panel) and (Asp1-COO-, His6, His13, His14) (right panel). (From P. Faller. "Copper and Zinc Binding to Amyloid-Beta: Coordination, Dynamics, Aggregation, Reactivity and Metal-Ion Transfer." 2009. *Chembiochem* 10: 2837–2845; and P. Faller and C. Hureau. "Bioinorganic Chemistry of Copper and Zinc Ions Coordinated to Amyloid-β Peptide." 2009. *Dalton Trans* 1080–1094. With permission from John Wiley and Sons.)

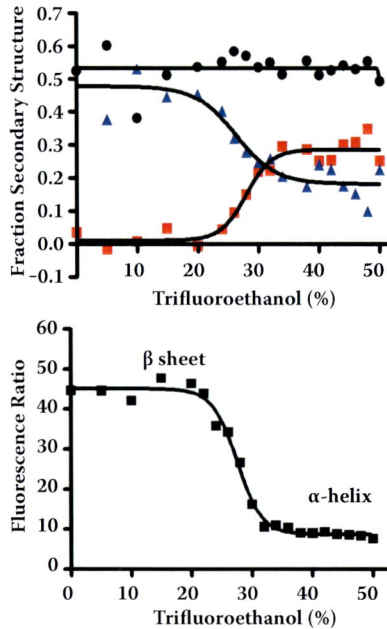

FIGURE 2.1 Conformational dynamics of Pronucleon™ Peptide Probe. Top panel: Circular dichroism measurements reveal the conformationally dynamic behavior of the Pronucleon peptide. Addition of increasing concentrations of the organic solvent trifluoroethanol induced a conformational switch in the Pronucleon peptide from largely alpha-helical structure (blue triangles) to β-sheet structure (red squares). Random coil structure (black circles) remained unchanged over the course of the experiment. Bottom panel: Conversion of the Pronucleon peptide from alpha-helix to β-sheet correlated with an increase in fluorescent excimer emission (reported as the fluorescence ratio of excimer: monomer signal).

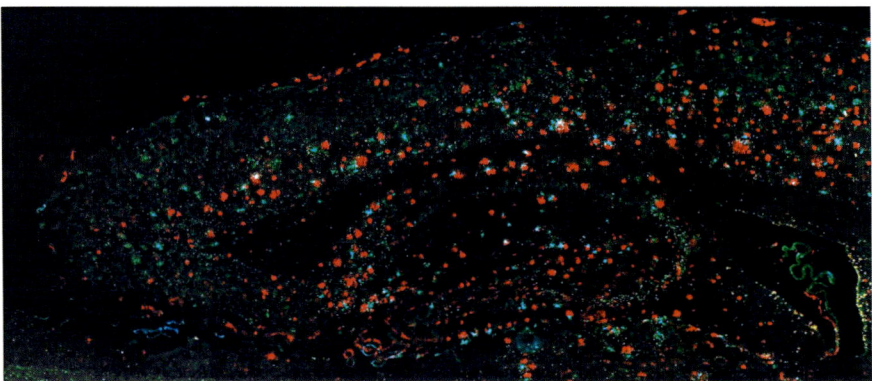

FIGURE 3.2 Fluorescent micrograph of brain histopathology of reactive Pronucleon™ peptide probes (blue) following intravenous administration in a transgenic mouse model (Tg2576) of Alzheimer's disease. The micrograph is a typical image from a sagittal section of mouse brain in late stage (>10 months) disease. The mice were sacrificed 15 minutes following injection. The sections are co-stained with monoclonal antibodies to Aβ (6E10) (red).

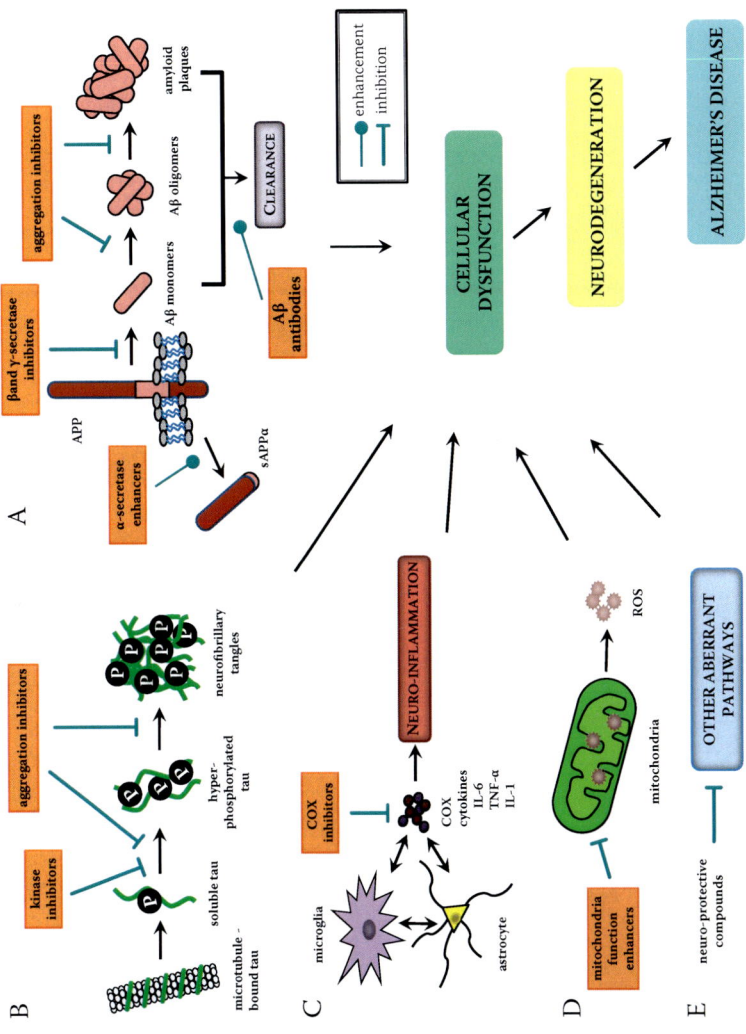

FIGURE 4.1 Proposed Alzheimer's disease pathogenesis and potential therapeutic targets. All pathways are interconnected; one may facilitate or give rise to another. Additionally, all pathways may originate from one unifying factor, such as genetic disposition; (A) amyloidogenic pathway; (B) hyperphosphorylated tau aggregation; (C) cyclo-oxygenase (COX) and cytokine-induced neuro-inflammatory mechanisms; (D) mitochondria dysfunction and production of reactive oxygen species (ROS), which distribute to other neural regions; and (E) other aberrant pathways that can be blocked by neuroprotective agents such as statins and docosahexanoic acid.

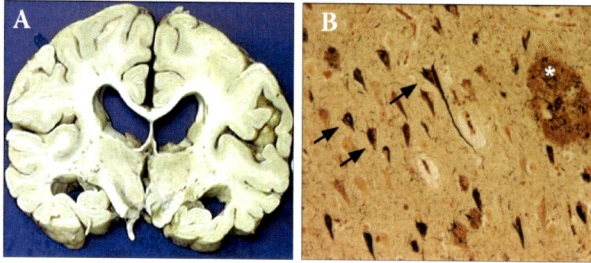

FIGURE 6.1 Gross and histopathological hallmarks of Alzheimer's disease (AD). (A) A coronal slice demonstrates enlarged ventricles, a thinned cortical ribbon, and atrophy of hippocampi. (B) A silver-stained section of the hippocampal pyramidal layer CA1 reveals numerous neurofibrillary tangles (arrows) and a prominent neuritic plaque (*). (Photos courtesy of Dr. Brent Harris, Director of Neuropathology, Georgetown University Medical Center.)

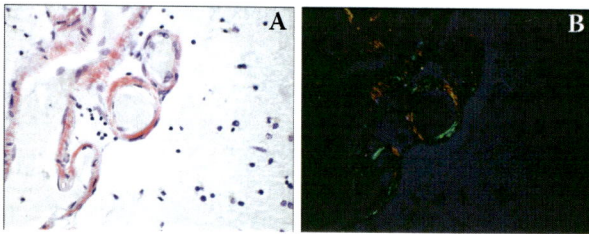

FIGURE 6.2 A Congo red–stained section highlights amyloid deposition within the wall of a small arteriole (orange/red) on brightfield microscopy (A) and demonstrates apple green birefringence by polarized light microscopy. (Photos courtesy of Dr. Brent Harris, Director of Neuropathology, Georgetown University Medical Center.)

Downs
Familial AD mutations
ApoE4 > 3 > 2
Aging

APP turnover

Aβ accumulation
Aβ oligomers, fibrils
amyloid plaques

low Aβ, high tau
levels in CSF

positive amyloid
imaging scan

neurotoxicity
neurofibrillary tangles

mild cognitive impairment
microgliosis and astrocytosis
inflammation
focal encephalopathy
neuronal morbidity
synaptic and neurotransmitter loss

focal
hypometabolism on
FDG-PET

memantine
donepezil
rivastigmine
galantamine

neuronal mortality
brain atrophy
white matter rarefaction
dementia
death

atrophy, white matter
changes on MRI

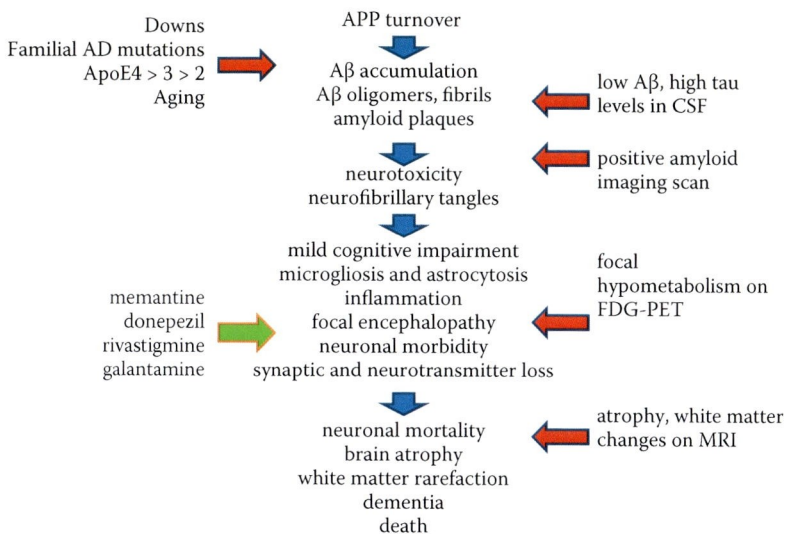

FIGURE 6.3 The amyloid cascade hypothesis of AD. Similar to most proteins, APP undergoes a rapid and constant turnover in cells throughout life; Aβ is a minor catabolite of normal APP proteolysis, and results from β- and then γ-secretase cleavage of APP. With aging, normal clearance mechanisms of Aβ begin to fail, leading to the progressive accumulation and deposition of neurotoxic Aβ/amyloid aggregates in brain parenchyma of certain regions, causing sporadic AD. Aβ monomers spontaneously alter their predominantly α-helical structure (to a conformation with a greater percentage of β-pleated sheet) and form dimers, trimers, oligomers, fibrils, and finally, the large neuritic plaques found on appropriately stained brain sections under microscopy (and apparent by amyloid PET imaging scans). The accumulation of Aβ oligomers and neuroinflammation result in a neurotoxic milieu that is visible as temporoparietal hypometabolism on FDG-PET imaging, reflecting an underlying focal metabolic encephalopathy. Accelerants of the amyloid cascade include Downs (trisomy 21) and mutations in APP, PS1, or PS2 associated with familial AD (all of which promote Aβ generation or aggregation), and possessing the ApoE4 genotype (which promotes Aβ deposition and impairs neuroplastic responses to brain injury). Current FDA-approved drug therapies for AD target relatively downstream events, thus having only modest, temporary, and palliative (symptomatic) benefits. Newer therapies now in clinical trials include passive and active anti-amyloid immunotherapies designed to promote CNS Aβ/amyloid clearance. Thus, by targeting the putative underlying cause of AD, these therapies may have disease-modifying effects. Abnormal diagnostic studies typically found in individuals with AD are shown on the right. Positive amyloid PET imaging may precede FDG-PET abnormalities and prove useful in detection of AD in the earliest stages.

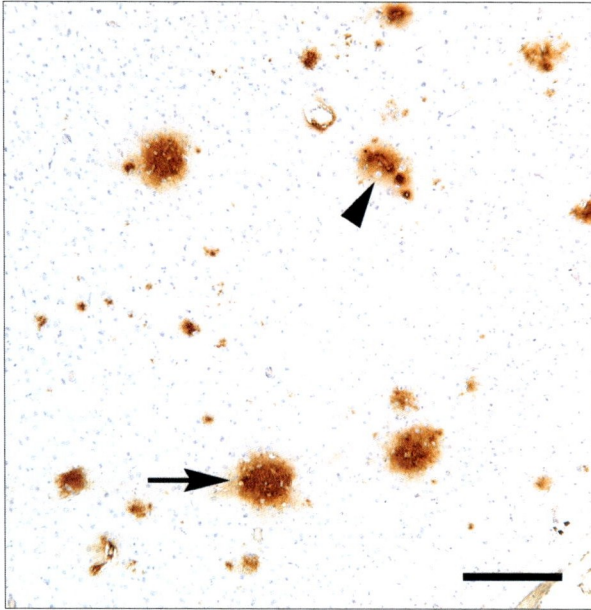

FIGURE 7.1 Aβ-immunostained senile plaques (one is marked by an arrow) and cerebral β-amyloid angiopathy (arrowhead) in the prefrontal neocortex of a >30-year-old rhesus monkey (*Macaca mulatta*). The Aβ peptide has the same amino acid sequence in humans and all nonhuman primates studied to date. However, cerebral β-amyloid angiopathy is more common in monkeys than in humans, and its incidence varies among species and among individuals within a species (Walker and Cork, 1999). Antibody 6E10 with a hematoxylin counterstain; Bar = 200 μm.

2 Emerging Principles and Biomarkers in In Vitro Diagnostics for Alzheimer's Disease

Renee D. Wegrzyn and Alan S. Rudolph

CONTENTS

2.1 DIAGNOSTICS: THE STATE OF THE ART

The extending life expectancy of the global population has led to a significant increase in the number of age-related diseases that are diagnosed and treated each year. Among these age-related diseases, Alzheimer's disease is the most common form of dementia affecting the elderly. The predominant risk factor for developing Alzheimer's disease is age. Various estimates indicate that the incidence of Alzheimer's disease begins to increase after the age of 65 and reaches a prevalence of 25–50% by age 85 (Hebert et al., 2003; Evans et al., 1989). Alzheimer's disease represents a growing global healthcare and socioeconomic burden that continues to expand in the absence of reliable diagnostics and therapeutic interventions. It is estimated that in 2010 there were 35.6 million people living with dementia worldwide at a cost of more than $600 billion dollars. Each year, the number of individuals living with dementia is increasing. In the five years between 2005 and 2010, the total number of individuals living with dementia grew by 18%. With such increases in the total number of dementia cases each year and an overall increase in life expectancy, it is projected that the total cost to manage dementia will increase 85% by 2030 (Wilmo and Price, 2010).

Currently, the diagnosis of Alzheimer's disease is concomitant with the manifestation of dementia-related cognitive symptoms as outlined by the current diagnostic criteria indicated in the *Diagnostic and Statistical Manual of Mental Disorders Fourth Edition* (DSM-IV), the National Institute of Neurological and Communicative Disorders and Stroke and the Alzheimer's Disease and Related Disorders Association (NINCDS-ADRDA), and the *International Statistical Classification of Diseases Tenth Edition* (ICD-10). In order to reach a diagnosis of Alzheimer's disease, clinicians typically perform a detailed review of a patient's medical history, test for episodic memory loss, measure cognitive impairment through neuropsychological tests such as the Mini-Mental State Exam (MMSE) and Alzheimer's Disease Assessment Scale-cognitive subscale (ADAS-cog), and exclude other neurological or physiological disorders through blood tests and brain imaging techniques (Growdon, 1999; Blennow et al., 2006). Using these methods, patients are categorized across a continuum of disease states of increasing severity from mild cognitive impairment (MCI), a state in which some cognitive decline is present but the criteria for dementia are not fulfilled, to mild, moderate, and severe Alzheimer's disease. Once diagnosed with MCI, approximately 40–60% of patients ultimately develop Alzheimer's disease within 5 years (DeCarli, 2003; Petersen, 2004).

The underlying molecular pathology that is associated with the onset of Alzheimer's disease is gradual and cumulative. A preclinical phase that precedes disease diagnosis in the clinic is thought to begin more than 10 years prior to symptomatic presentation of Alzheimer's disease (Morris and Price, 2001; Blennow, 2004; Blennow et al., 2006). Once patients are symptomatic, experienced clinicians can achieve diagnostic accuracy rates of 80–90%, especially in the context of multiple longitudinal visits of a patient to the clinic. Despite decades of research devoted to the investigation of reliable diagnostic techniques, the definitive diagnosis of Alzheimer's disease relies exclusively on postmortem histological confirmation of Alzheimer's disease pathology (Masters et al., 2006; Frank et al., 2003; McKhann et al., 1984). It can be argued, however, that because progressive pathological neurodegenerative changes manifest during the preclinical stages of Alzheimer's disease (Price et al., 2001), it should theoretically be possible to derive dependable antemortem diagnostic capabilities in the form of molecular biomarkers that are associated with these changes and are indicative of disease.

The potential impact of an antemortem diagnostic for Alzheimer's disease is enormous and far-reaching. For patients and caregivers, definitive diagnosis can offer answers to unknown symptoms and behaviors, provide appropriate treatment and care options for those suffering from the illness, and provide an opportunity to plan for the future. In the absence of effective diagnostics, Alzheimer's disease can be misdiagnosed for other disorders such as depression, unfavorable drug interactions, or other dementias. For physicians, proper diagnosis at a very basic level may enable rule-in/rule-out diagnosis for disease. For regulatory agencies and drug developers, effective Alzheimer's disease diagnostics or biomarkers that can serve as measures of clinical trial success will assist decision-making processes.

Alzheimer's disease is a progressive disease and biomarkers that can indentify not only the presence of disease but also disease severity and progression can offer new opportunities to properly administer critical care. The ability to identify individuals with Alzheimer's disease as early as possible in disease progression, when therapeutic intervention is more likely to be effective and before severe neuropathology is present, is critical not only for treatment of patient using existing therapies, but also for the completion of successful clinical trials for the development of new therapies.

Drug discovery and development for the treatment of Alzheimer's disease would greatly benefit from biomarkers that are predictive of clinical outcomes (Frank and Hargreaves, 2003) to inform the selection of effective drug candidates, monitor dose safety and efficacy on treated cohorts, and identify or confirm the mechanisms of drug action in hopes of developing treatments that go beyond symptomatic relief and are disease modifying (Hampel et al., 2010). The ability to monitor disease progression longitudinally during patient treatment will also be key to the development of effective Alzheimer's disease therapies. Useful biomarkers that assist the progression of drug discovery and development for treatment of Alzheimer's disease do not necessarily aid in clinical diagnosis of disease. For example, since Alzheimer's is a complex disease, biomarkers that confirm the existence of target molecules for a given therapeutic will be useful in selecting patients for clinical trial enrollment. Indeed, the lack of reliable biomarkers that can report any of these key criteria has contributed to several recent failures of Alzheimer's disease therapeutic clinical trials (Zetterberg et al., 2010). Researchers are still pursuing a surrogate endpoint biomarker for Alzheimer's disease, that is, a biomarker that is intended to substitute for a clinical endpoint that is characteristic of a patient's medical status and prognosis. Without a requirement for the sophisticated imaging equipment that is required for several brain imaging techniques for disease diagnosis, the development of reliable biomarkers that can aid in Alzheimer's disease diagnosis may be the best option for early disease detection and widespread adoption in the clinic.

In this chapter, we explore existing and emerging in vitro biomarker-based methodologies for the diagnosis of Alzheimer's disease focusing on genetic, biochemical, and conformational strategies. In vivo imaging diagnostic approaches are covered in more detail in the following chapter (Chapter 3, "Imaging Biomarkers for Diagnosis, Prognosis, and Treatment of Alzheimer's Disease").

2.2 GENETIC BIOMARKERS

Several genetic markers that are associated with the familial (hereditary) and sporadic forms of Alzheimer's disease have been employed to assist clinicians in determining patients who may be at risk of developing Alzheimer's disease. The familial form of Alzheimer's disease is a rare autosomal dominant disorder that is typically associated with an early onset of disease before age 65. The majority of familial Alzheimer's disease cases are linked to mutations in the presenilin genes presenilin 1 (*PSEN1*) and presenilin 2 (*PSEN2*) (Sherrington et al., 1995; Levy–Lahad et al., 1995a, 1995b), though a small number of cases have been reported to be associated with mutations in the amyloid precursor protein (APP) (Goate et al., 1991). Gene copy number variation (and subsequent change in gene dosage) is also a likely contributor in some cases of early-onset Alzheimer's disease, most notably in the case of patients with Down's syndrome who carry an extra copy of the APP. These individuals typically exhibit advanced pathological features of Alzheimer's disease, including senile plaques and neurofibrillary tangles, after the age of 35 (Oliver and Holland, 1986; Lai and Williams, 1989).

The vast majority of Alzheimer's disease cases are associated with late disease onset (after the age of 65) and are genetically complex. The ε4 mutation of the *APOE* gene, which encodes Apolipoprotein E, is one of the most significant genetic risk factors for the development of sporadic Alzheimer's disease (Strittmatter et al., 1993; Raber et al., 2004). ApoE can be found in amyloid plaques and tangles, and had been shown to bind Aβ (Namba et al., 1991; Strittmatter et al., 1993). The ApoE4 protein is less efficient than other ApoE variants in maintenance of membrane integrity, cholesterol transport, and response to neuronal cell injury (Poirier, 1994). Populations that are *APOE* ε4 heterozygotes have a two- to threefold higher incidence of Alzheimer's disease, and *APOE* ε4 homozygotes have more than a tenfold greater incidence of the disease (Farrer et al., 1997). Meta-analyses conducted to probe the published genetic association studies for Alzheimer's disease indicate that several other genes have been shown to have association with Alzheimer's disease, but most have only modest contributions when compared to the *APOE* ε4 allele (Blomqvist et al., 2006; Bertram et al., 2007).

Based on published estimates, the *APOE* ε4 allele is estimated to account for only about half of Alzheimer's disease heritability, leaving open a significant opportunity to identify additional factors that may contribute to the genetic variance of Alzheimer's disease (Ashford and Mortimer, 2002; Saykin et al., 2010). Researchers who investigate the genetics of Alzheimer's disease have recently focused on genomewide association studies. Approaches such as gene expression analysis are not ideal for Alzheimer's research since neuropathological tissue samples can only be obtained postmortem; however, there have been some notable recent successes in transcriptome analysis and microRNA analysis in blood mononuclear cells of patients with Alzheimer's disease (Maes et al., 2007; Schipper et al., 2007; Maes et al., 2009) that may eventually offer insight into disease diagnosis and prognosis using readily accessible patient blood samples.

The results of genomewide association studies conducted by Alzheimer's disease researchers have been assembled in the publicly available AlzGene database (http://www.alzgene.org/TopResults.asp) (Bertram et al., 2007). The AlzGene database is continuously updated with new study data and analyzed to provide a current summary of the leading candidate genes that are implicated in Alzheimer's disease. As of publication of this manuscript, more than 650 genes and nearly 3000 polymorphisms investigated in more than 1300 candidate gene studies for Alzheimer's disease could be found in the AlzGene database, where the top hit remains *APOE*. A list of the top ten AlzGene results as of submission of this manuscript can be found in Table 2.1.

Alzheimer's disease genomewide association studies are still in their infancy and so far mostly only relatively weak associations have been demonstrated. In order to increase the statistical power of these approaches, researchers can increase sample size, expand genetic sequencing coverage, and combine gene-association study results with other phenotypic measures including biochemical biomarkers, neuroimaging, and expression profiling to create larger data sets that lend themselves to meta-analyses. For example, increasing the sample size to several thousand subjects per cohort for genomewide association studies recently led to the identification of several novel genetic loci that are associated with Alzheimer's disease susceptibility including *CLU*, *PICALM*,

TABLE 2.1

Top Ten AlzGene Results for Alzheimer's Disease Associated Genes as of Submission of Manuscript

Ranking	Gene	Protein
1	APOE	Apolipoprotein E
2	BIN1	Bridging integrator 1
3	CLU	Clusterin (Apolipoprotein J)
4	ABCA7	ATP-binding cassette, subfamily A (ABC1), member 7
5	CR1	Complement component (3b/4b) receptor 1
6	PICALM	Phosphatidylinositol binding clathrin assembly protein
7	MS4A6A	Membrane-spanning 4-domains, subfamily A, member 6A
8	CD33	CD33 (transmembrane receptor)
9	MS4A4E	Membrane-spanning 4-domains, subfamily A, member 4E
10	CD2AP	CD2-associated protein

Source: Data from Alzheimer Research Forum, http://www.alzgene.org/TopResults.asp.

and *CR1* (see Table 2.1) (Harold et al., 2009; Lambert et al., 2009). Encouraging results have also emerged from a staged approach to genomewide association studies. In these studies, initial results from a meta-analysis conducted in the first stage using four large Alzheimer's disease data sets were tested against additional data sets in each subsequent stage in order to seek genetic variants that persist through multiple meta-analyses with high statistical stringencies (while specifically excluding *APOE*, *CLU*, and *PICALM* genes). The results of the studies identified new variants (*MS4A6A/ MS4A4E*, *EPHA1*, *CD33*, and *CD2AP*) or corroborated previous findings (*ABCA7* and *BIN1*) of gene variants that are associated with an increased risk for Alzheimer's disease (Hollingworth et al., 2011; Naj et al., 2011). In sum, data from nearly 20,000 Alzheimer's patients and nearly 40,000 controls for a total of more than two million single nucleotide polymorphisms were analyzed, making these studies the largest undertaken to date to determine novel genes associated with Alzheimer's disease.

The rapidly increasing availability and throughput of emerging genome sequencing technologies holds promise for continued progress in genomewide association studies and even targeted resequencing of existing samples to strengthen conclusions. The integration of genomewide association study results with multidimensional data sets, such as the Alzheimer's Disease Neuroimaging Initiative (ADNI), which combines imaging studies with genetic and biochemical biomarker investigation, will likely contribute to the identification of novel rare genetic variants or pathways of multiple genes acting in concert that contribute to Alzheimer's disease pathology and may eventually serve as useful antecedent biomarkers for the disease. Some initial encouraging results have been reported using such multidimensional data analysis approaches including the assessment of the association of genetic polymorphisms with each of five cerebrospinal fluid (CSF) protein biomarkers to reveal four candidate genes relating to Alzheimer's disease including one novel gene (Kim et al., 2011), the association of several gene alleles (*ACE*, *APOE*, *BDNF*, *DAPK1,* and *TF*) with Aβ levels in CSF (Kauwe et al., 2009), the discovery of a polymorphism associated with phosphorylated tau levels in CSF (Cruchaga et al., 2010), as well as a study that probes the association of multiple known Alzheimer's disease gene polymorphisms with tissue neuropathology and cognitive function proximate to death (Shulman et al., 2010).

2.3 BIOCHEMICAL BIOMARKERS

Many current research efforts that aim to identify protein or biochemical biomarkers of Alzheimer's disease focus on targets that reflect the underlying pathology of the disease. This is a rather daunting task considering that the brain tissue that succumbs to neurodegeneration directly can only be tested after patient death. As a consequence, the discovery of biomarkers that may enable the development of antemortem Alzheimer's disease diagnostics focuses on targets present in blood, CSF, and even urine that can serve as either direct or indirect indicators of the pathological changes that are taking place in the brain. Decades of research in Alzheimer's disease pathogenesis has helped to define many of the biomarkers targeted for diagnostic development. Alzheimer's disease biomarker discovery and development may be directed by the existing scientific information that has identified emerging biomarkers (although this introduces bias), or advances in high throughput protein analysis methodologies may be leveraged by researchers to study a patient's entire blood or CSF proteome profile in search of novel biomarkers or biomarker panels that may facilitate diagnosis or report drug efficacy.

The most commonly accepted hypothesis that describes the progression of Alzheimer's disease and its subsequent pathology depicts a cascade of events triggered by an imbalance in the production and clearance of the amyloid β (Aβ) protein in the brain. As increasing amounts of Aβ accumulate in the brain, soluble Aβ undergoes conformational changes that enrich β-sheet structures making the protein aggregation-prone with a propensity to adopt oligomeric and larger polymeric structures that are deposited as amyloid plaques in the brain (Hardy and Selkoe, 2002; Jarrett et al., 1993). Also consistent with the progression of Alzheimer's disease is the appearance of neurofibrillary tangles composed of hyperphosphorylated versions of the axonal microtubule-binding protein tau. Hyperphosphorylated tau eventually destabilizes microtubules and compromises neuronal function (Grundke-Iqbal et al., 1986; Nukina and Ihara, 1986; Iqbal et al., 2005). The accumulation and deposition of misfolded Aβ and hyperphosphorylated tau are accompanied by loss of synaptic integrity and progressive neuronal impairment leading to cognitive dysfunction (Blennow et al., 2006), though the exact mechanism by which this occurs is debated. While variants of Aβ and tau are clearly emerging as the leading diagnostic biochemical biomarkers for Alzheimer's disease, other factors that may contribute to Alzheimer's pathology may provide clues for additional biomarker candidates include indicators of oxidative stress and inflammation.

Aβ, the major component of brain plaques in Alzheimer's disease, can also be found circulating in CSF and plasma. The quantitation of Aβ in CSF using immunoassay methodologies has led to the development of diagnostic procedures reporting diagnostic accuracy upward of 75% in some cases (Blennow, 2004; Jensen et al.,

1999; Lewczuk et al., 2004), whereas the diagnostic efficacy of Aβ levels in plasma has yielded some conflicting or meager results that require further study (Assini et al., 2004; Pesaresi et al., 2006; Sobow et al., 2005; Giedraitis et al., 2007). There are several isoforms of the Aβ protein ranging from 38 to 43 amino acids in length that are produced after cleavage and processing of the amyloid precursor protein (APP) by β-secretase and γ-secretase. The most abundant isoforms of Aβ are Aβ40 and Aβ42. Aβ42 is more aggregation-prone than Aβ40 and its utility as a biomarker is linked to this activity. Decreased levels of Aβ42 in CSF and plasma are indicative of disease, presumably due to the sequestration of Aβ42 into amyloid aggregates in the brain consistent with the *amyloid sink* hypothesis. As such, Aβ42 or the ratio of Aβ42/Aβ40 levels in CSF have emerged as biomarkers with the potential to predict the progression of MCI to Alzheimer's disease (Fagan et al., 2007; Hansson et al., 2006; Li et al., 2007) and report plaque burden in the brain (Cairns et al., 2009). There has been some progress in the development of Aβ biomarkers in blood plasma, but Aβ levels in plasma do not seem to correlate with CSF levels, and plasma Aβ biomarker measures thus far do not reach the predictive value for disease progression as observed for these biomarkers in CSF (Fagan et al., 2009; Mehta et al., 2001; Vanderstichele et al., 2000; Graff-Radford et al., 2007; Mayeux et al., 1999; Perrin et al., 2009). While Aβ variants are perhaps the best studied biomarkers in the pursuit of minimally invasive diagnostic indicators of Alzheimer's disease, a lack of consensus results across studies and the significant overlap of the concentration of Aβ variants across study cohorts, leaves open opportunities for the development of more reliable diagnostic biomarkers with greater clinical applicability.

Tau and phosphorylated tau biomarkers in CSF have also been used to discriminate subjects with Alzheimer's disease from age-matched controls (Vandermeeren et al., 1993) and there are studies that support the use of tau and phosphorylated tau as prognostic biomarkers to predict the conversion of MCI subjects to dementia of the Alzheimer's type when applied together with Aβ 42 CSF biomarker measures (Fagan et al., 2007; Hansson et al., 2006; Li et al., 2007). A recent study revealed that once patients are symptomatic for Alzheimer's disease, there appear to be only very minor changes in tau and Aβ levels over time as measured in longitudinal studies over several years (Buchhave et al., 2009), perhaps because once onset of symptoms occurs, the disease pathology is already in advanced stages. These changes within each group are insignificant when compared to the differences between healthy controls and Alzheimer's disease subjects, supporting the notion that the most dramatic changes in these biomarker levels occurs before patients manifest symptoms in the clinic. The very minor changes described in CSF levels of Aβ and tau over time in Alzheimer's patients in this study also opens the possibility that these biomarkers could be used as relatively sensitive tools or surrogates to monitor the efficacy of clinical treatments that target the pathological events that can be reported using these biomarkers. However, some conflicting results have been reported for other longitudinal studies during the last decades (Seppala et al., 2010; Bouwman et al., 2007; Blennow et al., 2007; Zetterberg et al., 2007; Kanai et al., 1998; Sunderland et al., 1999) emphasizing that additional investigation, expansion of study cohorts, and standardization of study protocols may need to be achieved before a final determination can be made regarding the beneficence of longitudinal biomarker data in the diagnosis of Alzheimer's disease.

Beyond Aβ and tau derivatives, several new biomarkers are beginning to emerge as useful tools for the diagnosis and characterization of disease state for Alzheimer's either as completely novel and independent biomarkers, or as new biomarkers that enhance the clinical accuracy of Alzheimer's diagnosis using the more traditional biomarkers of Aβ and tau derivatives. One recent example of the latter includes the identification of four CSF biomarkers (NrCAM, YKL-40, chromogranin A, and carnosinase I) that enhance the diagnostic accuracy of Alzheimer's disease when measured together with Aβ42 and tau levels (Perrin et al., 2011).

Although still in the early stages of discovery and in need of expanded clinical validation, several emergent biomarkers are associated with the immune system and inflammation response. For example, some initial encouraging results were observed for a panel of 18 biomarkers comprised of signaling molecules in blood plasma. These biomarkers were indicative of a systemic inflammatory state associated with Alzheimer's disease, and were able to help identify patients with MCI that would later progress to a more advanced Alzheimer's disease state (Ray et al., 2007). Some additional exploratory experiments that are also noteworthy in the category of immune-related biomarkers include an analysis of Aβ antigen–antibody dissociation in serum that could differentiate between Alzheimer's samples and healthy controls (Gustaw et al., 2008).

2.4 CONFORMATIONAL BIOMARKERS

One of the hallmark features of amyloid disease progression is aggregate and conformational change in the amyloid species present in the brain and periphery. These have been extensively reviewed in other chapters in this book with regard to specific physicochemical dynamics as these aggregation and structural changes to amyloid protein occur, with particular focus on amyloid Aβ42 and its aggregate structure as plaque and as an oligomeric species. These changes have provided the basis for many efforts to exploit these conformationally dynamic events as biomarkers to diagnose early signs of disease and the prognosis for progression of disease.

One of the earliest reports of exploiting increasing conformational order of amyloid species to diagnose Alzheimer's disease was based on direct biophysical measurement of amyloidogenic species in cerebrospinal fluid using fluorescence correlation spectroscopy (Pitschke et al., 1998). In this study, the conformational order of amyloid protein was measured following the addition of fluorescently labeled Aβ reporter peptides to the CSF of Alzheimer's and age-matched control patients based on the hypothesis that amyloidogenic Aβ multimers present in the CSF of diseased patients could catalyze the polymerization of newly added Aβ in measureable amounts. This report showed statistically relevant separation of normal from disease samples based on the increased conformational order in the Alzheimer's group over normals.

Multimeric structures, including dimeric Ab, that impair long-term potentiation and memory storage, have been isolated from the brain (Shankar et al., 2008). A recent study focused on the identification of oligomeric Ab species in the cellular membrane-containing fraction of blood. Based on the hypothesis that oligomeric Ab structures better correlate with disease progression than heavy plaque burden in the brain (Rowe et al., 2007; Lue et al., 1999; McLean et al., 1999), this study demonstrated that oligomeric Ab species in the blood measured by surface-enhanced laser desorption ionization time of flight (SELDI-TOF) mass spectrometry indicated that the blood of Alzheimer's disease patients had significantly higher levels of Ab monomer and oligomer (specifically dimers) than healthy controls. In addition, the levels of monomer and oligomer also correlated with increased cognitive impairment and level of Ab in the brain (Villemagne et al., 2010), indicating a promising next step in the identification of new conformational biomarkers in the blood with clinical relevance in the study of Alzheimer's disease.

Most strategies to exploit conformational order as a strategy for developing diagnostic biomarkers for amyloid protein and Alzheimer's disease have focused on the development of antibodies that recognize structural motifs specific to amyloid aggregates (Glabe, 2008; Kayed et al., 2007; Xia et al., 2009; Georganopoulou et al., 2005; Sarsoza et al., 2009). Antibodies have been used to probe the conformational dynamics of amyloid aggregation and demonstrate specificity to structural epitopes that are shared as conformational order increases. Such conformation-specific antibodies have been reported to distinguish oligomer structures categorized into prefibrillar and fibrillar states (Glabe, 2008). The use of antibodies to monomeric amyloid species has also been used to map epitopes as aggregation proceeds and has been reported to detect b-sheet rich conformational forms of PrP in mouse and human peripheral blood from animals with transmissible spongiform encephalopathy (TSE) and humans with sporadic and variant Creutzfeldt-Jakob disease (CJD) (Lehto et al. 2006; Guntz et al., 2010).

Another strategy for creating a diagnostic for amyloid structural and aggregate forms has been the use of sequence-matched peptides that report on amyloid folding events that accompany the secondary structural changes to increasing β-sheet-rich character as the protein aggregates. Our group has employed synthetic peptide chemistry to link fluorophores to a peptide backbone to form what are termed *Pronucleon*™ *peptide probes* that report conformational changes as these moieties are brought in close proximity to each other as folding and conformational order increases (Pan et al., 2007). We have selected the fluorophore pyrene to conjugate to the termini of Pronucleon peptides to leverage the dramatic shift in the fluorescent emission spectrum that is observed when the pyrenes are distant (*monomeric* emission) or in close proximity (*excimeric* emission) for measurement of conformational changes. Our group has used circular dichroism measurements to demonstrate the conformational dynamics of these engineered Pronucleon peptide probes (Figure 2.1, and Wegrzyn, Nuss, and Rudolph, unpublished data).

The increase in excimer signal from pyrene-labeled Pronucleon peptides as a result of the conformational changes in the probe in the presence of conformationally rich target protein can be followed temporally in high-throughput microtiter plates, forming the basis for the development of diagnostic tests. Measurable changes in Pronucleon peptide fluorescent emissions are dependent on both the dose and structural state of the conformational target. The increase in pyrene excimer signal takes place over a period of hours and can be measured with commercial

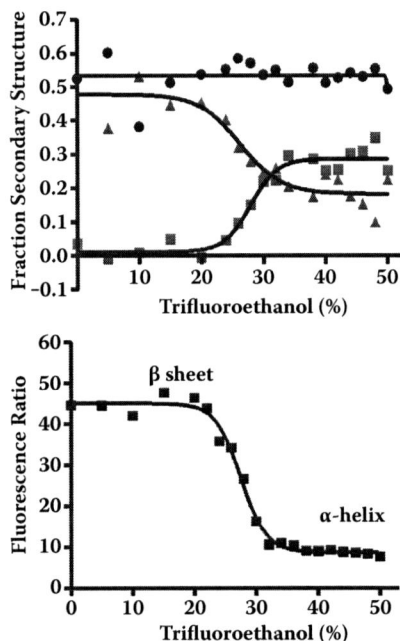

FIGURE 2.1 (See color insert.)   Conformational dynamics of Pronucleon™ Peptide Probe. Top panel: Circular dichroism measurements reveal the conformationally dynamic behavior of the Pronucleon peptide. Addition of increasing concentrations of the organic solvent trifluoroethanol induced a conformational switch in the Pronucleon peptide from largely alpha-helical structure (blue triangles) to β-sheet structure (red squares). Random coil structure (black circles) remained unchanged over the course of the experiment. Bottom panel: Conversion of the Pronucleon peptide from alpha-helix to β-sheet correlated with an increase in fluorescent excimer emission (reported as the fluorescence ratio of excimer: monomer signal).

diagnostic equipment. The earliest pursuit of diagnostic strategies using this concept was demonstrated for TSE showing the ability to distinguish prion conformational order increases in animal and human disease from both brain and blood samples (Pan et al., 2007; Tcherkasskaya et al., 2005).

Pronucleon peptide probes have been used to develop assay methodologies to explore the amyloid conformational state of known structural and aggregate states. For amyloid Aβ42 and 40, we have demonstrated that Pronucleon probes exhibit an increase in b-sheet structure when mixed with fibrous preparations of synthetic Aβ in vitro. The observed increase in pyrene excimer formation is measured over a period of hours and exhibits a dose-dependent response to increasing amounts of Ab40 and Ab42 fiber using published methods for fiber formation. It is speculated that the increase in fluorescence is a result of the direct binding of Pronucleon probes to fibers. Preliminary results support this hypothesis as Pronucleon probes are typically soluble under normal assay conditions but are able to be separated quantitatively into a low-speed centrifugation pellet in the presence of Ab fibers (Wegrzyn and Rudolph, unpublished data).

More recently, our efforts have focused on Pronucleon probes that report on presence and conformational state of earlier pathological states of amyloid aggregation, specifically oligomeric species. New designs of conformational probes have been developed that react with less ordered amyloid aggregates in early stages of assembly. These designs have recognized that the oligomeric state compared to fibers may be more disordered and fluid, and as a result may require probes that can respond and report to more disordered conformational states. The design of such probes has proceeded with amino acid sequence selection and pyrene coordination to specific sites that will facilitate spectroscopic changes upon binding to oligomers. The increased fluidity of the oligomer compared to fiber results in the increased disorder of the probes as measured by fluorescence changes in the probe. Such probes have demonstrated the dose-dependent change in response to synthetic oligomers in solution (Wegrzyn, Moll, and Rudolph, unpublished data). Future studies will focus on the ability of these probes to target oligomeric species in vivo.

2.5 CONCLUSIONS

The translation of emerging Alzheimer's disease biomarkers into effective tools for use in research labs, therapeutic development and clinical trials, regulatory agencies, and the clinic will positively impact patients at all stages of disease. Prior to the development of overt symptoms, the most effective biomarkers will be able to screen patients for risk and identify individuals that may benefit from preventative strategies. Early detection of disease and pathology, potentially decades prior to onset of symptoms, will enable early therapeutic intervention and disease treatment according to the measured disease profile of each patient. Once a definitive diagnosis is made and patients are undergoing treatment, biomarkers will enable longitudinal monitoring of patient response to treatment and facilitate decision making with respect to adjustment in treatment course. Importantly, the efficacy and quantitative value of the biomarkers must be validated using appropriately large sample sets and advanced analysis techniques to achieve statistical significance.

Perhaps the most promising diagnostic approaches will emerge from combined approaches that leverage advancements in genetic biomarkers, and biochemical and conformational biomarkers in blood and CSF, combined with robust neuroimaging strategies. The development of multimodal techniques that employ biomarkers to aid in the successful diagnosis of Alzheimer's disease will require the standardization of biomarkers (or biomarker panels) to be used in the clinic. Current challenges faced by Alzheimer's disease clinical researchers, including interlaboratory variation in the measurement of biomarkers (Mattson et al., 2010), and the difficulty in identifying and targeting conformationally dynamic pathological intermediates, must first be overcome.

ACKNOWLEDGMENTS

We thank Roxanne Duan, Jonathan Moll, Jonathan Nuss, and Andrew Nyborg, for excellent technical assistance and support.

REFERENCES

Ashford, J. W., and Mortimer, J. A. 2002. Non-familial Alzheimer's disease is mainly due to genetic factors. *J Alzheimer's Dis* 4: 169–177.

Assini, A., Cammarata, S., Vitali, A., e. al. 2004. Plasma levels of amyloid beta-protein 42 are increased in women with mild cognitive impairment. *Neurology* 63: 828–831.

Bertram, L., McQueen, M. B., Mullin, K., et al. 2007. Systematic meta-analyses of Alzheimer disease genetic association studies: the AlzGene database. *Nat Genet* 39: 17–23.

Blennow, K. 2004. Cerebrospinal fluid protein biomarkers for Alzheimer's disease. *NeuroRx* 1: 213–225.

Blennow, K., de Leon, M. J., and Zetterberg, H. 2006. Alzheimer's disease. *Lancet* 368: 387–403.

Blennow, K., Zetterberg, H., Minthon, L., et al. 2007. Longitudinal stability of CSF biomarkers in Alzheimer's disease. *Neurosci Lett* 419: 18–22.

Blomqvist, M. E., Reynolds, C., Katzov, H., et al. 2006. Towards compendia of negative genetic association studies: an example for Alzheimer disease. *Hum Genet* 119: 29–37.

Bouwman, F. H., van der Flier, W. M. Schoonenboom, N. S., et al. 2007. Longitudinal changes of CSF biomarkers in memory clinic patients. *Neurology* 69: 1006–1011.

Buchhave, P., Blennow, K., Zetterberg, H., et al. 2009. Longitudinal study of CSF biomarkers in patients with Alzheimer's disease. *PLoS One* 4(7), doi:10.1371/journal.pone.0006294.

Cairns, N. J., Ikonomovic, M. D., Benzinger, T., et al. 2009. Absence of Pittsburgh compound B detection of cerebral amyloid beta in a patient with clinical, cognitive, and cerebrospinal fluid markers of Alzheimer disease: a case report. *Arch Neurol* 66: 1557–1562.

Cruchaga, C., Kauwe, J. S., Mayo, K., et al. 2010. SNPs associated with cerebrospinal fluid phospho-tau levels influence rate of decline in Alzheimer's disease. *PLoS Genet* 6(9), doi:10.1371/journal.pgen.1001101.

DeCarli, C. 2003. Mild cognitive impairment: Prevalence, prognosis, aetiology, and treatment. *The Lancet Neurology* 2: 15–21.

Evans, D. A., Funkenstein, H. H., Albert, M. S., et al. 1989. Prevalence of Alzheimer's disease in a community population of older persons higher than previously reported. *JAMA* 262: 2551–2556.

Fagan, A. M., Head, D., and Shah, A. R. 2009. Decreased cerebrospinal fluid Abeta(42) correlates with brain atrophy in cognitively normal elderly. *Ann Neurol* 65: 176–183.

Fagan, A. M., Roe, C. M., Xiong, C., et al. 2007. Cerebrospinal fluid tau/beta-amyloid(42) ratio as a prediction of cognitive decline in nondemented older adults. *Arch Neurol* 64: 343–349.

Farrer, L. A., Cupples, L. A., Haines, J. L., et al. 1997. Effects of age, sex, and ethnicity on the association between apolipoprotein E genotype and Alzheimer disease: A meta-analysis. APOE and Alzheimer Disease Meta Analysis Consortium. *JAMA* 278: 1349–1356.

Frank, R., and Hargreaves, R. 2003. Clinical biomarkers in drug discovery and development. *Nat Rev Drug Discov.* 2: 566–580.

Frank, R. A., Galasko, D., Hampel, H., et al. 2003. Biological markers for therapeutic trials in Alzheimer's disease. Proceedings of the biological markers working group; NIA initiative on neuroimaging in Alzheimer's disease. *Neurobiol Aging* 24:521–536.

Georganopoulou, D. G., Chang, L., Nam, J-M., et al. 2005. Nanoparticle-based detection in cerebral spinal fluid of a soluble pathogenic biomarker for Alzheimer's disease. *Proc Natl Acad Sci USA* 102: 2273–2276.

Giedratis, V., Sundelof, J., Irizarry, M. C., et al. 2007. The normal equilibrium between CSF and plasma amyloid beta levels is disrupted in Alzheimer's disease. *Neurosci Lett* 427: 127–131.

Glabe, C. G. 2008. Structural classification of toxic amyloid oligomers. *J Biol Chem* 283: 29639–29643.

Goate, A., Chartier-Harlin, M. C., Mullan, M., et al. 1991. Segregation of a missense mutation in the amyloid precursor protein gene with familial Alzheimer's disease. *Nature* 349: 704–706.

Graff-Radford, N. R., Crook, J. E., Lucas, J., et al. 2007. Association of low plasma Abeta42/Abeta40 ratios with increased imminent risk for mild cognitive impairment and Alzheimer disease. *Arch Neurol* 64: 354–362.

Growdon, J. H. 1999. Biomarkers of Alzheimer disease. *Arch Neurol.* 56: 281–283.

Grundke-Iqbal, I., Iqbal, K., Tung, Y. C., et al. 1986. Abnormal phosphorylation of the microtubule-associated protein tau (tau) in Alzheimer cytoskeletal pathology. *Proc Natl Acad Sci USA* 83: 4913–4917.

Guntz, P., Walter, C., Schosseler P., et al. 2010. Feasibility study of a screening assay that identifies the abnormal prion protein PrPTSE in plasma: Initial results with 20,000 samples. *Transfusion* 50: 989–995.

Gustaw, K. A., Garrett, M. R., Lee, H. G., et al. 2008. Antigen-antibody dissociation in Alzheimer disease: A novel approach to diagnosis. *J Neurochem* 106: 1350–1356.

Hampel, H., Frank, R., Brioch, K., et al. 2010. Biomarkers for Alzheimer's disease: Academic, industry and regulatory perspectives. *Nature Rev Drug Disc* 9: 560–574.

Hansson, O., Zetterberg, H., Buchhave, P., et al. 2006. Association between CSF biomarkers and incipient Alzheimer's disease in patients with mild cognitive impairment: A follow-up study. *Lancet Neurol* 5: 228–234.

Hardy, J., and Selkoe, D. J. 2002. The amyloid hypothesis of Alzheimer's disease: Progress and problems on the road to therapeutics. *Science* 297: 353–356.

Harold, D., Abraham, R., Hollingworth, P., et al. 2009. Genome-wide association study identifies variants at CLU and PICALM associated with Alzheimer's disease. *Nat Genet* 41: 1088–1093.

Hebert, L. E., Scherr P. A., Bienias J. L., et al. 2003. Alzheimer disease in the US population: Prevalence estimates using the 2000 census. *Arch Neurol* 60: 1119–1122.

Hollingworth, P., Harold, D., Sims, R., et al. 2011. Common variants at ABCA7, MS4A6A/MS4A4E, EPHA1, CD33 and CD2AP are associated with Alzheimer's disease. *Nat Genet* 43: 429–435.

Iqbal, K., Alonso Adel, C., Chen, S., et al. 2005. Tau pathology in Alzheimer disease and other tauopathies. *Biochim Biophys Acta* 1739: 198–210.

Jarrett, J. T., Berger, E. P., and Lansbury, P. T., Jr. 1993. The carboxy terminus of the beta amyloid protein is critical for the seeding of amyloid formation: Implications for the pathogenesis of Alzheimer's disease. *Biochemistry* 32: 4693–4697.

Jensen, M., Schroder, J., Blomberg, M., et al. 1999. Cerebrospinal fluid A beta42 is increased early in sporadic Alzheimer's disease and declines with disease progression. *Ann Neurol* 45: 504–511.

Kanai, M., Matsubara, E. Isoe, K., et al. 1998. Longitudinal study of cerebrospinal fluid levels of tau, A beta1-40, and A beta1-42(43) in Alzheimer's disease: A study in Japan. *Ann Neurol* 44: 17–26.

Kauwe, J. S., Wang, J., Mayo, K., et al. 2009. Alzheimer's disease risk variants show association with cerebrospinal fluid amyloid beta. *Neurogenetics* 10: 13–17.

Kayed, R., Head, E., Sarsoza, F., et al. 2007. Fibril specific, conformation dependent antibodies recognize a generic epitope common to amyloid fibrils and fibrillar oligomers that is absent in prefibrillar oligomers. *Mol Neurodegener* 2: 18.

Kim, S., Swaminathan, S., Shen, L., et al. 2011. Genome-wide association study of CSF biomarkers Abeta 1-42, t-tau, and p-tau181p in the ADNI cohort. *Neurology* 76: 69–79.

Lai, F., and Williams, R .S. 1989. A prospective study of Alzheimer disease in Down syndrome. *Arch Neurol* 46: 849–853.

Lambert, J. C., Heath, S., Even, G., et al. 2009. Genome-wide association study identifies variants at CLU and CR1 associated with Alzheimer's disease. *Nat Genet* 41: 1094–1099.

Lehto, M. T., Peery, H. E., and Cashman, N. R. 2006. Current and future molecular diagnostics for prion diseases. *Expert Review of Molecular Diagnostics* 6: 597–611.

Levy–Lahad, E., Wasco, W., Poorkaj, P., et al. 1995a. Candidate gene for the chromosome 1 familial Alzheimer's disease locus. *Science* 269: 973–977.

Levy–Lehad, E., Wijsman, E. M., Nemens, E., et al. 1995b. A familial Alzheimer's disease locus on chromosome 1. *Science* 269: 970–973.

Lewczuk, P., Esselmann, H., Otto, M., et al. 2004. Neurochemical diagnosis of Alzheimer's dementia by CSF Abeta42, Abeta42/Abeta40 ratio and total tau. *Neurobiol Aging* 25: 273–281.

Li, G., Sokal, I., Quinn, J. F., et al. 2007. CSF tau/Abeta42 ratio for increased risk of mild cognitive impairment: A follow–up study. *Neurology* 69: 631–639.

Lue, L. F., Kuo, Y. M., Roher, A. E., et al. 1999. Soluble amyloid beta peptide concentration as a predictor of synaptic change in Alzheimer's disease. *Am J Pathol* 155: 853–862.

Maes, O. C., Chertkow, H. M., Wang, E., et al. 2009. MicroRNA: Implications for Alzheimer disease and other human CNS disorders. *Curr Genomics* 10: 154–168.

Maes, O. C., Xu, S., Yu, B., et al. 2007. Transcriptional profiling of Alzheimer blood mononuclear cells by microarray. *Neurobiol Aging* 28: 1795–1809.

Masters, C. L., Cappai, R., Barnham, K. J., et al. 2006. Molecular mechanisms for Alzheimer's disease: Implications for neuroimaging and therapeutics. *J Neurochem* 97: 1700–1725.

Mattson, N., Blennow, K., and Zetterberg, H. 2010. Inter-laboratory variation in cerebrospinal fluid biomarkers for Alzheimer's disease: United we stand, divided we fall. *Clin Chem Lab Med* 48: 603–607.

Mayeux, R., Tang, M. X., Jacobs, D. M., et al. 1999. Plasma amyloid beta-peptide 1-42 and incipient Alzheimer's disease. *Ann Neurol* 46: 412–416.

McKhann, G., Drachman, D., Folstein, M., et al. 1984. Clinical diagnosis of Alzheimer's disease: Report of the NINCDS-ADRDA Work Group under the auspices of Department of Health and Human Services Task Force on Alzheimer's Disease. *Neurology* 34: 939–944.

McLean, C. A., Cherny, R. A., Fraser, F. W., et al. 1999. Soluble pool of Abeta amyloid as a determinant of severity of neurodegeneration in Alzheimer's disease. *Ann Neurol* 46: 860–866.

Mehta, P. D., Pirttila, T., Patrick, B. A., et al. 2001. Amyloid beta protein 1-40 and 1-42 levels in matched cerebrospinal fluid and plasma from patients with Alzheimer disease. *Neurosci Lett* 304: 102–106.

Morris, J. C., and Price, A. L. 2001. Pathologic correlates of nondemented aging, mild cognitive impairment, and early-stage Alzheimer's disease. *J Mol Neurosci* 17: 101–118.

Naj, A. C., Jun, G., Beecham, G. W., et al. 2011. Common variants at MS4A4/MS4A6E, CD2AP, CD33 and EPHA1 are associated with late–onset Alzheimer's disease. *Nat Genet* 43: 436–441.

Namba, Y., Tomonaga, M., Kawasaki, H., et al. 1991. Apolipoprotein E immunoreactivity in cerebral amyloid deposits and neurofibrillary tangles in Alzheimer's disease and kuru plaque amyloid in Creutzfeldt-Jakob disease. *Brain Res* 541: 163–166.

Nukina, N., and Ihara, Y. 1986. One of the antigenic determinants of paired helical filaments is related to tau protein. *J Biochem* 99: 1541–1544.

Oliver, C., and Holland, A. J. 1986. Down's syndrome and Alzheimer's disease: A review. *Psychol Med* 16:307–322.

Pan, T., Sethi, J., Nelsen, C, et al. 2007. Detection of misfolded prion protein in blood with conformationally sensitive peptides. *Transfusion* 47: 1418–1425.

Perrin, R. J., Craig-Schapiro, R., Malone, J. P., et al. 2011. Identification and validation of novel cerebrospinal fluid biomarkers for staging early Alzheimer's disease. *PLoS One* 6(1), doi:10.1371/journal.pone.0016032.

Perrin R. J., Fagan, A. M., and Holtzman, D. M. 2009. Multimodal techniques for diagnosis and prognosis of Alzheimer's disease. *Nature* 461: 916–922.

Pesaresi, M., Lovati, C., Bertora, P., et al. 2006. Plasma levels of beta–amyloid (1-42) in Alzheimer's disease and mild cognitive impairment. *Neurobiol Aging* 27: 904–905.

Petersen, R. C. 2004. Mild cognitive impairment as a diagnostic entity. *J Intern Med* 256: 183–194.

Pitschke, M., Prior, R., Haupt, M., et al. 1998. Detection of single amyloid β–protein aggregates in the cerebrospinal fluid of Alzheimer's patients by fluorescence correlation spectroscopy. *Nat Med* 4:832–834.

Poirier, J. 1994. Apolipoprotein E in animal models of CNS injury and in Alzheimer's disease. *Trends Neurosci* 17: 525–530.

Price, J., Ko, A, Wade, M., et al. 2001. Neuron number in the entorhinal cortex and CA1 in preclinical Alzheimer's disease. *Arch Neurol* 58: 1395–1402.

Raber, J., Huang, Y., and Ashford, J. W. 2004. ApoE genotype accounts for the vast majority of AD risk and AD pathology. *Neurobiol Aging* 25: 641–650.

Ray, S., Britschgi, M., Herbert, C., et al. 2007. Classification and prediction of clinical Alzheimer's diagnosis based on plasma signaling proteins. *Nat Med* 13: 1359–1362.

Rowe, C. C., Ng, S., Ackermann, U., et al. 2007. Imaging beta-amyloid burden in aging and dementia. *Neurology* 68: 1718–1725.

Sarsoza, F., Saing, T., Kayed, R., et al. 2009. A fibril-specific, conformation-dependent antibody recognizes a subset of Ab plaques in Alzheimer disease, Down syndrome and Tg2576 transgenic mouse brain. *Acta Neuropathol* 118: 505–517.

Saykin, A. J., Shen, L., Foroud T. M., et al. 2010. Alzheimer's disease neuroimaging initiative biomarkers as quantitative phenotypes: Genetics core aims, progress, and plans. *Alzheimer's Dement* 6: 265–273.

Schipper, H. M., Maes, O. C., Chertkow, H. M., et al. 2007. MicroRNA expression in Alzheimer blood mononuclear cells. *Gene Regul Syst Bio* 1: 263–274.

Seppala T. T., Herukka, S. K., Hanninen, T., et al. 2010. Plasma Abeta42 and Abeta40 as markers of cognitive change in follow-up: A prospective, longitudinal, population-based cohort study. *J Neurol Neurosurg Psychiatry* 81: 1123–1127.

Shankar, G. M., Li, S., Mehta, T. H., et al. 2008. Amyloid-beta protein dimers isolated directly from Alzheimer's brains impair synaptic plasticity and memory. *Nat Med* 14: 837–842.

Sherrington, R., Rogaev, E. I., Liang, Y., et al. 1995. Cloning of a gene bearing missense mutations in early-onset familial Alzheimer's disease. *Nature* 375: 754–760.

Shulman, J. M., Chibnik, L. B., Aubin, C., et al. 2010. Intermediate phenotypes identify divergent pathways to Alzheimer's disease. *PLoS One* 5(6), doi:10.1371/journal.pone.0011244.

Sobow, T., Flirski, M., Kloszewska, I., et al. 2005. Plasma levels of alpha beta peptides are altered in amnestic mild cognitive impairment but not in sporadic Alzheimer's disease. *Acta Neurobiol Exp* 65: 117–124.

Strittmatter, W. J., Weisgraber, K. H., Huang, D. Y., et al. 1993. Binding of human apolipoprotein E to synthetic amyloid beta peptide: Isoform-specific effects and implications for late-onset Alzheimer disease. *Proc Natl Acad Sci USA* 90: 8098–8102.

Sunderland, T., Wolozin, B., Galasko, D., et al. 1999. Longitudinal stability of CSF tau levels in Alzheimer patients. *Biol Psychiatry* 46: 750–755.

Tcherkasskaya, O., Davidson, E. A., Schmerr, M. J., et al. 2005. Conformational biosensor for diagnosis of prion diseases. *Biotechnol Lett* 27: 671–675.

Vandermeeren, M., Mercken, M., Vanmechelen, E., et al. 1993. Detection of tau proteins in normal and Alzheimer's disease cerebrospinal fluid with a sensitive sandwich enzyme-linked immunosorbent assay. *J Neurochem* 61: 1828–1834.

Vanderstichele, H., Van Kerschaver, E., Hesse, C., et al. 2000. Standardization of measurement of beta-amyloid(1-42) in cerebrospinal fluid and plasma. *Amyloid* 7:245–258.

Villemagne, V. L., Perez, K. A., Pike, K. E., et al. 2010. Blood-borne amyloid-b dimer correlates with clinical markers of Alzheimer's disease. *J Neurosci* 30: 6315–6322.

Wilmo, A., and Price, M. 2010. *World Alzheimer's Report 2010: The Global Economic Impact of Dementia*. London UK: Alzheimer's Disease International, http://www.alz.co.uk/research/files/World AlzheimerReport2010.pdf.

Xia, W., Yang, T., Shankar, G., et al. 2009. A specific enzyme-linked immunosorbent assay for measuring β-amyloid protein oligomers in human plasma and brain tissue of patients with Alzheimer disease. *Arch Neurol* 66: 190–199.

Zetterberg, H., Mattsson, N., Blennow, K., et al. 2010. Use of theragnostic markers to select drugs for phase II/III trials for Alzheimer disease. *Alzheimer's Res Ther* 2: 32.

Zetterberg, H. Pedersen, M., Lind, K., et al. 2007. Intra-individual stability of CSF biomarkers for Alzheimer's disease over two years. *J Alzheimer's Dis* 12: 255–260.

3 Imaging Biomarkers for Diagnosis, Prognosis, and Treatment of Alzheimer's Disease

Daniel M. Skovronsky and Giora Z. Feuerstein

CONTENTS

3.1 INTRODUCTION

Alzheimer's disease (AD) is one of the most studied illnesses in contemporary medicine as its medical burden on elderly populations, societies at large, and national health services is daunting (Lovestone, 2009; Weiner and Lipton, 2009). The lack of disease-modifying prophylactic and therapeutic agents and the difficulties in diagnosing people at risk to develop AD, or already at preclinical, very early cognitive, or neuropsychiatric stages, continues to impose major medical challenges as it becomes clear that limited therapeutic benefits can be garnered when probable AD is diagnosed clinically. AD patients present substantial unmet medical need as disease-modifying agents have not been realized in spite of several decades of intense research and attempts for clinical development of therapeutic agents consuming billions of dollars. Over this background, leading researchers and institutes from academia, government, and industry have emphasized the need for focused efforts on translational medicine and biomarker discovery, development, and validation for AD (Khachaturian et al., 2010; Hampel et al., 2010; Petanceska et al., 2009). Indeed, major efforts are underway to identify biomarkers (genetic, genomic, biochemical, physiological) that might serve disease risk assessment, disease progression, and response to treatment. At this time, several biomarker studies are undergoing validation as surrogate biomarkers that may allow drug registration for treatment, diagnosis of subclinical disease, or identification of very early (pre-minimal cognitive impairment) MCI (Hampel et al., 2010; Borroni et al., 2006). Some of the difficulties in this regard are clearly the result of still insufficient understanding of the mechanisms that trigger the pathological processes of AD, maintain and amplify these processes along with temporal and confounding factors across the decades of AD evolution. Contemporary knowledge on putative mechanisms of AD focus on extracellular amyloid beta (Aβ) and the intracellular pathology associated with tau proteins (Kim et al., 2011; Shaw et al., 2011; Brunden et al., 2009), although many other molecular pathways (such as oxygen radicals, inflammatory mediators, neurotransmitters) continue to be studied (Shaw et al., 2011).

The quest for biomarkers that report on brain structure, functions, and molecular and biochemical processes that typify AD and its variant manifestations, have yielded many strategies based on various technologies and approaches. The structural approach utilizes imaging of brain volume/structure at regions of interest using x-rays, high resolution computed tomography (CT) scans, or magnetic resonance imaging (MRI). The functional approaches use methods that report on neuronal functions such as metabolic activity ([18]FDG-glucose), functional MRI (fMRI) (elicited neuronal activity), or electrophysiological procedures. The molecular approaches focus on the putative molecular mechanisms that are suspected to play a cardinal role in neuronal degeneration and synaptic inhibition/destruction. It appears that contemporary leading strategies consider multimodal technologies and their biomarker derivatives in the form of imaging and biochemical biomarkers (Ewers et al., 2010; Jack, Wist et al., 2010; Hu et al., 2010; Landau et al., 2010). In search of disease biomarkers, and especially disease-modifying biomarkers that could predict AD initiation and early progression, the Aβ cascade elements have taken central stage over the past two decades. The human APP protein and its protease cleavage products (especially Aβ(1-40)/(1-42), their aggregates and fibers) have been analyzed in biological specimens obtained from AD patients (and counterpart experimental models of AD) and have been intensely studied for correlation with the AD in cross-sectional and longitudinal studies. Most notable are efforts led by the consortium of academia, government, and industry (Alzheimer's Disease Neuroimaging Initiative, ADNI), which focuses on delivery of a validated biomarker-driven, "road map" for AD therapeutic development and clinical trials.

In parallel, efforts to track brain Aβ cascade elements via imaging biomarkers have been advanced into clinical studies. Thus, certain small organic molecules (e.g., Pittsburgh Compound B or [PIB]) have been shown to associate with AD plaque when transformed into positron emission tomography (PET)-imaging tools. Such imaging agents have shown high sensitivity in predicting definitive AD corroborating to AD postmortem pathology. Longitudinal PET imaging of brain Aβ have also emerged in some mild cognitive impairment (MCI) studies that show potential (Foster, 2009; Jack, Knopman et al., 2010). Since Aβ oligomers/aggregates (Aβ-OLM/AGG) have been shown to bear direct toxicities to neurons (Watson et al., 2005), monitoring these elements could also be important in assessing Aβ burden and AD evolution, as well as monitoring the efficacy of anti-Aβ drugs that inhibit Aβ monomer synthesis (thereby potentially reducing the oligomer and aggregate burden in the brain and cerebrospinal fluid [CSF]).

In summary, intense efforts to develop biomarkers that provide sensitive, accurate, and reproducible information at onset, progression, mechanism, and drug responses have taken center stage in AD early diagnosis, treatment, and prognosis of AD.

3.2 VOLUMETRIC BRAIN IMAGING IN ALZHEIMER'S DISEASE: COMPUTERIZED TOMOGRAPHY AND MAGNETIC RESONANCE IMAGING

3.2.1 COMPUTERIZED TOMOGRAPHY (CT)

Chronic degenerative diseases are invariably associated with structural changes in the brain, both at macroscopic and microscopic levels. Such is also the case in AD where loss of brain tissue/volume at large, and disparate structural changes over the decades of disease, become prominent features in both the *in life* (antemortem) and postmortem inspection of the brain. Imaging of these changes is an integral part of dementia and AD diagnosis, management, and prognosis via multimodal technological approaches.

Magnetic resonance imaging (MRI) and computerized tomography (x-ray based, CT) are the two leading techniques to assess structural changes in brain tissue, albeit with some fundamental differences and complementarities. CT provides images that are of particular usefulness in assessing bone structure, brain calcification, volume and configuration of the brain ventricular system, as well as lesions within this system, and brain sulci formations. Application of CT in evaluation of dementias is still considered of value in the era of fast progression of MRI, although it has largely taken a "backseat" in dementia (e.g., AD) structural imaging research (Brenner and Hall, 2007).

3.2.2 MAGNETIC RESONANCE IMAGING (MRI)

MRI has numerous advantages as the preferred imaging technology in AD. MRI enables the reader to discern, in superior resolution, grey matter from white matter and identify areas of hyperintensities in the aging brain. Furthermore, MRI provides significantly better three-dimensional images that provide both coronal and sagittal images of small brain regions of particular interest to cognitive function such as the hippocampus. Flexibility in parameters of data acquisition furthers the visual accuracy and details as compared to CT.

While the utility of MRI in dementia and AD medical management is undisputable, there are certain limitations in its utility. One prominent issue is the need to eliminate patients who carry ferromagnetic implants. While interferences by such foreign materials in routine imaging are minimal, exclusion of patients suspected to carry such foreign bodies might require x-ray in addition to detailed history. MRI is particularly hazardous for patients carrying pacemakers. Scanner claustrophobia due to the confining space in the scanner imposes some difficulties that in certain cases require open scanners or CT. It needs to be acknowledged that MRI takes more time and is more expensive.

As mixed dementias become more common with age, assessment of the vascular component of the cognitive/dementia situation can be aided with MRI (Scheider et al., 2007). Structural imaging is sensitive to cerebrovascular diseases. However, the high sensitivity of MRI to changes in water content results in overestimation or white matter abnormalities. Fluid-attenuated inversion recovery (FLAIR) in addition to T-2 weighted MRI is needed for accurate assessment. It is important to note that evidence of cerebrovascular disease on imaging is insufficient to exclude AD as it is considered by experts that AD pathology is often the primary factor for cognitive decline in older persons with cerebrovascular diseases (Fein et al., 2000). Gradient echo MRI showing cortical microhemorrhages typical of cerebral amyloid angiopathy also provide indirect evidence for AD. Although MRI is best to identify vascular lesions, F18-PET (FDG-PET, see the next section) can help discern the cognitive consequences of such lesions.

3.3 FUNCTIONAL AND MOLECULAR IMAGING IN DEMENTIA: FDG-PET

Brain metabolic activity at resting and activated states has been used extensively for the past two decades in research and clinical evaluation of many brain disorders, including various forms of dementias. Since glucose is the sole source of energy for neurons, it closely tracks synaptic activity. Glucose uptake into neurons (dendrites, axons, synapses) can be monitored with a glucose derivative, 6-deoxy-glucose, which can be up-taken into these neuronal structures but cannot be further metabolized. When this glucose derivative is tagged with a positron emission isotope (such as F18), the accumulation rate and extent can be noninvasively monitored by PET within minutes. Fluorodeoxyglucose (FDG) has therefore become an important technology to assess a patient's brain metabolism. The metabolic state registered (indirectly) via ^{18}F-PET signals report on the functional intactness and integrity of brain areas of interest. In normal persons at rest, brain metabolism shows disparate activities in various brain regions with basal ganglia, thalamus, cerebellum, and brain cortex showing augmented metabolic states over brain stem regions and white matter. FDG-PET is a very sensitive method to track neuronal damage and synaptic malfunction. Dementia states are associated with global decline in glucose hypometabolism that carries distinct regional patterns underlined by the disease and in association with symptoms. Thus individual differences in regional FDG-PET signals represent, with high fidelity, symptoms associated with the afflicted brain region. Significant hypometabolic FDG-PET signals in the frontal regions are likely to be present in dementia manifested in behavioral disturbances. In this regard, dementia-associated FDG-PET hypometabolic recording is considered to represent mostly the "synaptic traffic" rather than neuronal efficiency.

In practice, the utility of FDG-PET imaging finds an important role in the differential diagnosis of dementias, such as differentiation of AD from frontotemporal dementia (FTD), because of the clear contrasting patterns of hypometabolism (Foster et al., 2007). The test is recognized for its utility and reimbursed by many health care management facilities and Medicare as a supplemental tool needed for optimization of dementia patients' management (Hodges and Patterson, 2007). FDG-PET also provides objective evidence supporting a neurodegenerative condition. In such cases, a clear hypometabolic pattern better defines the patient's diagnostic and prognostic status. FDG-PET imaging in AD has consistent regional patterns: frequently early hypometabolic state can be identified in the cingulated gyrus, followed by the associated parietal and posterior temporal cortical regions with further spread as the disease progresses into frontal, and in fact global, hypometabolic state. The visual (occipital) cortex is relatively spared and so also the brain stem and cerebellum.

Since synaptic loss (rather than neurons and axons) is a hallmark of early Alzheimer's disease, FDG-PET might be especially suitable to identify early disease stages in individuals at risk, such as people with compelling genetic/familial background or apoE4 homozyge genotype. Furthermore, many nondemented individuals identified with MCI have FDG-PET metabolic signals similar to AD and are more likely to develop AD over time (Anchist et al., 2005).

In summary, FDG-PET imaging technology has advanced from an experimental research tool to a useful part of dementia patients' management, including diagnosis, differential diagnosis, and prognostic aid along with other imaging and medical practices in dementia management.

3.4 AMYLOID PLAQUES AS A TARGET FOR IMAGING

Both of the widely used neuropathological criteria for postmortem diagnosis of Alzheimer's disease (Mirra et al., 1991; NIA Reagan Working Group, 1997) rely on the presence of brain neuritic plaques as a required diagnostic feature. The Consortium to Establish a Registry for Alzheimer's Disease (CERAD) diagnostic criteria provides guidelines for categorization of neuritic amyloid plaque burden as *none, sparse, moderate,* or *frequent* (Mirra et al., 1991; Mirra et al., 1993). The CERAD criteria describe the use of these categories (taking into account the patient's symptoms, other neuropathologies, and age at death) to generate a neuropathologic diagnosis (Mirra et al., 1991). In patients who die with dementia, frequent or moderate plaque burden is considered indicative of the diagnosis of AD (definite AD or probable neuropathologic AD), and lack of neuritic plaques (i.e., none) precludes the pathologic diagnosis of AD (Mirra et al., 1991).

The National Institute on Aging and the Reagan Institute Working Group on Diagnostic Criteria for the Neuropathological Assessment of Alzheimer's Disease published updated criteria for postmortem diagnosis of AD in 1997, commonly referred to as the NIA-Reagan criteria (NIA Reagan, 1997). These criteria also relied on the CERAD methodology for categorization of neuritic amyloid plaque burden and converted these categories to neuropathologic diagnoses, taking into account the patients' neurofibrillary tangle burden. In patients with a CERAD frequent plaque score and neocortical neurofibrillary tangles, NIA-Reagan criteria assign a "high likelihood that dementia is due to AD." In patients with a CERAD moderate plaque score and limbic neurofibrillary tangles, NIA-Reagan criteria assign an "intermediate likelihood that dementia is due to AD." In patients with a CERAD plaque score of sparse or low, NIA-Reagan criteria assign a "low likelihood that dementia is due to AD" (NIA Reagan, 1997).

Thus, detection of neuritic amyloid plaques at autopsy is a required criterion for postmortem diagnosis of AD, with the presence of frequent to moderate plaques at autopsy being considered consistent with a diagnosis of AD (NIA Reagan, 1997). Given the central role that amyloid plaque detection plays in postmortem diagnosis, development of in vivo techniques for amyloid plaque detection by molecular imaging has been an important goal for the AD research field (Klunk and Mathis, 2008; Wolk and Klunk, 2009). Indeed, the advent of techniques for in vivo imaging of amyloid plaques has been highlighted as a major breakthrough in clinical neuroscience (Rabinovici and Jagust, 2009).

3.4.1 ^{11}C-PIB

While the first attempt to image amyloid plaques in vivo used a labeled anti-Ab antibody (Friedland et al., 1997), the first successful amyloid-specific imaging agent was ^{11}C-Pittsburgh Compound B, commonly known as ^{11}C-PiB (Klunk et al., 2004). ^{11}C-PiB is a derivative of thioflavin-T (Figure 3.1), which binds specifically and sensitively to the fibrillar beta-amyloid aggregates that comprise amyloid plaques (Klunk et al., 2005). The ^{11}C radiolabel allows for detection by PET; however, the use of ^{11}C-PiB is limited to research centers with on-site cyclotrons and radiopharmaceutical manufacturing due to the 20-minute half-life of [11]C.

PET studies in humans using ^{11}C-PiB show a significant difference in signal between subjects clinically diagnosed with AD and cognitively normal controls with increased retention of tracer in AD subjects as compared to controls. Retention of

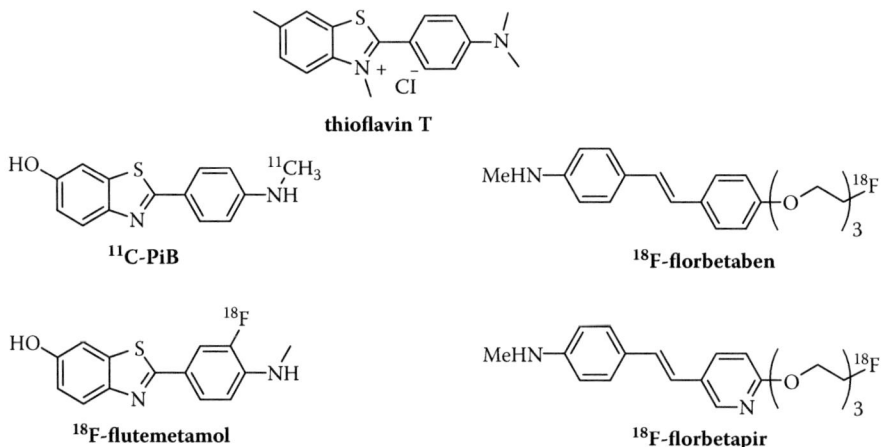

FIGURE 3.1 Chemical structure of thioflavin T, 11C-PiB, ^{18}F-flutemetamol, ^{18}F-florbetaben, and 18F-florbetapir.

[11]C-PiB in AD subjects is particularly high in neocortical regions known to be affected by amyloid plaques, including prefrontal cortex, posterior cingulate/precuneus, lateral parietal regions, and lateral temporal cortex (Klunk et al., 2004; Rowe et al., 2007).

While most cognitive normal subjects have negative ^{11}C-PiB PET scans, AD-like patterns of uptake can be found in a significant proportion of cognitively normal elderly subjects (Mintun et al., 2006; Rowe et al., 2007), suggesting that PET scans are detecting amyloid plaques in these individuals. Indeed, the prevalence of amyloid-positive PET scans in cognitively normal subjects ranges from 10% to 30%, depending on age, which closely matches the prevalence of moderate-to-frequent neuritic amyloid plaques documented in the autopsy literature (Mintun et al., 2006; Aizenstein et al., 2008; Reiman et al., 2009; Braak and Braak, 1997). Interestingly, cross-sectional analysis has shown a correlation between amyloid burden assessed on PET scan and poorer cognitive performance as measured by memory testing (Villemagne et al., 2008; Reiman et al., 2009; Pike et al., 2007). Longitudinal studies confirm that cognitively normal individuals who are amyloid positive are more likely to have had declining cognitive test scores over the preceding years and to progress to symptomatic AD (Villemagne et al., 2008; Morris et al., 2009; Storandt et al., 2009). Thus, the weight of current data suggests that amyloid in cognitively normal subjects is associated with subclinical decreases of memory performance, leading some to hypothesize that amyloid in cognitively normal subjects may suggest incipient AD (Rabinovici and Jagust, 2009).

In subjects with MCI, a bimodal distribution of amyloid levels can be seen, with a significant fraction of MCI patients (40–80%) showing AD-like retention of ^{11}C-PiB and others showing no appreciable ^{11}C-PiB retention (Forsberg et al., 2008; Jack et al., 2008; Rowe et al., 2007; Wolk and Klunk, 2009; Pike et al., 2007). As in cognitively normal individuals, studies show a negative correlation between amyloid burden on PET scan and episodic memory scores at baseline (Forsberg et al., 2008; Mormino et al., 2009; Pike et al., 2007). Indeed, patients with MCI who are amyloid positive on PET scan are at increased risk for clinical progression and conversion to AD as compared to those who are amyloid negative (Okello et al., 2009; Forsberg et al., 2008).

The development of ^{11}C-PiB has demonstrated proof of concept for amyloid imaging. Its use in research laboratories around the world has opened new avenues for investigation, allowing for the first time, longitudinal studies exploring the role of amyloid in aging. However, the short half-life of [11]C ($T_{1/2} = 20$ minutes) limits its use to academic research centers with PET cyclotrons and radiochemistry facilities. To overcome this obstacle, three different amyloid imaging agents labeled with [18]F ($T_{1/2} = 110$ minutes) are now in late-stage development (Figure 3.1). The longer half-life of ^{18}F has permitted the widespread availability of ^{18}F-FDG through regional production at commercial cyclotrons and distribution to local imaging centers. A similar approach may be possible for distribution of ^{18}F-labeled amyloid imaging agents (Jagust, 2010).

3.4.2 ^{18}F-FLUTEMETAMOL

[18]F-flutemetamol (also known as 18F-GE067) is an ^{18}F-labeled derivative of Pittsburgh Compound B (Koole et al., 2009). Phase I clinical trials showed that ^{18}F-flutemetamol

had acceptable radiation dosimetry (Koole et al., 2009), and significant differences in brain retention could be quantified between AD subjects and controls (Nelissen et al., 2009). In a Phase II clinical trial, 27 subjects with AD and 15 healthy volunteers were scanned with ^{18}F-flutemetamol (Vandenberghe et al., 2010). Scans from 25 of 27 AD subjects were rated as positive, and scans from 14 of 15 healthy volunteers were rated as negative. In the Phase II trial, ^{18}F-flutemetamol images were acquired for 30 minutes, beginning 85 minutes following injection and were co-registered with MRIs for quantitative analysis. There were good correlations between ^{18}F-flutemetamol scans and ^{11}C-PiB scans in patients who had both studies for most regions analyzed; however, in pons and subcortical white matter, ^{18}F-flutemetamol showed more pronounced retention than did ^{11}C-PiB, possibly due to higher nonspecific white-matter binding (Vandenberghe et al., 2010). Multiple ongoing Phase III trials, sponsored by GE Healthcare, are reported on ClinicalTrials.gov (NCT01028053, NCT01165554).

3.4.3 ^{18}F-FLORBETABEN

[18]F-florbetaben (also known as 18F-AV-1 or 18F-BAY94-9172) is an ^{18}F-labeled stilbene derivative initially developed by Hank Kung and colleagues at the University of Pennsylvania (Zhang et al., 2005). In a Phase I trial of ^{18}F-florbetaben, 15 patients with AD, 15 healthy elderly controls, and five individuals with frontotemporal lobar degeneration (FTLD) were studied. All AD patients showed increased tracer retention, consistent with the reported postmortem distribution of amyloid plaques. Most healthy controls and FTLD patients showed only nonspecific white-matter binding, although three controls and one FTLD patient had significant uptake in frontal and precuneus cortex. In a second Phase I trial (O'Keefe et al., 2009), ^{18}F-florbetaben was shown to have acceptable radiation dosimetry. In a Phase II clinical trial, 81 patients with AD and 69 healthy controls were imaged with ^{18}F-florbetaben, and scans were visually interpreted by three blinded raters (Barthel et al., 2011). Eighty percent of the AD patients showed positive scans, and 91% of the controls showed negative scans based on median visual reads. Inter-reader agreement, as measured by Kappa, was 0.56 or greater (where 1.0 indicates perfect agreement). In the Phase II trial, the primary analysis was conducted on ^{18}F-florbetaben images that were acquired for 20 minutes, beginning 90 minutes following injection; however, other time points (including a 15-minute scan acquired 45 minutes following injection) were explored with similar results. An ongoing Phase III trial, sponsored by Bayer, is reported on ClincialTrials.gov (NCT01070838).

3.4.4 ^{18}F-FLORBETAPIR

[18]F-florbetapir (also known as 18F-AV-45) is an ^{18}F-labeled styryl-pyridine derivative initially developed by Hank Kung and colleagues at the University of Pennsylvania (Zhang et al., 2007). The compound shows high binding affinity and specificity for amyloid plaques in vitro (Choi et al., 2009). In a Phase I trial of ^{18}F-florbetapir, 16 patients with AD and 16 cognitively normal healthy controls were studied. PET scans showed significant discrimination among AD patients and controls using quantitative methods (Wong et al., 2010). In a second Phase I

trial (Lin et al., 2010), ^{18}F-florbetapir was shown to have acceptable radiation dosimetry. A total of 269 subjects received ^{18}F-florbetapir in two Phase I and three Phase II studies. A pooled Phase I/Phase II analysis of these subjects showed that AD, MCI, and older health controls participants differed significantly in mean cortical florbetapir uptake with 81% of AD subjects, 40% of MCI subjects, and 21% of cognitively normal subjects showing significant amyloid levels (Fleisher et al., 2011). Among cognitively normal controls, percent positivity increased linearly by age decile and was highest in APOE ε4 carriers (Fleisher et al., 2011). A Phase III clinical trial of ^{18}F-florbetapir was conducted to determine if PET imaging with this compound accurately predicted the presence of amyloid pathology in the brain at autopsy. The study involved 152 subjects who were imaged, of whom 35 came to autopsy within 12 months. In these 35 subjects (15 of whom met pathologic criteria for AD), there was a significant correlation between ^{18}F-florbetapir PET results and the presence and quantity of amyloid pathology at autopsy as measured by immunohistochemistry and silver stain neuritic plaque score (Clark et al., 2011). A control group of 74 younger cognitively normal individuals was also enrolled in this study, and 100% had scans rated as negative. In the Phase II and III trials, ^{18}F-florbetapir images were acquired for 10 minutes, beginning 50 minutes following injection. A New Drug Application (NDA) was submitted for ^{18}F-florbetapir by Avid Radiopharmaceuticals, and a Food and Drug Administration (FDA) advisory panel gave conditional support for approval contingent on additional training for radiologists (Ledford, 2011). Multiple ongoing trials, including the Alzheimer's Disease Neuroimaging Initiative and several therapeutic trials that evaluate ^{18}F-florbetapir as a potential biomarker, are reported on ClinicalTrials.gov (e.g. NCT01231971).

3.4.5 ROLE OF AMYLOID PET IMAGING IN EMERGING DIAGNOSTIC CRITERIA FOR AD

New research criteria for diagnosis of AD were published by Dubois and colleagues in 2007 (Dubois et al., 2007) and updated in 2010 (Dubois et al., 2010). These criteria rely on evidence of both specific memory changes and in vivo markers of Alzheimer's pathology (including amyloid imaging or other biomarkers) for the clinical diagnosis of AD dementia or prodromal AD (depending on clinical severity). In addition, the criteria provide for identification of a preclinical state of AD called *asymptomatic at-risk state for AD* by in vivo evidence of amyloidosis in the brain (Dubois et al., 2010).

Similarly, the National Institute on Aging–Alzheimer's Association workgroup has published new guidelines for diagnosis of AD (McKhann et al., 2011), diagnosis of MCI due to AD (Albert et al., 2011), and for defining preclinical stages of AD (Sperling et al., 2011). The AD guidelines define a new diagnosis, "Probable AD dementia with evidence of the AD pathophysiological process," which requires biomarker evidence of AD pathophysiology, including amyloid PET imaging (McKhann et al., 2011). Biomarker use is not advocated for routine diagnosis but rather is suggested as an optional clinical tool for use when deemed appropriate by the clinician. For the diagnosis of MCI due to AD and preclinical AD, biomarker evidence of AD pathology (e.g., amyloid PET imaging) is recommended for use for research criteria, for example, to define subjects for enrollment in clinical trials (Sperling et al., 2011; Albert et al., 2011).

3.5 AMYLOID BETA CASCADE ELEMENTS (AGGREGATE) IMAGING

The recognition that Aβ cascade elements, such as oligomers and aggregates, might play an important role in the evolution of AD plaque (insoluble amyloid fiber formation), neuronal death (direct neurotoxicity), and synaptic dysfunction has compelled research on means to identify and modulate Aβ oligomers and aggregate formation. Moreover, efforts to devise a way to monitor brain oligomers and aggregate burden that might complement biochemical biomarkers of the amyloid cascade have recently yielded new opportunities. Such an example is the engineering of peptides that have the propensity to more selectively bind to Aβ aggregates and oligomers. This technology, termed Pronucleon™, generates unique Aβ-sequence derivatives by rational design and modeling (See Chapter 2 for complete description). Addition of pyrenated moieties at the N- and C-termini allows the cardinal property, that is, monitoring the selectivity of the designed peptide for binding to Aβ-OLM/AGG as measured by fluorescence methods. The selectivity of these designed Pronucleon peptides toward Aβ-OLM/AGG is a unique property not shared by other known methods, which is further evidence that the association of these probes with amyloid Aβ aggregates has come from preclinical models of disease. Pronucleon probes have been injected intravenously into transgenic (Tg2576) mice that express human forms of the amyloid precursor protein, exhibit amyloid plaque formation in the brain, and show impaired learning and memory functions compared to wild-type mice. In mice with late-stage disease, it was shown that Pronucleon probes crossed the blood–brain barrier and associated with plaque structures that cross-react with monoclonal antibodies to the

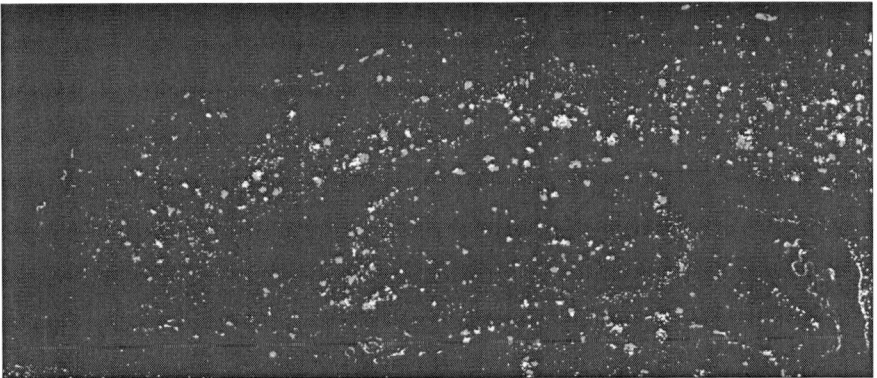

FIGURE 3.2 (See color insert.) Fluorescent micrograph of brain histopathology of reactive Pronucleon™ peptide probes (blue) following intravenous administration in a transgenic mouse model (Tg2576) of Alzheimer's disease. The micrograph is a typical image from a sagittal section of mouse brain in late stage (>10 months) disease. The mice were sacrificed 15 minutes following injection. The sections are co-stained with monoclonal antibodies to Aβ (6E10) (red).

N-terminus of Ab, and also exhibit some independent staining of punctate structures that may represent other aggregates or oligomers that are components of Alzheimer's pathology (Figure 3.2, and Wegrzyn, Nyborg, Duan, and Rudolph, unpublished data). These data, depicted in Figure 3.2, provide compelling evidence that Pronucleon peptides can access the brain and identify plaques no less than standard methods.

In summary, these preliminary data suggest that monitoring of Aβ oligomers and aggregates might be feasible using new tools and compounds that specifically recognize Aβ cascade elements that could afford early detection of augmented burden of Aβ *mid-cascade* toxic element at the time when plaques and fibers are sparse and are not likely to be consistently detectable.

3.6 SUMMARY

Amyloid PET imaging is rapidly becoming a core neuroimaging tool for research of brain aging and dementia (Rabinovici and Jagust, 2009). The initial catalyst for this field was the development of ^{11}C-PiB, which has proved to be a critical research tool (Villemagne et al., 2008). Now there are three new ^{18}F-labeled amyloid imaging agents, designed for widespread application, that are in late-stage clinical development for dementia diagnosis and prediction of progression in MCI (Jagust, 2010). New guidelines and diagnostic criteria are being developed to help guide the appropriate use of these new research tools (Dubois et al., 2010; McKhann et al., 2011).

REFERENCES

Aizenstein, H. J., Nebes, R. D., and Saxton, J. A., et al. 2008. Frequent amyloid deposition without significant cognitive impairment among the elderly. *Arch Neurol* 65(11): 1509–1517.

Albert, M. S., Dekosky, S. T., and Dickson, D., 2011. The diagnosis of mild cognitive impairment due to Alzheimer's disease: Recommendations from the National Institute on Aging-Alzheimer's Association workgroups on diagnostic guidelines for Alzheimer's disease. *Alzheimer's Dement* 7(3): 270–279.

Anchist, D., Borroni, B., Franceschi, M., et al. 2005. Heterogeneity of brain glucose metabolism in mild cognitive impairment and clinical progression of to Alzheimer disease. *Arch Neurol* 62(11): 1728–1733.

Bathel, H., Gertz, H. J., Dresel, S., et al. 2011. Cerebral amyloid-β PET with florbetaben ((18)F) in patients with Alzheimer's disease and healthy controls: a multicentre phase 2 diagnostic study. *Lancet Neurol* 10(5): 424–435.

Borroni, B., Di Luca, M., and Padovani, A. 2006. Predicting Alzheimer dementia in mild cognitive impairment patients: Are biomarkers useful? *Eur J Pharmacol* 545(1): 73–80.

Braak, H., and E. Braak. 1997. Diagnostic criteria for neuropathologic assessment of Alzheimer's disease. *Neurobiol Aging* 18(4 Suppl): S85–88.

Brenner, D. J., and E. J. Hall. 2007. Computed tomography: An increasing source of radiation exposure. *N Eng J Med* 357(22): 2277–2284.

Brunden, K. R., Trojanowski, J. Q., and Lee, V. M. 2009. Advances in tau–focused drug discovery for Alzheimer's disease and related tauopathies. *Nat Rev Drug Discov* 8(10): 783–793.

Choi, S. R., Golding, G., Zhuang, Z., et al. 2009. Preclinical properties of 18F-AV-45: A PET agent for Abeta plaques in the brain. *J Nucl Med* 50(11): 1887–1894.

Clark, C. M., Schneider, J. A., Bedell, B. J., et al. 2011. Use of florbetapir-PET for imaging beta-amyloid pathology. *JAMA* 305(3): 275–283.

Dubois, B., Feldman, H. H., Jacova, C., et al. 2007. Research criteria for the diagnosis of Alzheimer's disease: Revising the NINCDS-ADRDA criteria. *Lancet Neurol* 6(8): 734–746.

Dubois, B., Feldman, H. H., Jacova, C., et al. 2010. Revising the definition of Alzheimer's disease: a new lexicon. *Lancet Neurol* 9(11): 1118–1127.

Ewers, M., Walsh, C., Trojanowski, J. Q., et al. 2010. Prediction of conversion from mild cognitive impairment to Alzheimer's disease dementia based upon biomarkers and neuropsychological test performance. *Neurobiol Aging*, December 13, http://www.ncbi.nlm.nih.gov/pubmed/21159408 [E-pub ahead of print].

Fein, G., Di Sclafani, V., Tanabe, J., et al. 2000. Hippocampal and cortical atrophy predict dementia in subcortical ischemic vascular disease. *Neurology* 55(11): 1626–1635.

Fleisher, A., Chen, K., Liu, X, et al., 2011 Florbetapir-PET imaging of cortical amyloid in Alzheimer's disease and mild cognitive impairment. *Arch Neurol* July 11, http://www.ncbi.nlm.nih.gov/pubmed/21747008 [E-pub ahead of print].

Forsberg, A., Engler, H., Almkvist, O., et al. 2008. PET imaging of amyloid deposition in patients with mild cognitive impairment. *Neurobiol Aging* 29(10): 1456–1465.

Foster, N. L. 2009. Neuroimaging. In *Textbook of Alzheimer Disease and Other Dementias*, ed. M. F. Weiner and A. M. Lipton. Washington, DC: American Psychiatric Publishing.

Foster, N. L., Heidebrink, J. L., Clark, C. M., et al. 2007. FGD-PET improves accuracy in distinguishing frontotemooral dementia and Alzheimer disease. *Brain* 130(10): 2616–2635.

Friedland, R. P., Kalaria, R., Berridge, M., et al. 1997. Neuroimaging of vessel amyloid in Alzheimer's disease. *Ann N Y Acad Sci* 826: 242–247.

Hampel, H., Frank, R., Broich, K., et al. 2010. Biomarkers for Alzheimer's disease: Academic, industry and regulatory perspective. *Nat Rev Drug Discov* 9(7): 560–574.

Hodges, J. R., and Patterson, K. 2007. Semantic dementia: A unique clinic-pathological syndrome. *Lancet Neurol* 6(11): 1004–1014.

Hu, W. T., McMillan, C., Libon, D., et al. 2010. Multimodal predictors for Alzheimer disease in nonfluent primary progressive aphasia. *Neurology* 75(7): 595–602.

Jack, C. R. Jr., Knopman, D. S., Jagust, W. J., et al. 2010. Hypothetical model of dynamic biomarkers of the Alzheimer's pathological cascade. *Lancet Neurol* 9(1): 119–128.

Jack, C. R. Jr., Lowe, V. J., Senjem, M. L., et al. 2008. 11C PiB and structural MRI provide complementary information in imaging of Alzheimer's disease and amnestic mild cognitive impairment. *Brain* 131(3): 665–680.

Jack, C. R., Jr., Wiste, H. J., Vemuri, P., et al. 2010. Brain beta-amyloid measures and magnetic resonance imaging atrophy both predict time-to-progression from mild cognitive impairment to Alzheimer's disease. *Brain* 133(11): 3336–3348.

Jagust, W. J. 2010. Amyloid imaging: Coming to a PET scanner near you. *Ann Neurol* 68(3): 277–278.

Khachaturian, Z. S., Barnes, D., Einstein, R., et al. 2010. Developing a national strategy to prevent dementia: Leon Thal Symposium 2009. *Alzh & Dem* 6(2): 89–97.

Kim, S., Swaminathan, S., Shen, L., et al. 2011. Genome-wide association study of CSF biomarkers Abeta1-42, t-tau, and p-tau181p in the ADNI cohort. *Neurology* 76(1): 69–79.

Klunk, W. E., Engler, H., Nordberg, A., et al. 2004. Imaging brain amyloid in Alzheimer's disease with Pittsburgh Compound-B. *Ann Neurol* 55(3): 306–319.

Klunk, W. E., Lopresti, B. J., Ikonomovic, M. D., et al. 2005. Binding of the positron emission tomography tracer Pittsburgh compound-B reflects the amount of amyloid-beta in Alzheimer's disease brain but not in transgenic mouse brain. *J Neurosci* 25(46): 10598–10606.

Klunk, W. E., and Mathis, C. A. 2008. The future of amyloid-beta imaging: A tale of radionuclides and tracer proliferation. *Curr Opin Neurol* 21(6): 683–687.

Koole, M., Lewis, D. M., Buckley, C., et al. 2009. Whole-body biodistribution and radiation dosimetry of 18F-GE067: A radioligand for in vivo brain amyloid imaging. *J Nucl Med* 50(5): 818–822.

Landau, S. M., Harvey, D., Madison, C. M., et al. 2010. Comparing predictors of conversion and decline in mild cognitive impairment. *Neurology* 75(3): 230–238.

Ledford, H. 2011. Alzheimer's-disease probe nears approval. *Nature* 469(7331): 458.

Lin, K. J., Hsu, W. C., Hsiao, I. T., et al. 2010. Whole-body biodistribution and brain PET imaging with [18F]AV-45, a novel amyloid imaging agent: A pilot study. *Nucl Med Biol* 37(4): 497–508.

Lovestone, S. 2009. Biomarkers in brain diseases. *Annals N Y Acad Sci* 1180: vii.

McKhann, G. M., Knopman, D. S., and Chertkow, H., 2011. The diagnosis of dementia due to Alzheimer's disease: Recommendations from the National Institute on Aging-Alzheimer's Association workgroups on diagnostic guidelines for Alzheimer's disease. *Alzheimer's Dement* 7(3): 263–269.

Mintun, M. A., Larossa, G. N., Sheline, Y. I., et al. 2006. [11C]PIB in a nondemented population: Potential antecedent marker of Alzheimer disease. *Neurology* 67(3): 446–452.

Mirra, S. S., Hart, M. N., and Terry, R. D. 1993. Making the diagnosis of Alzheimer's disease. A primer for practicing pathologists. *Arch Pathol Lab Med* 117(2): 132–144.

Mirra, S. S., Heyman, A., McKeel, D., et al. 1991. The Consortium to Establish a Registry for Alzheimer's Disease (CERAD). Part II. Standardization of the neuropathologic assessment of Alzheimer's disease. *Neurology* 41(4): 479–486.

Mormino, E. C., Kluth, J. T., Madison, C. M., et al. 2009. Episodic memory loss is related to hippocampal-mediated beta-amyloid deposition in elderly subjects. *Brain* 132(5): 1310–1323.

Morris, J. C., Roe, C. M., Grant, E. A., et al. 2009. Pittsburgh compound B imaging and prediction of progression from cognitive normality to symptomatic Alzheimer disease. *Arch Neurol* 66(12): 1469–1475.

National Institute on Aging, and the Reagan Institute Working Group on Diagnostic Criteria for the Neuropathological Assessment of Alzheimer's Disease. 1997. Consensus recommendations for the postmortem diagnosis of Alzheimer's disease. Neurobiol Aging 18(4 Suppl): S1–2.

Nelissen, N., Van Laere, K., Thurfjell, L., et al. 2009. Phase 1 study of the Pittsburgh compound B derivative 18F-flutemetamol in healthy volunteers and patients with probable Alzheimer disease. *J Nucl Med* 50(8): 1251–1259.

O'Keefe, G. J., Saunder, T. H., Ng, S., et al. 2009. Radiation dosimetry of beta-amyloid tracers 11C-PiB and 18F-BAY94-9172. *J Nucl Med* 50(2): 309–315.

Okello, A., Koivunen, J., Edison, P., et al. 2009. Conversion of amyloid positive and negative MCI to AD over 3 years: An 11C-PIB PET study. *Neurology* 73(10): 754–760.

Petanceska, S., Ryan, L., Silverberg, N., et al. 2009. Commentary on "a roadmap for the prevention of dementia II. Leon Thal Symposium 2008." Alzheimer's disease translational research programs at the National Institute on Aging. *Alzheimer's Dement* 5(2): 130–132.

Pike, K. E., Savage, G., Villemagne, V. L., et al. 2007. Beta-amyloid imaging and memory in non–demented individuals: Evidence for preclinical Alzheimer's disease. *Brain* 130(11): 2837–2844.

Rabinovici, G. D., and Jagust, W. J. 2009. Amyloid imaging in aging and dementia: Testing the amyloid hypothesis in vivo. *Behav Neurol* 21(1): 117–128.

Reiman, E. M., Chen, K., Bandy, D., et al. 2009. Fibrillar amyloid-beta burden in cognitively normal people at 3 levels of genetic risk for Alzheimer's disease. *Proc Natl Acad Sci USA* 106(16): 6820–6825.

Rowe, C. C., Ng, S., Ackermann, U., et al. 2007. Imaging beta-amyloid burden in aging and dementia. *Neurology* 68(20): 1718–1725.

Scheider, J. A., Arvanitakis, Z., Bang, W., et al. 2007. Mixed brain pathologies account for most dementia cases in community dwelling older persons. *Neurology* 69(24): 2197–2204.

Shaw, L. M., Vanderstichele, H., Knapik-Czajka, M., et al. 2011. Qualification of the analytical and clinical performance of CSF biomarker analyses in ADNI. *Acta Neuropathol* 121(5): 597–609.

Sperling, R. A., Aisen, P. S., Beckett, L. A., et al. 2011. Toward defining the preclinical stages of Alzheimer's disease: Recommendations from the National Institute on Aging-Alzheimer's Association workgroups on diagnostic guidelines for Alzheimer's disease. *Alzheimer's Dement* 7(3): 280–292.

Storandt, M., Mintun, M. A., Head, D., et al. 2009. Cognitive decline and brain volume loss as signatures of cerebral amyloid-beta peptide deposition identified with Pittsburgh compound B: Cognitive decline associated with Abeta deposition. *Arch Neurol* 66(12): 1476–1481.

U.S. National Institutes of Health. "Assess the Prognostic Usefulness of Flutemetamol (18F) Injection for Identifying Subjects With Amnestic Mild Cognitive Impairment Who Will Convert to Clinically Probable Alzheimer's Disease." http://clinicaltrials.gov/ct2/show/NCT01028053

U.S. National Institutes of Health. "Phase III Study of Florbetaben (BAY94-9172) PET Imaging for Detection/Exclusion of Cerebral β-amyloid Compared to Histopathology." http://clinicaltrials.gov/ct2/show/NCT01020838

U.S. National Institutes of Health. "Positron Emission Tomography (PET) Imaging of Brain Amyloid Compared to Post-Mortem Levels." http://clinicaltrials.gov/ct2/show/NCT01165554

U.S. National Institutes of Health. "Positron Emission Tomography (PET) Amyloid Imaging of the Brain in Healthy Young Adult Subjects." http://clinicaltrials.gov/ct2/show/NCT01265394

Vandenberghe, R., Van Laere, K., and Ivanoiu, A., 2010. 18F–flutemetamol amyloid imaging in Alzheimer disease and mild cognitive impairment: A phase 2 trial. *Ann Neurol* 68(3): 319–329.

Villemagne, V. L., Fodero-Tavoletti, M. T., Pike, K. E., et al. 2008. The ART of loss: Abeta imaging in the evaluation of Alzheimer's disease and other dementias. *Mol Neurobiol* 38(1): 1–15.

Villemagne, V. L., Pike, K. E., Darby, D., et al. 2008. Abeta deposits in older non-demented individuals with cognitive decline are indicative of preclinical Alzheimer's disease. *Neuropsychologia* 46(6): 1688–1697.

Watson, D., Castan, E., Kokjohn, T. A., et al. 2005. Physicochemical characteristics of soluble oligomeric Ab and their pathologic role in Alzheimer's disease. *Neurology Research* 27: 869–881.

Weiner, M. F., and Lipton, A. M., eds. 2009. *Textbook of Alzheimer Disease and Other Dementias*. Washington, DC: American Psychiatric Publishing.

Wolk, D. A., and Klunk, W. 2009. Update on amyloid imaging: From healthy aging to Alzheimer's disease. *Curr Neurol Neurosci Rep* 9(5): 345–352.

Wong, D. F., Rosenberg, P. B., Zhou, Y., et al. 2010. In vivo imaging of amyloid deposition in Alzheimer disease using the radioligand 18F-AV-45 (Flobetapir F 18). *J Nucl Med* 51(6): 913–920.

Zhang, W., Kung, M. P., Oya, S., et al. 2007. 18F-labeled styrylpyridines as PET agents for amyloid plaque imaging. *Nucl Med Biol* 34(1): 89–97.

Zhang, W., Oya, S., Kung, M. P., et al. 2005. F-18 stilbenes as PET imaging agents for detecting beta–amyloid plaques in the brain. *J Med Chem* 48(19): 5980–5988.Ôb

4 The Current Status of Alzheimer's Disease Treatment: Why We Need Better Therapies and How We Will Develop Them

Krista L. Lanctôt, Ida Kircanski, Sarah A. Chau, and Nathan Herrmann

CONTENTS

4.1 INTRODUCTION

In 2050, the number of older people in the world will surpass the number of younger people for the first time in history (United Nations, 2002). Alzheimer's disease (AD) is an illness of the aging population and is currently one of the leading causes of death. It is the most common form of dementia, accounting for about 60% to 80% of cases (Alzheimer's Association, 2010). An estimated 35.6 million people worldwide are living with AD and other types of dementias, a number expected to almost double every 20 years (Alzheimer's Disease International, 2010). The annual worldwide costs of dementia are estimated to be US\$604 billion (Alzheimer's Disease International, 2010). This progressive and fatal neurodegenerative disorder is steadily leading to a public health crisis in developed countries around the world.

The last two decades of clinical research in AD have resulted in the regulatory approval of only five drug treatments, including four cholinesterase inhibitors (tacrine, donepezil, rivastigmine, and galantamine) and an N-methyl-d-aspartate (NMDA)-receptor antagonist (memantine). Tacrine is rarely prescribed due to significant risks of hepatocellular death (Knapp et al., 1994; Watkins et al., 1994; Blackard et al., 1998) and questionable efficacy (Food and Drug Administration, 1991). The remaining four therapies are considered to be symptomatic treatments, improving cognition or functional ability for a limited period of time, rather than halting or reversing the advancement of the disease. These medicines consistently demonstrate small, but statistically significant effects on primary outcomes in trials of AD. While donepezil is used for all stages of severity in the United States, rivastigmine and galantamine are indicated for mild to moderate AD, and memantine for moderate to severe AD (Birks, 2006; McShane et al., 2006). Evidence shows that the three cholinesterase inhibitors demonstrate similar levels of efficacy, and that no one treatment is considerably better than another (Birks, 2006; Lanctôt et al., 2003).

Much research throughout the last decade has focused on the discovery of disease-modifying drugs. Of the myriad agents that have undergone clinical testing, none have successfully demonstrated disease modification in AD. The focus of research has also shifted toward discovering more effective symptomatic treatments than those currently available, as well as examining the cognitive changes occurring in the early or presymptomatic stages of the disease, in the hopes of establishing preventative therapies.

Despite achieving encouraging results in preclinical phases of testing, potential drug treatments have thus far failed on primary endpoints. In order to meet our objectives in the years to come, it is imperative that we review current clinical trial methodologies. Specifically, there is a need to critically examine the standard outcome measures pertaining to the four commonly assessed domains (cognition, global status, function, and behavior).

Once the aging brain begins to undergo pathological changes within the neuronal infrastructure leading to neuronal loss, it is difficult to reverse these changes and prevent further neurodegeneration. It is likely that disease-modifying treatments would be most effective if administered for a long period of time, starting in the early or prodromal stages of the disease trajectory. It is uncertain whether current outcome scales would detect changes occurring in response to such agents, as they may be administered too early in the disease process. Additionally, deficiencies in standard scales, such as the reduced sensitivity to change across disease severities, may limit the interpretation of clinically meaningful treatment effects and impede successful drug development.

4.2   EVOLVING DIAGNOSTIC CRITERIA

One of the first and most influential guidelines regarding clinical diagnostic criteria in AD was created by the National Institute of Neurological and Communicative Disorders and Stroke (NINCDS) and the Alzheimer's Disease and Related Disorders Association (ADRDA) in 1984 (McKhann et al., 1984). These criteria divide patients into categories for possible, probable, and definite AD based on relevant factors, such as presenting symptoms or family history. A task force created by the National Institute on Aging and the Alzheimer's Association recently revisited these criteria and proposed that patients be classified as having probable AD dementia, possible AD dementia, or possible and probable AD dementia, wherein the first two classifications are intended for clinical purposes and the third for research settings (McKhann et al., 2011). Other widely used diagnostic criteria include the *Diagnostic and Statistical Manual of Mental Disorders*, 4th edition (*DSM-IV*-TR) of the American Psychiatric Association (American Psychiatric Association, 2000) and the *International Classification of Diseases* (*ICD*-10) from the WHO (World Health Organization, 1992). *DSM-5* criteria are currently underway and are expected to be released in 2013 (First, 2010).

4.3   HEALTH REGULATORY GUIDELINES

Methodological concerns that evolved during the tacrine trials in the 1980s gave rise to guidelines and interim reports published by the Food and Drug

Administration (FDA), detailing a standardized approach to clinical investigations in dementia (Schmitt and Wichems, 2006). Those documents emphasized the inclusion of a concurrent control group, randomization, and double-blinding as critical components of systematic testing procedures. As cognitive decline embodies the core characteristic of AD, an externally validated cognitive measure was required for staging and demonstrating efficacy of the putative compound. Aside from cognitive benefits, evidence of a clinically meaningful effect was declared necessary. A measure of global change was thus mandatory in trials of AD. Phase 3 trials were required to recruit a minimum of 1000 patients, of which one third were to receive a dose at or above the median recommended dose for at least 6 months.

Since then, multiple sets of guidelines for AD have been published in the United States and Europe. In 2008, the European Medicines Agency (EMA) issued a guideline document addressing diagnostic criteria, assessment of therapeutic efficacy, pharmacokinetic measures, and evaluation of safety in this population (European Medicines Agency, 2008). The EMA states that improvement of symptoms upon treatment with an antidementia agent should be measured using outcomes in cognition and activities of daily living (ADL) (coprimary endpoints), as well as a global assessment of change (secondary endpoint). In addition, clinical studies in AD should be at least six months in duration, and the treatment effect should be presented in terms of the proportion of patients who achieve a clinically meaningful benefit.

Recent years have led to advances in technology, especially regarding the detection of biomarkers indicative of AD. Biomarkers have the potential to enhance sensitivity and specificity for AD, especially in the early stages of the clinical course (DeKosky et al., 2011). Researchers have outlined potential revisions for clinical diagnostic criteria, which incorporate the use of molecular and biochemical biomarkers and imaging techniques (DeKosky et al., 2011; McKhann et al., 2011). At the present time, primary endpoints in trials of AD are expected to remain clinical in nature. Thus, magnetic resonance imaging, positron emission tomography, and cerebrospinal fluid assays can only act as supporting evidence for clinical measures (DeKosky et al., 2011). According to European guidelines for the development of antidementia drugs (European Medicines Agency, 2008), the claim that an agent possesses disease-modifying capabilities can only be substantiated if clinical improvement on standard scales is demonstrated in combination with molecular or neuroimaging data, depicting evidence of biological modification (such as a delay in brain atrophy).

4.4 CURRENT OUTCOME MEASURES

Treatment groups in clinical research studies are often compared in terms of change on psychometric scales specific to the following four domains: cognition, activities of daily living, global assessment of change, and behavior. The usefulness of these psychometric scales is evaluated using historically accepted criteria. Satisfactory measurement tools should be externally validated, be sensitive to small changes across the range of disease severity, have good inter-rater and test–retest reliability, and exhibit minimal floor, ceiling, and practice effects over time. It is also important that the tests have a short duration, be standardized across diverse cultures, and be available in many languages (European Medicines Agency, 2008; Black et al., 2009).

At present, the scales most commonly used to measure cognitive changes are the Alzheimer's Disease Assessment Scale-cognitive subscale (ADAS-Cog) (Mohs and Cohen, 1988), the Mini-Mental Status Examination (MMSE) (Folstein et al., 1975), and the Severe Impairment Battery (SIB) (Saxton et al., 1990). For activities of daily living or self-care, the complete 23-item or modified 19-item Alzheimer's Disease Cooperative Study Activities of Daily Living (ADCS-ADL$_{19 \text{ or } 23}$) (Galasko et al., 1997) and the Disability Assessment for Dementia (DAD) scale (Gelinas et al., 1998) are most often employed, while global status is usually measured by the Clinician's Interview-Based Impression of Change plus Caregiver Input (CIBIC-Plus) (Joffres et al., 2000), Alzheimer's Disease Cooperative Study–Clinical Global Impression of Change (ADCS-CGIC) (Schneider et al., 1997) or Clinical Dementia Rating (CDR) (Berg, 1988). Behavioral disturbances are most frequently assessed using the Neuropsychiatric Inventory (NPI) (Cummings et al., 1994; Cummings, 1997).

4.4.1 COGNITION

The ADAS-Cog scale (Mohs and Cohen, 1988) is the gold standard for the evaluation of cognitive function in clinical trials of dementia, particularly for patients with mild to moderate severity. This scale includes components of memory, language, attention, and constructional and ideational praxis (Connor and Sabbagh, 2008). It originally consisted of 11 items, but has since been revised to contain additional items, such as digit-cancellation, maze completion, and delayed recall in word-learning tasks, in order to improve validity and sensitivity to detecting impairment across a range of severities (Mohs et al., 1997; Mohs and Cohen, 1988). The total score ranges from 0 to 70 (a higher score indicates poorer cognitive performance). The ADAS-Cog has been shown to be both valid and reliable (Rosen et al., 1984; Weyer et al., 1997), and is generally considered more comprehensive than the alternative cognitive measurement tools (Graham et al., 2004).

Despite its many advantages, the ADAS-Cog has several notable limitations. Past studies have demonstrated that factors such as gender (males achieve slightly better scores) and age (younger age is correlated with better scores), as well as level of education, influence ADAS-Cog performance (Weyer et al., 1997; Doraiswamy et al., 1995). Thus, the level of impairment in individuals with higher education may not be distinguishable from those with no impairment and less education (Graham et al., 2004). Designing a cognitive battery that is standardized across gender, age, and level of education would be ideal.

A comprehensive review by Chiu and Lam (2007) provides a discussion of culture and region-specific factors that may affect performance on the ADAS-Cog, such as literacy levels, relevance of specific items, test-taking skills, motivation, and differences in word imagery. The changing definition of a clinically meaningful result across different nations is also discussed. Many developing countries lack the funds and resources required for using biomarkers as a diagnostic criterion, and therefore rely solely on traditional outcome scales (Chiu and Lam, 2007). As a result, it is of critical importance that outcome scales be available in different languages and be standardized across many cultures to allow for meaningful and unbiased comparisons.

In addition, one study conducted by Connor and Sabbagh (2008) using 26 raters at a clinical trials meeting demonstrated significant variation in the way raters administer and score the items on the ADAS-Cog. A lack of consistency and reliability has the potential to confound the comparison of outcome measures between clinical trials.

Perhaps the most commonly noted limitation of the ADAS-Cog is its susceptibility to floor and ceiling effects (Black et al., 2009). A recent study (Cano et al., 2010) reported substantial ceiling effects in 7 out of 11 items in mild to moderate AD patients, while another (Sevigny et al., 2010) noted ceiling effects in spoken language ability and comprehension, among other items in mild AD. These findings implicate a reduced sensitivity of the ADAS-Cog to detect impairment in AD patients, especially in those with mild AD or mild cognitive impairment (MCI). Additionally, as patients progress to the severe stages of their disease, their loss of language and motor function may subject their performance to floor effects.

The SIB was designed specifically for patients who are not able to complete regular neuropsychological testing due to severe cognitive impairment (Saxton et al., 1990). This 100-point instrument consists of 57 questions and has been extensively implemented in clinical research studies of AD (Reisberg et al., 2003; Winblad et al., 2006; Tariot et al., 2004). The SIB can be divided into several subscales, including language, orientation, praxis, memory, social skills, visuospatial perception, construction, and attention (Boller et al., 2002). It has also been validated in various languages and is considered to have good inter-rater and test–retest reliability (Verny et al., 1999; Panisset et al., 1992; Llinas Regla et al., 1995; Pippi et al., 1999).

The SIB takes approximately 30 minutes to complete (Boller et al., 2002). A short form was also developed, as this length of administration time may be approaching the attention limit of some patients, particularly those with increased agitation (Saxton et al., 2005). This version was recently evaluated in a sample of 264 nursing home patients with moderate to severe dementia, and proved to have sufficient inter-rater and test–retest reliability (de Jonghe et al., 2009).

A third scale commonly used in clinical research for screening and description of severity, is the MMSE (Folstein et al., 1975). It is scored on a scale of 0–30, where a higher score indicates less cognitive impairment. As a general rule, patients belong to one of four categories, including intact functioning (MMSE score between 26–30), mild dementia (score 21–25), moderate dementia (score 11–20), or severe dementia (score ≤10) (Mungas, 1991). The reliability and construct validity of this test have been affirmed (Folstein et al., 1975; Tombaugh and McIntyre, 1992). However, the sensitivity of this test is commonly disputed. The MMSE seems to have a high sensitivity for moderate to severe levels of impairment, but low sensitivity for detecting change at mild levels of impairment (Espinoza, 2001; Tombaugh and McIntyre, 1992).

Similar to the ADAS-Cog, performance on the MMSE is thought to be influenced by several noncognitive factors. A population-based survey of community-dwelling Mexican Americans found that factors including age, marital status, immigrant status, years of education, and language of interview were related to test scores

(Black et al., 1999). Gender, however, does not seem to influence performance on the MMSE (Tombaugh and McIntyre, 1992).

The MMSE was not intended as a diagnostic test, but rather as a complementary screening test to assess the degree of cognitive impairment in the context of a comprehensive physician's assessment. It is useful for tracking cognitive changes over time (Tombaugh and McIntyre, 1992).

4.4.2 INDEPENDENT FUNCTION AND SELF-CARE

Persons afflicted with AD typically experience a steady loss of independence when performing everyday activities. This decline in self-care and functional abilities is progressive and ultimately incapacitating. Activities of daily living (ADL) are usually divided into instrumental ADL (IADL), such as handling money or cleaning, and the simpler, basic ADL (BADL), such as toileting and eating. Several scales are used to track functional decline in terms of IADL and BADL, including the ADCS-ADL (Galasko et al., 1997) and the DAD (Gelinas et al., 1998).

The ADCS-ADL inventory is a structured interview developed by the Alzheimer's Disease Cooperative Study group. Galasko and colleagues initially tested 45 items in 242 AD patients and 64 elderly controls, and of those, 23 items were eventually selected for use. This version is scored from 0–78, where a score of 78 represents no impairment (Livingston et al., 2004). A 19-item version was later designed for use in patients with moderate to severe AD only (Galasko et al., 2005).

The DAD scale was specifically developed for community-dwelling individuals with dementia, but has since been used as a clinical research tool in trials of AD. It has established content, construct validity, and reliability (inter-rater, test–retest, internal consistency) and takes approximately 15 minutes to complete. The domains assessed include components of BADL and IADL, as well as leisure activities, initiation, planning, and effective performance of an intended action.

A review produced by the Alzheimer's Association Research roundtable meeting in 2009 concluded that current functional scales overemphasize measurement of BADL and IADL, while ineffectively testing social function, such as the capability for social interaction, degree of withdrawal, or confidence in social settings (Black et al., 2009). Moreover, functional scales are largely dependent on informant interviews, introducing an inherent source of bias due to the subjective opinions and interpretations of the informants, recall bias, and a lack of clinician judgment.

4.4.3 GLOBAL ASSESSMENT OF CHANGE

Assessments of global change are built on the notion that any change detected by an experienced physician is clinically meaningful. These scales generally possess little structure and are not sensitive enough to detect small (clinically insignificant) changes in overall function. Thus, they have lower inter-rater reliability than their counterparts (Schneider et al., 1997).

The ADCS-CGIC (Schneider et al., 1997) is one of the principal scales used to measure global change. It is intended for determining a patient's overall functioning, and examines 15 different subject areas pertaining to social engagement, daily functioning, cognition, and behavior, using input from both the patient and caregivers. Patients, assessed at baseline and follow-up, are assigned a score from 1 to 7, wherein 1 indicates a marked improvement, 4 indicates no change, and 7 designates a significant worsening. The CGIC contains more structure than other global measures, such as the CIBIC-Plus, and therefore exhibits better inter-rater reliability and validity (Schneider et al., 1997).

Another widely used global measure, the CIBIC-Plus, includes data on changes in disease severity, cognition, behavior, function, general appearance, and history of the patient (Joffres et al., 2000). Good face and predictive validity were demonstrated, as scores on the CIBIC-Plus were associated with that of the CDR, Global Deterioration Scale (GDS), and MMSE. A reasonable sensitivity to change over 24- to 30-week clinical trials was also shown (Schneider et al., 1997). In order to diminish the risk of bias, the CIBIC was originally proposed to include an interview with the patient only. However, information given by caregivers was later included, as patients with AD are not considered independently reliable sources.

The CDR (Berg, 1988) is also frequently used for global assessment, as well as staging. The CDR was developed as a result of the Memory and Aging project in 1977. Multiple items, including memory, orientation, judgment and problem solving, community affairs, hobbies, and personal care are rated on a scale of 0–3 by the patient or an appropriate caregiver. This scale is considered the most structured of the global assessments and has good sensitivity toward clinically meaningful change (Black et al., 2009).

4.4.4 BEHAVIOR

Behavioral disturbances, including agitation, aggression, apathy, or hallucinations are common in patients with AD. These symptoms are known to increase caregiver burden, and significantly contribute to both direct and indirect costs of patient care (Herrmann et al., 2006). Despite their importance, regulatory authorities do not require agents to demonstrate efficacy in treating behavioral abnormalities. As a result, treatment effect on behavior is not always incorporated as an outcome measure. When it is included, the NPI (Cummings et al., 1994; Cummings, 1997) is most often used as a measurement scale.

The NPI consists of 12 subscales representing various domains, including agitation/aggression, disinhibition, anxiety, irritability/lability, delusions, hallucinations, dysphoria, euphoria, apathy, and aberrant motor activity. A significant advantage of this test is that the severity and frequency of each behavioral symptom is incorporated into the final score. This type of assessment is reflective of a patient's overall behavior and is easy to interpret. The NPI has reasonable content validity, as well as test–retest and inter-rater reliability (Cummings et al., 1994). As this test relies on information provided by caregivers, it is exposed to a certain degree of subjectivity. The lack of clinician judgment and specificity to the range of dementia severities are commonly cited limitations (David et al., 2010).

Deficiencies in the NPI as a behavioral assessment have been described in a review by Gauthier et al. (2010). At times, a substantial change in only one or two individual domains is not enough to produce a change in the total score, while minor changes on a large number of domains may considerably affect the total score. Therefore, the total NPI score may sometimes misrepresent a true shift in behavioral patterns (Gauthier et al., 2010). It is also useful to analyze NPI symptom domains on an individual basis, since agents with more selective properties may produce effects on a limited number of subdomains (Gauthier et al., 2010).

In 2010, the widely used NPI was revised by the NPI-C Research Group (de Medeiros et al., 2010). The revised version, called the NPI-Clinician (NPI-C) rating scale, includes expanded domains and items, as well as a clinician-rating methodology. The authors noted several limitations of the traditional NPI as a rationale for designing the NPI-C, including a lack of depth of individual NPI domains (limiting their utility in the assessment of individual neuropsychiatric symptoms), data acquisition from informants or caregivers only (versus direct patient observation), uncertain reliability of individual items as opposed to global domain ratings, a decreased sensitivity to change compared to assessments that include a clinician's judgment, and a limited number of items specific for moderate or severe AD (de Medeiros et al., 2010). Most items on the NPI-C were found to have good inter-rater reliability, as well as convergent validity for clinician ratings (de Medeiros et al., 2010).

A common alternative scale to the NPI is the Behavioral Pathology in Alzheimer's Disease Rating Scale (BEHAVE-AD) (Reisberg et al., 1987). Scales assessing individual neuropsychiatric symptoms have also been developed, such as the Cohen-Mansfield Agitation Inventory (CMAI) (Cohen-Mansfield and Libin, 2004) and the Cornell Scale for Depression in Dementia (CSDD) (Alexopoulos et al., 1988).

4.5 BIOMARKERS IN CLINICAL TRIALS

Although neuropsychological tests of cognition and function are the standard in clinical trials of AD drugs, there is an increasing call for the incorporation of biomarkers in evaluating trial outcomes. In the development of candidates and during the preclinical stage, biomarkers may serve as a means to assess drug pharmacokinetics and pharmacodynamics, ultimately defining effects at varying doses. In clinical practice, biomarkers may be utilized to create a more powerful set of diagnostic tools available for physicians. Recently, NINCDS-ADRDA criteria for AD have been revised to include neuroimaging, cerebrospinal fluid, and genetic testing (DeKosky et al., 2011). Given the detectable differences in specific biomarker presentation between patients at the early stages of dementia and healthy individuals, diagnosis can be made for presymptomatic AD. For the MCI population, this could signify a more dependable means of identifying those at high risk for progressing to AD. With respect to clinical trials, biomarkers are being used to monitor drug candidate effects on disease pathology and patient safety as secondary outcomes. While trials using cognitive, functional, or global assessments as primary endpoints have been successful in validating drugs that provide symptomatic relief, they have thus far failed to identify disease-modifying treatments. Neuropsychological tests may not possess the sensitivity required to detect disease-modifying effects within the given time frame of current trial designs, thus potentially giving credence to the use of biomarkers. The goal of research in this field is to establish biomarkers as reliable surrogate endpoints for measuring efficacy more accurately.

4.5.1 Neuroimaging Biomarkers

Brain imaging techniques can illustrate the anatomical changes that accompany the progression of Alzheimer's disease. Clinical studies have employed structural magnetic resonance imaging (MRI), functional MRI (fMRI), magnetic resonance spectroscopy (MRS), and positron emission tomography (PET) as secondary endpoints. Structural MRIs reveal atrophy, an indication of neuronal loss, in specific regions depending on the type of dementia (Small, 2008). Regional neural processing can be measured with blood oxygen level–dependent (BOLD) fMRI to determine activation deficits that may be unrelated to atrophy (Logothetis, 2002). Brain biochemical and metabolic information can be obtained from MRS and glucose-consumption from PET. Radioligands specific for AD-related proteins such as Aβ can also be used with PET to examine pathological accumulation. Imaging results may provide differential diagnoses and distinguish between treatment arms in drug trials.

4.5.1.1 Structural MRI

The high spatial resolution of MRIs provides reliable data on the structure of brain regions that are compromised in AD. Atrophy of the hippocampus has been primarily implicated in AD when compared with healthy controls (Duara et al., 2008; Jack et al., 2000) and shows strong correlations with decline in cognition (Fleischman et al., 2005). The sensitivity of the hippocampal volume as a biomarker has been reported to be 76–84% with a specificity of approximately 90% (Laakso et al., 1998; Morinaga et al., 2010). Cortical thickness, as well, had a high specificity (90%) in differentiating AD patients with controls (Lerch et al., 2008). Whole brain volume analysis can also differentiate AD patients and unaffected individuals, with patients demonstrating significantly greater and more rapid loss in total volume (Fox et al., 2000).

However, hippocampal reduction associated with normal aging introduces a confounding factor in distinguishing between healthy elderly and those with AD. Although, a longitudinal study revealed the value of hippocampal mapping in predicting conversion of MCI to AD following 3 years (Apostolova et al., 2006). Additionally, marked atrophy was found in cognitively normal elderly who eventually had a diagnosis of MCI 3 years following and AD 6 years following. In cognitively normal elderly, cortical thinning assessed by MRI was predictive of conversion to AD approximately a decade later (Dickerson et al., 2011). The data from this longitudinal study also suggest initial cortical thickness measurements could predict the time of dementia onset. Whole brain and hippocampal volume is currently being employed, as secondary endpoints, in phase II and III trials to assess whether the candidate drug can slow atrophy and related cognitive and functional deficits.

4.5.1.2 Functional MRI

Decreases in hippocampal activity quantified by fMRI mirrors the atrophy shown in structural imaging. In clinical studies with AD patients, treatment with cholinesterase inhibitors (ChEIs) changed activation in attention networks, including the dorsal visual pathway (Kircher et al., 2005; Bokde et al., 2009), and the hippocampus during a recognition task (Goekoop et al., 2006). Pairing fMRI with tasks evaluating the specific deficits present in AD provides a potential means of identifying related neural correlates and activation patterns. Further, changes in neural processing and recovery of closer-to-normal activation induced by treatments might represent an appropriate surrogate endpoint in late-phase trials.

4.5.1.3 Proton-MRS

The chemical composition of brain regions can be measured with proton-MRS (^{1}H-MRS) using the marker amino acid N-acetyl aspartate (NAA) to gauge mitochondria function (Moffett et al., 2007). Alzheimer's patients have reduced NAA levels, independent of atrophy, which is shown to increase with ChEI treatment (Jessen et al., 2006). Additionally, response to medication and NAA changes are correlated and low baseline NAA predicted positive treatment effects. This imaging technique may be a valuable complement to MRI information in multicenter studies where the technology is available.

4.5.1.4 PET

Cerebral glucose metabolism, an implicit indicator of synaptic function, is measured with ^{18}F-2-fluoro-2-deoxy-d-glucose (FDG)-PET. The uptake of radioligand FDG is reduced in cognitive regions such as temporoparietal, posterior cingulate, and frontal cortex (Yuan et al., 2010), and can distinguish AD from other neurodegenerative disorders (Mosconi, 2005). FDG-PET has a much higher sensitivity (93–94%) than MRI but lower specificity (73–78%) for AD compared with control (Silverman et al., 2011). In clinical trials, glucose metabolism improved in patients treated with ChEIs and phenserine, and furthermore, increased cortical activation was positively correlated with cognitive improvements (Mega et al., 2005; Stefanova et al., 2006; Kadir et al., 2008). The use of this technique in large-scale trials may be limited by costs and accessibility across centers.

The quantification of amyloid plaque burden in the brain can be performed with ^{11}C-labeled Pittsburgh Compound B (^{11}C-PiB), a radioligand with binding sites on Aβ sheets and not the soluble proteins (Lockhart et al., 2007). Greater binding of this compound is observed in AD patients compared with controls (Klunk et al., 2004). However, ^{11}C-PiB uptake does not increase during progression of AD, despite continued cognitive deterioration (Engler et al., 2006). Increases in ^{11}C-PiB uptake occur in prodromal AD but stabilize during the clinical stage of the disorder (Jack et al., 2009). Thus, this radioligand may be useful as a diagnostic marker, though its value as a surrogate endpoint is more unclear. Other amyloid-associated tracers with longer half-lives using the F18 isotope, such as florbetapir, are currently under investigation (Clark et al., 2011; Okamura and Yanai, 2010). Amyloid tracers provide an approach to measure the effects of drugs that target the amyloidogenic cascade.

4.5.2 BIOCHEMICAL BIOMARKERS

In order to examine the pathological events occurring in Alzheimer's disease, biochemical markers are studied in both preclinical and clinical research. Amyloid and tau pathology have been the most popular hypotheses of the underlying causes of the disorder and subsequently, a multitude of drug candidates currently under investigation target elements of these pathways. Biomarkers in the cerebrospinal fluid (CSF) and serum are measured, though the usefulness of plasma amyloid and tau protein levels is not well established. In clinical trials, biochemical biomarkers are widely used as a secondary endpoint; their value could also be a surrogate endpoint to track changes in pathways associated with the disease.

4.5.2.1 CSF Biomarkers

There are four well-established CSF biomarkers currently used in clinical trials: $A\beta40$, $A\beta42$, phosphorylated tau (p-tau), and total tau (t-tau). The $A\beta42$ or $A\beta42/A\beta40$ ratio is reduced in AD patients, which is intuitive given that the $A\beta42$ isoform, secreted from amyloid precursor protein (APP), is the main constituent of extracellular amyloid plaques in the brain (Olsson et al., 2005). $A\beta42$ reductions have exhibited 90–96% sensitivity and 77–80% specificity (Andreasen et al., 2001; Shaw et al., 2009) while the $A\beta42/A\beta40$ ratio showed 86% sensitivity and 60% specificity in discriminating AD patients from unaffected elderly. The neurofibrillary tangles composed of phosphorylated tau are another hallmark of AD. Increases in intracellular phosphorylated tau are indicative of AD pathology (Buerger et al., 2006), while total tau is a nonspecific marker of axonal damage, a fundamental aspect of neurodegeneration (Blennow et al., 1995). Total tau levels have been shown to be associated with disease severity (Andersson et al., 2007), an observation not found for $A\beta42$ (Stefani et al., 2006). Both t-tau and p-tau have demonstrated sensitivity and specificity between 80% and 90% (Hampel et al., 2008). The combination of tau and $A\beta$ quantification has excellent sensitivity in differentiating various types of dementia in the early stages of the disease (Fagan et al., 2007) and could enhance assessments of outcomes in clinical trials.

Other potential biomarkers either reflect different constituents of the amyloid cascade or other hypotheses of the causes of AD. A reassessment of the amyloid hypothesis identified elevated concentrations of soluble $A\beta$ oligomers, not polymeric aggregates, as the key factor of pathogenesis (Pimplikar, 2009). $A\beta$ oligomers, β-site amyloid precursor protein-cleaving enzymes (BACE1), and soluble nonaggregating isoforms of APP were also measured in some trials. Biomarkers mirroring events that accompany AD include neuroinflammatory markers such as cytokines and products of oxidative stress or mitochondrial dysfunction. These biomarkers hold promise for evaluating the effects of drug candidates that purport to target these pathways.

4.5.2.2 Serum Biomarkers

Peripheral biomarkers are not well established for diagnostic and outcome monitoring purposes. The blood–brain barrier (BBB) interferes with the amount of brain-derived biomarkers that can access the plasma, making it difficult to measure and convincingly link to AD pathogenesis. However, plasma $A\beta$ has been shown to be higher in familial AD (Kosaka et al., 1997), though these results do not translate to the more prevalent sporadic AD (Assini et al., 2004). Most studies, though, found serum Aβ measures unable to distinguish between AD patients and healthy controls. Similarly, candidate biomarkers of the inflammatory pathways and cholesterol metabolism have yet to be validated.

4.5.3 GENETIC BIOMARKERS

The interindividual variation in biomarkers points to substantial genetic variability, which can be explored in clinical trials to select patients likely to either develop the disease or respond, therefore decrease sample size. Mutations in genes such as APP, apolipoprotein E (APOE), and presenilin (PSEN) increase the risk of AD (Kauwe et al., 2009). Screens for APOE ε4 homozygosity have good predictive value for later development of AD (Coon et al., 2007). As disease-modifying treatments have been unsuccessful to date, early diagnosis and treatment prior to the manifestation of symptoms may improve prognosis. Additionally, determination of genetic disposition allows for the stratification of patients in order to observe diverse treatment effects. Accordingly, treatments may target a specific genetic population that is more responsive to a particular drug. Poirier et al. (1995) demonstrated that AD patients with the APOE ε4 variant did not show the marked cognitive improvements observed in noncarriers when given the ChEI tacrine. This illustrates an example where genotyping could be successfully employed to enhance treatment outcomes.

4.5.3.1 Monitoring Biomarkers in Clinical Trials

Combining different biomarkers may improve clinical trials by decreasing sample sizes and study timelines, providing better methods of assessing treatment-related change. The Alzheimer's Disease Neuroimaging Initiative (ADNI), a five year longitudinal prospective study that began in 2004, compared neuroimaging and CSF markers in healthy, AD, and MCI samples to evaluate their value as outcome measures. Results from ADNI indicate that MRI hippocampal volume was strongly correlated with CSF biomarkers, particularly phosphorylated tau levels, also strongly correlated with PiB uptake in the precuneal area (Apostolova et al., 2010). The close associations of these biomarkers imply that they measure either a single pathological event or many connected events. However, in order for biomarkers to be a truly validated means of evaluating outcomes, their relationships with primary cognitive and functional endpoints must be established. In MCI patients, CSF Aβ42, CSF tau, FDG-PET in regions of interest, and MRI hippocampal and ventricle volume were all correlated with scores on the ADAS-Cog (Beckett et al., 2010). In the same study, CSF tau and FDG-PET results were correlated with cognition on the ADAS-Cog in those with AD. For both populations, brain glucose metabolism measured by FDG-PET had strong correlations with ADAS-cog scores when corrected for joint effects of the other biomarkers (multivariate modeling). As changes in biomarkers appear to reflect changes in cognition, there is support for the use of biomarkers as surrogate endpoints in clinical trials. However, the procedure for imaging and type of MRI machines and PET radioligands used can differ across study sites, thereby introducing inconsistencies. The standardization of methods of obtaining and analyzing biomarkers must be appropriately addressed to ensure precision and accuracy.

4.6 AVAILABLE THERAPIES

4.6.1 Cholinesterase Inhibitors

Reduced acetylcholine neurotransmission due to loss of neurons in the basal forebrain and depletion of choline acetyltransferase (an acetylcholine-synthesizing enzyme) in the hippocampus and cortex are observed in AD pathology (Mangialasche et al., 2010). Given that acetylcholine functions within memory-associated areas of the brain, pathologically low levels of this neurotransmitter are thought to contribute to overall cognitive and functional decline. Moreover, correlations exist between cholinergic loss and severity of cognitive deficits (Perry et al., 1978; Sims et al., 1983). Currently approved treatments for AD work to inhibit the activity of acetylcholinesterase, an acetylcholine-hydrolyzing enzyme, thereby increasing acetylcholine levels in the central nervous system (CNS) in order to restore cognitive function (Kosasa et al., 2000). However, ChEIs may improve cognition via several other mechanisms: processing of APP by promotion of the α-secretase-mediated non-amyloidogenic pathway (Pakrasi and O'Brien, 2005), reduction of Aβ cytotoxicity, and expression of acetylcholine and its nicotinic receptors (Nordberg, 2006). Though ChEIs are indicated for symptomatic relief of AD, they may hold some capacity for inducing disease-modifying effects, which is unlikely to occur at late stages of the disorder.

The ChEIs approved in North America include donepezil, rivastigmine, and galantamine. In China, huperzine A, derived from club moss, is also used as antidementia medication due to its acetylcholinesterase inhibitor activity. It is also thought to possess protective effects against glutamatergic excitotoxicity, ischemia, hydrogen peroxide toxicity, and Aβ aggregation (Li et al., 2008). Some studies suggest that huperzine A appears to improve cognition, global status, daily function, and behavior in AD patients, though these trials are limited by small sample sizes and inadequate methodology (Li et al., 2008). The results of a recent phase II trial (Rafii et al., 2011) did not show evidence supporting the use of huperzine A for improving cognition in AD. While this compound is approved for mild-to-moderate AD in China, it is sold as a dietary supplement in the United States. Meta-analyses of randomized controlled trials (RCTs) on current ChEI drugs approved in the United States, Canada, and the European Union are reviewed in the following sections.

4.6.1.1 Donepezil

4.6.1.1.1 Pharmacology

Donepezil, the most commonly prescribed medication for AD, was approved by the FDA for mild-to-moderate AD in 1996 and severe AD in 2006 (Winblad, 2009). It is highly selective for acetylcholinesterase and binds reversibly and noncompetitively, blocking the binding of acetylcholine and subsequently preventing its hydrolysis. As a result of its long plasma half-life and minimal peripheral effects, donepezil is administered once daily (Mayeux and Sano, 1999). Additional proposed mechanisms include protective effects against glutamatergic toxicity and apoptosis, facilitation of nicotinic receptor expression, anti-Aβ expression and toxicity (Takada et al., 2003; Mangialasche et al., 2010).

4.6.1.1.2   Efficacy

In a Cochrane Collaboration meta-analysis, Birks and Harvey (2006) found that patients given 5 and 10 mg/day of donepezil for 12 to 24 weeks, showed improved scores on the ADAS-Cog, MMSE, and SIB. The study used an intent-to-treat last observation carried forward (ITT-LOCF) analysis to analyze differences between the treatment and placebo groups and additionally found no statistical heterogeneity. Interestingly, there were only marginal differences on scores between the 10 mg and 5 mg treatment arms. Larger dose-dependent effects were found in another meta-analysis by Ritchie et al. (2004), using scales of cognition (ADAS-Cog and MMSE) and global function (CIBIC-Plus, CDR-SB, CGIC, and GDS). Overall, larger doses (10 mg) produced greater improvements in cognitive outcome assessments compared with the smaller dose (5 mg); global outcomes had more moderate improvements. A clinical guideline (Raina et al., 2008) published by the American College of Physicians indicated statistical significance on cognition, global status, and behavior between donepezil (5–10 mg) and placebo-treated patients. A recent study of donepezil 23 mg daily for severely to moderately impaired AD patients found significant benefits for cognition (SIB) but not for global functioning (CIBIC-Plus) when compared with the typical 10-mg dose (Farlow et al., 2010). However, post hoc analysis from this RCT showed that greater impairment at baseline (MMSE ≤ 16) was associated with significantly better response to the higher dose for both cognition and global functioning.

Hansen et al. (2008) obtained similar results in their meta-analysis on RCTs for mild-to-moderate AD. That study also described 2 open-label trials directly comparing donepezil and galantamine. In the 52-week trial (Wilcock et al., 2003), no significant differences were found between the two drugs, while the 12-week trial (Jones et al., 2004) found cognitive and functional outcomes favoring donepezil. Similarly, a 2-year RCT (Bullock et al., 2005) found no differences in donepezil and rivastigmine for cognition and behavior. However, patients on rivastigmine performed better on tests of global status and function at the end of the 2 years. A 12-week open-label trial (Wilkinson et al., 2002) found no statistical significance in cognition between donepezil- and rivastigmine-treated patients. Thus, the time frame for comparative studies may need to be at least 6 months to convincingly demonstrate differences in efficacy.

Though donepezil proved to be beneficial in the controlled environment of the typical pivotal RCT with a specified time frame, long-term results from the AD2000 study of 565 AD patients (Courtney et al., 2004) suggested that progression to disability (loss of two basic or six instrumental activities of daily living) and rates of institutionalization were not different between donepezil and placebo. Similarly, this study concluded that the cost-effectiveness of this drug was also questionable. Subsequently, multiple commentaries highlighting the limitations of the methodologies employed in the AD2000 study were published (Standridge, 2004; Holmes et al., 2004a; Black et al., 2009; Akintade et al., 2004; Clarke, 2004; Howe, 2004; Schneider, 2004). Unfortunately, large trial biases due to patient selection and dropout limit the conclusions that can be drawn from that study. Results from all meta-analyses consistently suggest modest benefits in cognition in favor of donepezil, with a dose-dependent effect, though improvements in behavior disturbances have not been consistently demonstrated (Holmes et al., 2004b; Howard et al., 2007).

4.6.1.2 Rivastigmine

4.6.1.2.1 Pharmacology

Rivastigmine, unlike donepezil, possesses a pseudo-irreversible inhibitory effect as a result of its continued action on acetylcholinesterase long after plasma levels have dropped off (Polinsky, 1998). Acetylcholinesterase is inactivated for over 24 hours since the carbamyl moiety of rivastigmine remains bound to the active site despite hydrolysis and dissociation of the rivastigmine molecule. In contrast to donepezil, rivastigmine also significantly inhibits butyrylcholinesterase (Polinsky, 1998) found in both the CNS and periphery. In the temporal cortex, the activity of this enzyme is associated with cognitive decline (Farlow et al., 2005). In the plasma, the interaction between butyrylcholinesterase and rivastigmine may affect cerebral blood flow (Farlow et al., 2005; Crawford, 1998). However, drug–drug interactions in the periphery are not a huge concern as rivastigmine is not significantly metabolized by cytochrome P450s or bound to plasma proteins (Polinsky, 1998). Rivastigmine can be given orally (twice a day), which raises concern over compliance—a daily transdermal patch was approved by the FDA in 2000 to circumvent this issue (Emre et al., 2010).

4.6.1.2.2 Efficacy

A Cochrane Collaboration (Birks et al., 2009) review examined the effects of high (6–12 mg) and low (1–4 mg) daily doses of rivastigmine on patients of various AD severities. For both dose ranges, improvements were observed in cognition (ADAS-Cog) and global status (CIBIC-Plus and ADCS-CGIC). Behavioral disturbances, evaluated by the NPI, were not significantly different between rivastigmine and placebo. Also, for cognition (ADAS-Cog, MMSE), function (ADCS-ADL), behavior (NPI), and global change (ADCS-CGIC), no differences were found between small dose (9.8 mg/day) transdermal and oral (6–12 mg/day) administration. The larger 20-cm^2 (17.4mg/day) and smaller 10-cm^2 (9.8 mg/day) dose patch were comparable on all outcomes. In the Investigation of transDermal Exelon in ALzheimer's disease (IDEAL) trial, a trend toward a dose-dependent effect was observed—numerical improvements on ADAS-Cog scores were nonsignificantly larger for the 20-cm^2 patch (Grossman et al., 2009 Jul; Winblad et al., 2007b).

An analysis by Ritchie et al. (2004) described results similar to the Cochrane study, with an additional reported dose-dependent effect on cognition for the rivastigmine oral capsule. However, a meta-analysis completed by Raina et al. (2008) highlighted some inconsistencies; for cognition, improvements were observed on the ADAS-Cog (with evidence of heterogeneity) while the MMSE and SIB were not significant between treatment and placebo. Inconsistencies were also detected for functional ability: the Nurses' Observation Scale for Geriatric Patients (NOSGER) scores demonstrated benefits while Progressive Deterioration Scale (PDS) scores were insignificant. Rivastigmine did not significantly improve behavior outcomes.

Overall, the available studies suggest that rivastigmine does possess dose-dependent properties. Benefits were present on cognitive, global, and functional domains, with some inconsistencies across outcome scales. Behavior did not improve with rivastigmine treatment.

4.6.1.3 Galantamine

4.6.1.3.1 Pharmacology

Galantamine is a reversible and competitive ChEI with modulatory (allosteric) effects on the nicotinic acetylcholine receptors to amplify nicotinic transmission (Shimohama, 2009). Unlike rivastigmine, this compound is metabolized by cytochrome P450 (mainly CYP2D6 and CYP3A4) and excreted through the urine (Razay and Wilcock, 2008). The immediate release capsule is taken twice daily, absorbed quickly in the intestine, and reaches peak plasma levels within 1 to 2 hours due to its high bioavailability. The newer extended release preparation can be administered once daily.

4.6.1.3.2 Efficacy

In a meta-analysis of RCTs, Ritchie et al. (2004) found modest significant improvements on cognition (ADAS-Cog) and global status (CIBIC-Plus and CGI) for treatment with galantamine (8-36 mg) compared with placebo, although a dose-dependent effect was not detected. Similar observations were made in another meta-analysis (Raina et al., 2008), with further benefits found on functional (ADCS-ADL and DAD) and behavior (NPI) scales. Favorable results on cognitive, global, and function scales were, as well, found in a Cochrane Collaboration analysis (Loy and Schneider, 2006). For cognition, 6 months of treatment was more efficacious than 3 months of treatment.

Taken together, meta-analyses on galantamine for AD treatment had small but significant effect sizes on cognitive, global, functional, and behavioral domains with questionable dose-dependent effects.

4.6.1.4 Pooled Effects of Cholinesterase Inhibitors

4.6.1.4.1 Efficacy

A diverse number of meta-analyses have pooled results for all ChEIs. In a Cochrane meta-analysis (Birks, 2006), small yet significant effect sizes in cognition (ADAS-Cog and MMSE) and global state (CIBIC-Plus) were calculated for ChEI-treated versus placebo groups. In contrast, behavior (NPI) and activities of daily function (PDS) did not differ between treatment groups. Small effects for functional outcomes were exhibited in a study by Hansen et al. (2007), causing the authors to question the clinical relevance of the drugs. A specific examination of donepezil and galantamine on cognitive outcomes also yielded small effect sizes, once again raising the question of treatment effectiveness in the real world (Harry and Zakzanis, 2005). The ChEIs were found to improve behavioral and psychological symptoms of dementia, with greater efficacy observed in mild than severe AD patients (Campbell et al., 2008).

A quantification of the mean global responders to ChEI treatment, performed by Lanctôt et al. (2003), found significantly higher proportions of responders to treatment compared with placebo, with similar observations for low- and high-dose groups. These investigators also calculated 12 to be the number of patients needed to treat for an additional patient to have a global improvement.

The established efficacy of ChEIs on cognition (ADAS-Cog) and global status (CIBIC-Plus) found in RCTs was critiqued in a review by Kaduszkiewicz et al. (2005). The authors criticized the positive results found in these studies, pointing to methodological flaws such as missing ITT analyses, use of LOCF for incomplete data, and primary endpoints uncorrected for multiple comparisons. It was concluded that scientific bias may be contributing to the efficacy found in these RCTs. This review has been challenged by others in the field. Herrmann et al. (2007) commented that the previous authors failed to statistically amalgamate data from each included trial, thereby masking the strong consistency in positive results and dose-dependent relationship for ChEIs. Luckmann (2006) noted that excluding dropout patients after randomization and absence of multiple comparison corrections is not likely a huge concern in terms of bias. Also, Birks (2008) remarked that multiple comparison corrections are typically conducted in post hoc analyses rather than predetermined outcome analyses. It was additionally noted that estimation of bias can be performed for missing data.

4.6.2 MEMANTINE

4.6.2.1 Pharmacology
Memory impairment in AD is associated with Ca^{2+}-induced excitotoxicity due to elevated glutamate release and overactivation of the NMDA receptor (Witt et al., 2004). This is the premise for use of memantine, a specific, non-competitive NMDA receptor antagonist with moderate affinity (McShane et al., 2006; Gauthier et al., 2005). At pathological levels of glutamate, the rapid kinetics and voltage dependency of memantine permits better blocking of the NMDA receptor, while regular glutamate concentrations produce reduced antagonistic actions (Wenk et al., 2006). This drug was initially indicated for moderately severe to severe AD in Europe and eventually revised to include moderate-to-severe AD.

4.6.2.2 Efficacy
A meta-analysis conducted by Doody et al. (2007) reported that significant benefits for cognition, global status, function, and behavior in moderate to severe AD patients given memantine for 24–28 weeks. However, in contrast to other work, the authors also reported significant improvements on cognition and global status (but not function and behavior) for the mild-to-moderate AD sample as well. These authors concluded that memantine was effective for all AD stages. A critique of this study (Knopman, 2007) noted that three unpublished negative trials (two of which looked exclusively at mild to moderate AD) were not included in the analysis. A closer examination of these three trials found that combining the data (totaling over 1300 subjects) resulted in statistical significance in favor of memantine over placebo. This may be due to an increase in power as a consequence of a large sample size. Another critique (Schneider, 2007) pointed out concerns over the methodology, remarking that the statistical combination of the mild-to-moderate and moderate-to-severe groups to conclude efficacy across the entire spectrum was impractical and introduced bias.

A Cochrane Collaboration meta-analysis (McShane et al., 2006) examined the same RCTs as Doody et al. (2007) and found very small but significant improvements in cognition (SIB), global status (CIBIC-Plus), daily function (ADCS-ADL), and behavior (NPI) for memantine-treated patients with moderate to severe AD.

However, only cognition was statistically significant in the mild-to-moderate sample. Maidment et al. (2008) though, did find positive effects on behavioral disturbances, as measured by the NPI. Using an observed cases (OC) analysis of the available RCTs, Winblad et al. (2007a) found effect sizes favoring memantine on cognition, global status, daily function, and behavior. In a recent meta-analysis of RCTs, Schneider et al. (2011) stratified mild-to-moderate AD severity to examine the effects of memantine on each population; they found no benefit in any outcome for the mild population but very modest efficacy for cognition (ADAS-Cog) and global functioning (CIBIC-Plus) in the moderately impaired patients.

Taken together, efficacy in the moderate-to-severe population is well established, whereas benefits for mild-to-moderate patients do not appear to be consistent across the four domains of evaluation.

4.6.3 Long-Term Safety

The ChEIs and memantine have been proven to be safe and tolerable in large-scale clinical trials. However, RCTs do not accurately represent the real-world population on antidementia medications; many patients with comorbid disorders or using concomitant drugs are excluded from entry into trials to maintain homogeneity (Rothwell, 2005). Thus, large, naturalistic, long-term observational studies of diverse patient populations can provide valuable knowledge of the drug effects that cannot be uncovered in controlled studies with shorter time frames.

Lockhart et al. (2009) reviewed retrospective and prospective studies on observed adverse events (AEs) in samples on ChEIs. In a comparison of rivastigmine and donepezil, gastrointestinal (GI) AEs, such as diarrhea, vomiting, nausea, and abdominal cramps were more prominent in rivastigmine (Turon-Estrada et al., 2003). However, total incidences of AEs were similar for the two drugs, with the highest AE total observed in galantamine-treated patients (Pakrasi et al., 2003). In general, AE incidences associated with the cardiovascular and central nervous systems were much lower than GI for all ChEIs (Lockhart et al., 2009). However, a retrospective case-control study showed that ChEI-treated patients were more than twice as likely to be hospitalized due to bradycardia (Park-Wyllie et al., 2009). Similarly, in a retrospective study, Gill et al. (2009) found that compared with untreated cohorts, ChEI-treated dementia patients were at a higher risk for development of syncope or a brief loss of consciousness, a syndrome linked with bradycardia.

In contrast, prospective studies appear to favor donepezil. Total frequency of AEs (Mosello et al., 2004), particularly GI-related AEs, were lower in donepezil-treated patients compared with those on rivastigmine and galantamine (Fuschillo et al., 2004; Aguglia et al., 2004). Additionally, two studies found that donepezil was also associated with lower discontinuation rates, which corresponds to its popularity over the other two AD medications (Mosello et al., 2004; Lopez-Pousa et al., 2005).

The safety of memantine and the ChEIs in observational studies have yet to be compared directly. However, postmarketing surveillance (Calabrese et al., 2007) shows that AEs are generally low in patients on memantine monotherapy. In contrast to the GI-associated AEs found with ChEI treatment, the most prominent types of AEs were observed to be neurological and psychiatric in nature.

Evidence from observational studies indicate that the approved antidementia medications have a good safety profile in a naturalistic setting, thereby adding to the justification for their use as symptomatic therapy.

4.7 EMERGING THERAPIES

4.7.1 AMYLOID-TARGETED TREATMENTS

The amyloid hypothesis has historically dominated the proposed pathology of AD. Nonetheless, no anti-amyloid drugs have been successful in consistently demonstrating efficacy and gaining regulatory approval.

It was initially thought that the accumulation of polymeric Aβ subunits within the extracellular space leads to the formation of senile plaques and neuronal death (Selkoe, 1991; Hardy and Higgins, 1992). However, disease severity is not strongly correlated with plaque burden (Terry et al., 1991) and does not improve with plaque removal (Holmes et al., 2008).

Normally, the transmembrane protein APP is cleaved by α-secretase to produce a soluble, nonaggregate forming peptide (sAPPα) (Selkoe, 1996). In the amyloidogenic pathway (Figure 4.1A), APP undergoes proteolytic cleavage by β-secretase and γ-secretase to produce the hydrophobic Aβ fragment (Glenner and Wong, 1984a, 1984b). This fragment occurs in two main forms, one consisting of 40 amino acids (Aβ40) and the other containing 42 amino acids (Aβ42) (Cappai and Barnham, 2008). Aβ42 is less common, but more likely to aggregate and cause the formation of amyloid plaques (Cappai and Barnham, 2008).

It has been shown that mutations in the secretase-associated genes lead to an increase in Aβ42 (Kumar-Singh et al., 2006; Suzuki et al., 1994). As a result, researchers proposed that Aβ42 is the causal source of AD pathophysiology (Younkin, 1995), and that a decreased Aβ42/Aβ40 ratio may represent a novel treatment target. It was subsequently postulated that the disease mechanism is caused by soluble Aβ oligomers, rather than polymeric plaques (Pimplikar, 2009).

4.7.1.1 Decreasing Aβ Production

4.7.1.1.1 Stimulation of α-Secretase

α-secretase competes for the APP substrate with β-secretase to commence a nonamyloidogenic pathway, resulting in the formation of sAPPα, which is less likely to form aggregates. This protein has been found to have anti-apoptotic (Turner et al., 2003), as well as neuroprotective (Furukawa et al., 1996) and memory-enhancing (Meziane et al., 1998) properties.

Stimulating this enzyme provides a possible means of regulating AD pathogenesis. A select group of α-secretase stimulators are in early-phase testing trials. Etazolate promotes the production of sAPPα by activating the $GABA_A$ receptors (Marcade et al., 2008) and bryostatin-1 activates protein kinase C (PKC) thereby stimulating the α-secretase transduction pathway (Etcheberrigaray et al., 2004).

Alternative α-secretase stimulators mediate statins, hormones (estrogen, testosterone), and neurotransmitters (glutamate, serotonin) (Griffiths et al., 2008). At this time, there are no α-secretase stimulators in phase III clinical trials.

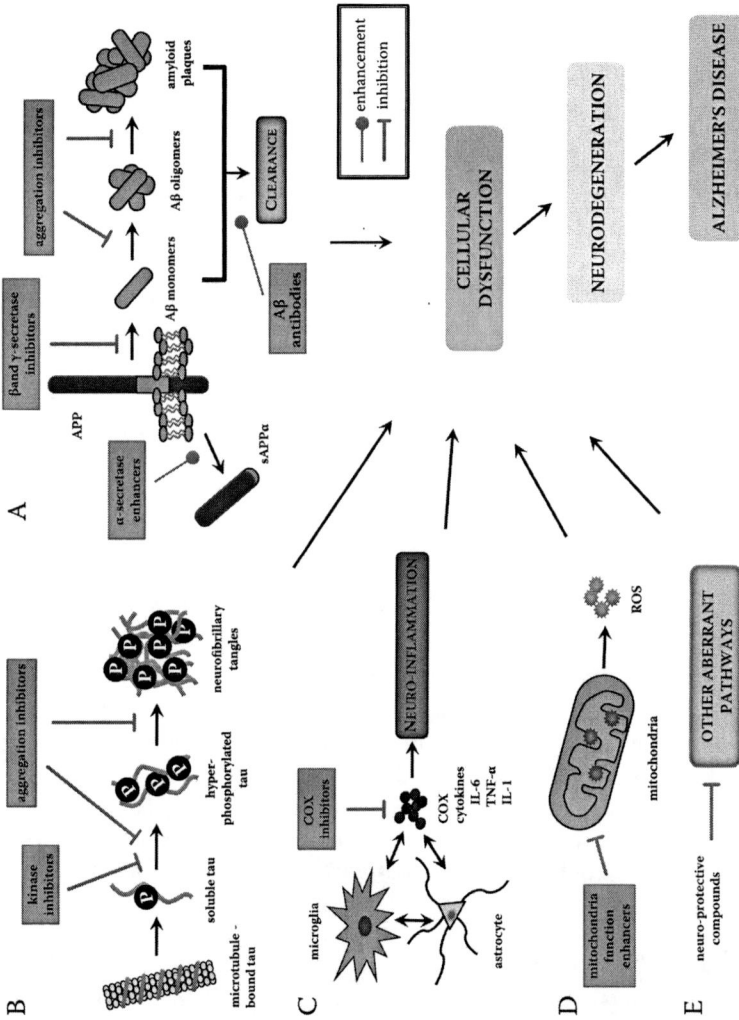

FIGURE 4.1 (See color insert.) Proposed Alzheimer's disease pathogenesis and potential therapeutic targets. All pathways are interconnected; one may facilitate or give rise to another. Additionally, all pathways may originate from one unifying factor, such as genetic disposition; (A) amyloidogenic pathway; (B) hyperphosphorylated tau aggregation; (C) cyclo-oxygenase (COX) and cytokine-induced neuro-inflammatory mechanisms; (D) mitochondria dysfunction and production of reactive oxygen species (ROS), which distribute to other neural regions; and (E) other aberrant pathways that can be blocked by neuroprotective agents such as statins and docosahexanoic acid.

4.7.1.1.2   Inhibition of β-Secretase

Insulin resistance has previously been proposed as a primary mechanism of AD (Watson and Craft, 2003; Craft, 2007), since diabetes increases the risk of dementia (Profenno et al., 2010; Forti et al., 2010). Rosiglitazone and pioglitazone are thiazolidinedione drugs that help to decrease insulin resistance. By stimulating nuclear peroxisome proliferator-activated receptor γ (PPARγ) these compounds are able to down-regulate β-secretase, and influence APP expression (Jiang et al., 2008).

A phase II trial of rosiglitazone (Risner et al., 2006) in 511 patients with mild to moderate AD showed significant benefits for cognition (as measured by the ADAS-cog) in patients without the (APOE ε4 allele compared with placebo. No such improvement was observed in APOE ε4-positive patients. Subsequent to this, a multi-national phase III RCT (Gold et al., 2010) (REFLECT-1) focusing on the APOE ε4-negative patients failed to demonstrate efficacy on primary outcomes in cognition (ADAS-cog) and global status (CIBIC-Plus). A possibility for is that rosiglitazone is actively transported out of the CNS upon crossing of the blood-brain-barrier (BBB) (Festuccia et al., 2008).

A phase II study in 29 patients evaluated the safety and efficacy of pioglitazone (Geldmacher et al., 2011). That RCT found reasonable safety and tolerability of pioglitazone, but insignificant clinical effects. Currently, there are no ongoing phase III trials of β-secretase inhibiting agents.

4.7.1.1.3   Inhibition of γ-Secretase

Aside from completing the final step in the production of Aβ, γ-secretase is involved in the cleavage of the Notch receptors (Lewis et al., 2003). Since the Notch receptor is vital to neural signaling and normal development (Hartmann et al., 2001), the utility of γ-secretase inhibitors is considerably limited.

The only γ-secretase inhibitor that has been extensively studied in trials of AD is semagacestat. Phase II trials have shown that doses up to 140 mg do not reduce the Aβ40 levels within the CSF (Fleisher et al., 2008; Siemers et al., 2006). Adverse effects including skin lesions and skin cancer were observed. In fact, semagacestat seemed to cause worsening of cognitive and daily function as compared to groups receiving the placebo (Eli Lilly and Company, 2010). More recently, two large phase III trials in over 2600 subjects were discontinued (IDENTITY & IDENTITY-2), as they did not demonstrate efficacy of primary endpoints. Second-generation inhibitors exhibiting a strong selectivity for APP are currently being tested in ongoing trials (Jacobsen et al., 2009; Soares et al., 2009 Jul; Grossman et al., 2009 Jul).

4.7.1.2   Reducing Aβ Aggregation

In recent years, the focus of disease-modifying research has shifted toward identifying compounds that prevent the aggregation of Aβ oligomers. As mentioned, it is now thought that soluble oligomers of Aβ, rather than large deposits of fibrillary Aβs, are associated with the neuro- and synaptotoxicity (Haass and Selkoe, 2007; Shankar et al., 2008; Gong et al., 2003) that is characteristic of AD pathogenesis.

A polyphenolic flavinoid found in green tea binds to Aβ42 and prevents the formation of oligomeric structures (Guo et al., 2010). This compound, epigallocatechin gallate (EGCg), seems to exert neuroprotective effects in vitro (Bastianetto et al.,

2006; Levites et al., 2003; Choi et al., 2001). EGCg is currently undergoing an 18-month phase II/III trial (SUN-AK) (ClinicalTrials.gov, Identifier: NCT00951834) examining the effects of this compound as an add-on treatment in early-stage AD.

Scyllo-inositol (Garzone et al., 2009 Jul) and clioquinol (Lannfelt et al., 2008) are also thought to decrease Aβ aggregation, but neither are currently being considered for a phase III investigation.

Tramiprosate (3-amino-1-propanesulfonic acid [3APS]) studied at the pre-clinical level demonstrated the ability to reduce plaque buildup in the brains and plasma of mice, by binding to Aβ40 and Aβ42. Upon binding, it prevented these molecules from achieving the conformational state required for oligomer and fibril assembly (Gervais et al., 2007). A phase II trial (Aisen et al., 2006) generated promising results by reducing the levels of Aβ42 in the CSF of patients receiving 150 mg/kg tramiprosate therapy over 3 months, as compared with the placebo. However, a phase III RCT (Alphase study) (Aisen et al., 2011) of 1052 patients with AD, receiving 100 mg, 150 mg, or placebo for 18 months showed no differences in clinical outcomes (ADAS-cog for cognition). A subsequent analysis (Saumier et al., 2009) showed improvements on individual items of the ADAS-Cog, includ-ing memory, language, and praxis. Further development of tramiprosate for AD was discontinued.

4.7.1.3 Promoting Clearance of Aβ

An additional approach derived from the Aβ hypothesis is making use of the immune system to facilitate the clearance of neurotoxic Aβ sediments. Four mechanisms of Aβ removal have been identified so far: antibody and phagocytosis by microglia (Schenk et al., 1999; Bard et al., 2000), interference and solubilization of Aβ (Frenkel et al., 2000; Bacskai et al., 2002), removal of soluble Aβ from the CNS by antibodies (peripheral sink hypothesis) (DeMattos et al., 2001), and antibody binding to prevent oligomer formation (Dodart et al., 2002).

Clearance facilitated by antibody binding can be achieved by active immunization with the full-length Aβ peptide and passive immunization with immunoglobulins raised against Aβ. Active immunization was associated with meningoencephalitis, believed to be due to cytotoxic pro-inflammatory T cell activation and resulting neu-roinflammation (Gilman et al., 2005). Vaccines that stimulate B cells were found to be tolerable in early phase trials (Wang et al., 2007; Schneeberger et al., 2009). Agents designed for passive immunization are being tested in ongoing phase III trials.

A humanized monoclonal antibody currently in the pipeline is solanezumab. This antibody binds soluble Aβ and was found to be tolerable in both phase I (Siemers et al., 2010) and phase II (Siemers et al., 2008 Jul; Goto et al., 2010 Jul) trials. A phase II RCT found that infusions of 100 and 400 mg in AD patients and healthy individuals produced a reduction in Aβ42 levels. However, these molecular modifi-cations were not accompanied by a clinical response in cognitive function (Siemers et al., 2008 Jul). Phase III trials of solanezumab (EXPEDITION) in AD patients for up to 19 months have yet to disclose their results (NCT00905372, NCT00904683). An open-label study is ongoing (NCT01127633).

A monoclonal antibody, bapineuzumab, was designed to have high affinity for the N-terminus of Aβ and contain a B cell epitope. A 1.5 mg/kg dose infusion of bapineuzumab was found to be safe, while a 5 mg/kg dose seemed to increase the risk of vasogenic edema in a phase I trial (Black et al., 2010). An 18-month phase II trial showed no cognitive benefits associated with 0.15–2 mg doses of bapineuzumab compared with placebo (Salloway et al., 2009). A subsequent exploratory analysis did suggest a pattern of cognitive improvement in the ITT population, as well as statistically significant cognitive improvement in study completers. A multinational 18-month phase III RCT of bapineuzumab in APOE ε4 carriers and noncarriers is underway (NCT00676143, NCT00667810). In addition, there will be a 2-year extension phase for long-term safety monitoring (NCT00996918, NCT00998764).

It is hypothesized that passive immunization can be achieved through the use of intravenous immunoglobulin (IVIg), which would decrease Aβ within the CSF and in turn lead to a rise in serum Aβ concentrations. Two early-phase trials were performed using nonspecific polyclonal antibodies obtained from human donors. Modest benefits to cognition were observed in mild to moderate AD patients (Dodel et al., 2004; Relkin et al., 2009). Another phase II trial generated similar findings in patients over 6 months. Due to the encouraging results achieved in these studies, a phase III RCT plans to enroll 360 patients with mild to moderate AD and monitor cognitive function, as well as global impression of change (NCT00818662).

4.7.2 TAU-TARGETED TREATMENTS

Perhaps the second-most influential hypothesis in AD pathology involves tau protein (Figure 4.1B). When hyperphosphorylated, tau proteins aggregate to form the tangles that define AD pathology. This cytoplasmic protein is associated with tubulin and stabilizes axonal microtubules during polymerization (Goedert et al., 2006). Upon hyperphosphorylation, it detaches from microtubules and forms neurofibrillary tangles in the shape of paired helices. The degree of cognitive dysfunction is associated with the quantity of tangles, termed *tangle load* (Thal et al., 2000). It has been postulated that the presence of these tangles results in a loss of cytoskeletal structure, and causes an accumulation of cytotoxic intraneuronal filaments resulting in cell death. Therefore, agents that inhibit tau hyperphosphorylation or promote filament disassembly represent possible treatment alternatives (Schneider and Mandelkow, 2008; Lee and Trojanowski, 2006).

Methylthioninium chloride (methylene blue) dissolves tau filaments in vitro (Wischik et al., 1996), but also targets neurotransmitters and mediates oxidation and mitochondrial function (Oz et al., 2009; Atamna and Kumar, 2010). One phase II trial of methylene blue in moderate AD patients (receiving 30-, 60-, and 100-mg dosing) demonstrated encouraging improvements on cognitive scales for the 60-mg dose at 50 weeks (Wischik et al., 2008). A phase III trial is being planned to assess the clinical efficacy of leuco-methylthioninium (LMTX).

Valproate and lithium are two compounds that inhibit glycogen synthase kinase-3 (GSK-3), which is known to regulate tau phosphorylation (Tariot and Aisen, 2009). A phase II RCT of lithium failed to show improvements in cognition in mild AD patients (Hampel et al., 2009). Similarly, a phase III trial of valproate (VALID)

(Tariot et al., 2009) did not demonstrate improvements in cognition or activities of daily living.

4.7.3 NEUROINFLAMMATION

The neuroinflammatory pathway (Figure 4.1C) is based on the notion that the characteristic features of AD, such as plaques and tangles, are correlated with the presence of inflammatory substances (cytokines and cyclo-oxygenase-2 [COX-2]) and activated microglia (Swardfager et al., 2010; McGeer and McGeer, 2007; Cagnin et al., 2001; Floyd, 1999). The neuroinflammatory basis for AD is further supported by the evidence pointing to the neuroprotective properties of nonsteroidal inflammatory drugs (NSAIDs) and their ability to decrease the risk of AD (McGeer et al., 1996; Szekely et al., 2004). Unfortunately, these drugs did not fare well in clinical research.

The efficacy of an antimalarial agent, hydroxychloroquine, which plays a role in inflammatory pathways involving lymphocytes, macrophages, and cytokine responses (Aisen and Davis, 1994) were explored. Similar to most of the other putative agents, it did not demonstrate significant improvements in cognition versus placebo (Van Gool et al., 2001).

Prednisone, a glucocorticoid with diverse immunosuppressant activity, was administered in a multicenter phase III trial lasting 52 weeks in 138 patients with AD. The 10-mg oral treatment did not produce significant differences on the cognitive domain compared to placebo, but some benefits in behavioral symptoms were identified (Aisen et al., 2000).

NSAIDs possessing a higher degree of selectivity were chosen for subsequent clinical investigations. Rofecoxib is an inhibitor of COX-2 and was examined in a phase III trial of 692 AD patients (Reines et al., 2004). Subjects on ChEI therapy were randomized to 25 mg of rofecoxib or placebo for 12 months. No benefits in cognition or daily function were noted. Similarly negative primary outcomes were seen in a 220-mg naproxen 12-month therapy was tested in a clinical trial of 351 patients (Aisen et al., 2003).

Indomethacin belongs to a class of nonselective NSAIDs, which exhibits anti-amyloidogenic properties. In one trial (Rogers et al., 1993), 44 participants suffering from AD received 100–150 mg of indomethacin for 6 months. The Cochrane Collaboration performed a reanalysis of the data, as the study reported a high dropout rate. That analysis did not find any significant differences in cognition between indomethacin therapy and placebo (Tabet and Feldman, 2002). Recruitment difficulties led to the discontinuation of a phase III trial of indomethacin in the Netherlands (de Jong et al., 2008). However, 12-month data were available on 51 patients, but failed to demonstrate improvements on primary outcomes.

Finally, another Notch-sparing NSAID affecting γ-secretase is tarenflurbil. However, this drug does not affect the COX enzyme (Eriksen et al., 2003; Morihara et al., 2002), and was proven to be tolerable in early phase trials at a dose up to 800 mg (Galasko et al., 2007; Wilcock et al., 2008). A phase II (Wilcock et al., 2008) trial established that tarenflurbil slowed decline on functional and global outcomes, but failed to have any effects on cognition. Subsequently, a phase III trial (Green et al., 2009) was initiated, but found no differences in the cognitive and functional domains.

4.7.4 MITOCHONDRIAL DYSFUNCTION PATHWAY

Studies have shown that mitochondrial dysfunction occurs in the early stages of the disease (Figure 4.1D), which can cause apoptosis and synaptotoxicity. It was further shown that soluble APP and Aβ proteins disturb mitochondrial operation and create oxidative stress (Hansson Petersen et al., 2008). The mitochondrial dysfunction hypothesis derived from this evidence represents an additional approach to resolving the pathological manifestation of AD.

Latrepirdine (dimebon) is thought to enhance mitochondrial function through the inhibition of permeability transition pores. Some researchers think that latrepirdine has neuroprotective properties by impeding Aβ-induced toxicity and stimulating the generation of ATP (Bachurin et al., 2001; Zhang et al., 2010). This agent also acts on a number of different pathways, including weak inhibition of acetylcholinesterase and butyrylcholinesterase, as well as involvement in NMDA signaling (Wu et al., 2008). Latrepirdine was tested in Russia, in the context of a phase II study of 183 AD patients receiving 20 mg three times a day. That study showed remarkable improvements in cognition and activities of daily living as compared with placebo (Doody et al., 2008). Unfortunately, those results could not be replicated in a large, multinational 6-month phase III trial (CONNECTION) sponsored by Pfizer (Medivation, 2010). The effects of latrepirdine therapy were negative on cognitive, functional, and global outcomes compared to placebo. Despite these disappointing results, another phase III trial (CONCERT) of latrepirdine is still ongoing (NCT00829374). It is projected that this study will enroll 1050 AD patients who are stable on donepezil.

4.7.5 OTHER APPROACHES

Additional approaches (Figure 4.1E) to the development of disease-modifying therapies are based on the observations of a lower AD incidence associated with the ingestion of various substances.

The relation between use of statins (cholesterol-reducing agents) and the incidence of AD remains uncertain, as the results of several studies appear to contradict each other (McGuinness et al., 2010; Rockwood et al., 2002; Jick et al., 2000; Arvanitakis et al., 2008; Tokuda et al., 2001; Benito-Leon et al., 2010). However, statins have been shown to possess anti-inflammatory and antioxidant properties, and perhaps more importantly, to decrease Aβ production (Hoglund and Blennow, 2007; Fassbender et al., 2001; Refolo et al., 2001). A trial (ADCLT) (Sparks et al., 2006) of 67 mild to moderate AD patients assigned to either 80 mg atorvastatin or placebo treatment found significant improvement on cognitive scales at 6 months. These results were contradicted by that of the phase III LEADe trial (Feldman et al., 2010) of 614 patients stable on donepezil, which showed that there were no substantial differences in cognition and global status between treatment arms. An alternative statin drug, thought to cross the BBB with more ease than atorvastin, is simvastatin (Tsuji et al., 1993; Sparks et al., 2002). A phase III RCT (CLASP) (NCT00053599) investigating the efficacy of 20–40 mg simvastatin over a period of 18 months is underway.

Studies have shown that a diet rich in omega-3 fatty acids decreases the risk of developing dementia (Kalmijn et al., 1997; Morris et al., 2003; Schaefer et al., 2006). Levels of the omega-3 fatty acid docosahexanoic acid (DHA) are significantly reduced in the brains of affected persons, as compared to healthy volunteers. The OmegAD study tested 1000 mg of EPAX1050TG (430 mg DHA and 150 mg EPA) over 6 months (Freund-Levi et al., 2006). Though good tolerability was demonstrated, the drug did not show efficacy on primary outcomes. However, a slowing of cognitive decline was observed in the mildest AD patients, suggesting that DHA may be helpful in early stage AD. An 18-month phase III study (Quinn et al., 2010) examining the effects of 510 mg of DHA was completed in 402 patients. Similarly, no improvements in cognition, global status, or activities of daily living were noted. In contrast to the result of the OmegAD study (Freund-Levi et al., 2006), a post hoc analysis did not reveal a delay in cognitive decline in mild AD patients receiving DHA, but it did find that APOE ε4 noncarriers experienced less cognitive decline.

4.8   FUTURE DIRECTIONS

Compounds claiming disease-modifying abilities in AD have thus far failed to produce effects that are clinically significant. At present, the symptomatic pharmacotherapies available to patients are considered to be marginally effective at best. Nevertheless, research in this field persists at a staggering rate. With each negative trial, it is increasingly evident that we must reevaluate our existing research models and endpoints, on both the preclinical and clinical levels.

Since AD is a complex and multifactorial disorder, future treatments will likely consist of combinations of drugs that possess both disease-modifying and symptom-reducing qualities. Therefore, while the currently prescribed drugs, such as the cholinesterase inhibitors, do not target disease-modifying processes, the search for improved symptomatic treatments of this kind continues to be of great importance. Over the last decade, efforts to target the traditional pathways, such as the amyloid-beta hypothesis, have been consistently ineffective. There is growing consensus that resources should be reallocated toward gaining a better understanding of the underlying disease mechanism and investigating the role of novel etiopathological factors. Development of preclinical models that more closely mirror the disease in humans could form the starting point for exploring these pathways effectively. Moving beyond the widely used transgenic mice models toward higher-order mammals and genetic variants to explore the hereditary forms of AD would be helpful in expanding preclinical horizons.

Current clinical trial methodologies should be strengthened by improving outcome measures. Scales possessing higher sensitivity and specificity for the currently used clinical outcomes allow for a more precise assessment of changes in condition. The development of standardized scales tailored toward subgroups of AD patients may also improve sensitivity in this population. Incorporating multiple biomarkers including CSF, serum, genetic, and neuroimaging markers will be particularly essential for studies of drugs with potential disease-modifying effects.

Overall, abandoning the one protein, one drug hypothesis, and using biochemical and imaging biomarkers in conjunction with improved clinical scales appears to be the way forward in the search for treatments that may provide relief to millions of people worldwide.

REFERENCES

Aguglia, E., Onor, M. L., Saina, M., and Maso, E. 2004. An open-label, comparative study of rivastigmine, donepezil and galantamine in a real-world setting. *Curr Med Res Opin* 20 (11): 1747–1752.

Aisen, P. S., and Davis, K. L. 1994. Inflammatory mechanisms in Alzheimer's disease: Implications for therapy. *Am J Psychiatry* 151 (8): 1105–1113.

Aisen, P. S., Davis, K. L., Berg, J. D., Schafer, K., Campbell, K., Thomas, R. G., Weiner, M. F., Farlow, M. R., Sano, M., Grundman, M., and Thal, L. J. 2000. A randomized controlled trial of prednisone in Alzheimer's disease. Alzheimer's Disease Cooperative Study. *Neurology* 54 (3): 588–593.

Aisen, P. S., Gauthier, S., Ferris, S., Saumier, D., Haine, D., Garceau, D., Duong, A., Suhy, J., Oh, J., Lau, W. C., and Sampalis, J. 2011. Tramiprosate in mild-to-moderate Alzheimer's disease: A randomized, double-blind, placebo-controlled, multi-centre study (the Alphase Study). *Arch Med Sci* 7 (1): 102–111.

Aisen, P. S., Saumier, D., Briand, R., Laurin, J., Gervais, F., Tremblay, P., and Garceau, D. 2006. A Phase II study targeting amyloid-beta with 3APS in mild-to-moderate Alzheimer disease. *Neurology* 67 (10): 1757–1763.

Aisen, P. S., Schafer, K. A., Grundman, M., Pfeiffer, E., Sano, M., Davis, K. L., Farlow, M. R., Jin, S., Thomas, R. G., and Thal, L. J. 2003. Effects of rofecoxib or naproxen vs placebo on Alzheimer disease progression: a randomized controlled trial. *JAMA* 289 (21): 2819–2826.

Akintade, L., Zaiac, M., Ieni, J. R., and McRae, T. 2004. AD2000: Design and conclusions. *Lancet* 364 (9441): 1214; author reply 1216–1217.

Alexopoulos, G. S., Abrams, R. C., Young, R. C., and Shamoian, C. A. 1988. Cornell Scale for depression in dementia. *Biol Psychiatry* 23 (3): 271–284.

Alzheimer's Association. 2010. Alzheimer's disease facts and figures. *Alzheimers Dement* 7 (2): 208–244.

Alzheimer's Disease International. *World Alzheimer Report 2010.* 2010. http://www.alz.co.uk/research/files/WorldAlzheimerReport2010.pdf (accessed May 10, 2011).

American Psychiatric Association. 2000. *Diagnostic and statistical manual of mental disorders*, 4th ed. Washington, DC: American Psychiatric Association.

Andersson, C., Blennow, K., Johansson, S. E., Almkvist, O., Engfeldt, P., Lindau, M., and Eriksdotter-Jonhagen, M. 2007. Differential CSF biomarker levels in APOE-epsilon4- positive and -negative patients with memory impairment. *Dement Geriatr Cogn Disord* 23 (2): 87–95.

Andreasen, N., Minthon, L., Davidsson, P., Vanmechelen, E., Vanderstichele, H., Winblad, B., and Blennow, K. 2001. Evaluation of CSF-tau and CSF-Abeta42 as diagnostic markers for Alzheimer disease in clinical practice. *Arch Neurol* 58 (3): 373–379.

Apostolova, L. G., Dutton, R. A., Dinov, I. D., Hayashi, K. M., Toga, A. W., Cummings, J. L., and Thompson, P. M. 2006. Conversion of mild cognitive impairment to Alzheimer disease predicted by hippocampal atrophy maps. *Arch Neurol* 63 (5): 693–699.

Apostolova, L. G., Hwang, K. S., Andrawis, J. P., Green, A. E., Babakchanian, S., Morra, J. H., Cummings, J. L., Toga, A. W., Trojanowski, J. Q., Shaw, L. M., Jack, C. R., Jr., Petersen, R. C., Aisen, P. S., Jagust, W. J., Koeppe, R. A., Mathis, C. A., Weiner, M. W., and Thompson, P. M. 2010. 3D PIB and CSF biomarker associations with hippocampal atrophy in ADNI subjects. *Neurobiol Aging* 31 (8): 1284–1303.

Arvanitakis, Z., Schneider, J. A., Wilson, R. S., Bienias, J. L., Kelly, J. F., Evans, D. A., and Bennett, D. A. 2008. Statins, incident Alzheimer disease, change in cognitive function, and neuropathology. *Neurology* 70 (19 Pt 2): 1795–1802.

Assini, A., Cammarata, S., Vitali, A., Colucci, M., Giliberto, L., Borghi, R., Inglese, M. L., Volpe, S., Ratto, S., Dagna-Bricarelli, F., Baldo, C., Argusti, A., Odetti, P., Piccini, A., and Tabaton, M. 2004. Plasma levels of amyloid beta-protein 42 are increased in women with mild cognitive impairment. *Neurology* 63 (5): 828–831.

Atamna, H., and Kumar, R. 2010. Protective role of methylene blue in Alzheimer's disease via mitochondria and cytochrome c oxidase. *J Alzheimers Dis* 20 Supplement 2: S439–452.

Bacskai, B. J., Kajdasz, S. T., McLellan, M. E., Games, D., Seubert, P., Schenk, D., and Hyman, B. T. 2002. Non-Fc-mediated mechanisms are involved in clearance of amyloid-beta in vivo by immunotherapy. *J Neurosci* 22 (18): 7873–7878.

Bard, F., Cannon, C., Barbour, R., Burke, R. L., Games, D., Grajeda, H., Guido, T., Hu, K., Huang, J., Johnson-Wood, K., Khan, K., Kholodenko, D., Lee, M., Lieberburg, I., Motter, R., Nguyen, M., Soriano, F., Vasquez, N., Weiss, K., Welch, B., Seubert, P., Schenk, D., and Yednock, T. 2000. Peripherally administered antibodies against amyloid beta-peptide enter the central nervous system and reduce pathology in a mouse model of Alzheimer disease. *Nat Med* 6 (8): 916–919.

Bastianetto, S., Yao, Z. X., Papadopoulos, V., and Quirion, R. 2006. Neuroprotective effects of green and black teas and their catechin gallate esters against beta-amyloid-induced toxicity. *Eur J Neurosci* 23 (1): 55–64.

Beckett, L. A., Harvey, D. J., Gamst, A., Donohue, M., Kornak, J., Zhang, H., and Kuo, J. H. 2010. The Alzheimer's Disease Neuroimaging Initiative: Annual change in biomarkers and clinical outcomes. *Alzheimers Dement* 6 (3): 257–264.

Benito-Leon, J., Louis, E. D., Vega, S., and Bermejo-Pareja, F. 2010. Statins and cognitive functioning in the elderly: A population-based study. *J Alzheimers Dis* 21 (1): 95–102.

Birks, J. 2006. Cholinesterase inhibitors for Alzheimer's disease. *Cochrane Database Syst Rev* (1): CD005593.

Birks, J. 2008. The evidence for the efficacy of cholinesterase inhibitors in the treatment of Alzheimer's disease is convincing. *Int Psychogeriatr* 20 (2): 259–292.

Birks, J., Grimley, E. J. , Iakovidou, V., Tsolaki, M., and Holt, F. E. 2009. Rivastigmine for Alzheimer's disease. *Cochrane Database Syst Rev* (2): CD001191.

Birks, J., and Harvey, R. J. 2006. Donepezil for dementia due to Alzheimer's disease. *Cochrane Database Syst Rev* 25 (1): CD001190.

Black, R., Greenberg, B., Ryan, J. M., Posner, H., Seeburger, J., Amatniek, J., Resnick, M., Mohs, R., Miller, D. S., Saumier, D., Carrillo, M. C., and Stern, Y. 2009. Scales as outcome measures for Alzheimer's disease. *Alzheimers Dement* 5 (4): 324–339.

Black, R. S., Sperling, R. A., Safirstein, B., Motter, R. N., Pallay, A., Nichols, A., and Grundman, M. 2010. A single ascending dose study of bapineuzumab in patients with Alzheimer disease. *Alzheimer Dis Assoc Disord* 24 (2): 198–203.

Black, S. A., Espino, D. V., Mahurin, R., Lichtenstein, M. J., Hazuda, H. P., Fabrizio, D., Ray, L. A., and Markides, K. S. 1999. The influence of noncognitive factors on the Mini-Mental State Examination in older Mexican-Americans: Findings from the Hispanic EPESE. Established Population for the Epidemiologic Study of the Elderly. *J Clin Epidemiol* 52 (11): 1095–1102.

Blackard, W. G., Jr., Sood, G. K., Crowe, D. R., and Fallon, M. B. 1998. Tacrine: A cause of fatal hepatotoxicity? *J Clin Gastroenterol* 26 (1): 57–59.

Blennow, K., Wallin, A., Agren, H., Spenger, C., Siegfried, J., and Vanmechelen, E. 1995. Tau protein in cerebrospinal fluid: A biochemical marker for axonal degeneration in Alzheimer disease? *Mol Chem Neuropathol* 26 (3): 231–245.

Bokde, A. L., Karmann, M., Teipel, S. J., Born, C., Lieb, M., Reiser, M. F., Moller, H. J., and Hampel, H. 2009. Decreased activation along the dorsal visual pathway after a 3-month treatment with galantamine in mild Alzheimer disease: A functional magnetic resonance imaging study. *J Clin Psychopharmacol* 29 (2): 147–156.

Boller, F., Verny, M., Hugonot-Diener, L., and Saxton, J. 2002. Clinical features and assessment of severe dementia. A review. *Eur J Neurol* 9 (2): 125–136.

Buerger, K., Ewers, M., Pirttila, T., Zinkowski, R., Alafuzoff, I., Teipel, S. J., DeBernardis, J., Kerkman, D., McCulloch, C., Soininen, H., and Hampel, H. 2006. CSF phosphorylated tau protein correlates with neocortical neurofibrillary pathology in Alzheimer's disease. *Brain* 129 (Pt 11): 3035–3041.

Bullock, R., Touchon, J., Bergman, H., Gambina, G., He, Y., Rapatz, G., Nagel, J., and Lane, R. 2005. Rivastigmine and donepezil treatment in moderate to moderately-severe Alzheimer's disease over a 2-year period. *Curr Med Res Opin* 21 (8): 1317–1327.

Cagnin, A., Brooks, D. J., Kennedy, A. M., Gunn, R. N., Myers, R., Turkheimer, F. E., Jones, T., and Banati, R. B. 2001. In-vivo measurement of activated microglia in dementia. *Lancet* 358 (9280): 461–467.

Calabrese, P., Essner, U., and Forstl, H. 2007. Memantine (Ebixa) in clinical practice: Results of an observational study. *Dement Geriatr Cogn Disord* 24 (2): 111–117.

Campbell, N., Ayub, A., Boustani, M. A., Fox, C., Farlow, M., Maidment, I., and Howards, R. 2008. Impact of cholinesterase inhibitors on behavioral and psychological symptoms of Alzheimer's disease: A meta-analysis. *Clin Interv Aging* 3 (4): 719–728.

Cano, S. J., Posner, H. B., Moline, M. L., Hurt, S. W., Swartz, J., Hsu, T., and Hobart, J. C. 2010. The ADAS-cog in Alzheimer's disease clinical trials: Psychometric evaluation of the sum and its parts. *J Neurol Neurosurg Psychiatry* 81 (12): 1363–1368.

Cappai, R., and Barnham, K. J. 2008. Delineating the mechanism of Alzheimer's disease: A beta peptide neurotoxicity. *Neurochem Res* 33 (3): 526–532.

Chiu, H. F., and Lam, L. C. 2007. Relevance of outcome measures in different cultural groups: Does one size fit all? *Int Psychogeriatr* 19 (3): 457–466.

Choi, Y. T., Jung, C. H., Lee, S. R., Bae, J. H., Baek, W. K., Suh, M. H., Park, J., Park, C. W., and Suh, S. I. 2001. The green tea polyphenol (-)-epigallocatechin gallate attenuates beta-amyloid-induced neurotoxicity in cultured hippocampal neurons. *Life Sci* 70 (5): 603–614.

Clark, C. M., Schneider, J. A., Bedell, B. J., Beach, T. G., Bilker, W. B., Mintun, M. A., Pontecorvo, M. J., Hefti, F., Carpenter, A. P., Flitter, M. L., Krautkramer, M. J., Kung, H. F., Coleman, R. E., Doraiswamy, P. M., Fleisher, A. S., Sabbagh, M. N., Sadowsky, C. H., Reiman, E. P., Zehntner, S. P., and Skovronsky, D. M. 2011. Use of florbetapir-PET for imaging beta-amyloid pathology. *JAMA* 305 (3): 275–283.

Clarke, N. 2004. AD2000: Design and conclusions. *Lancet* 364 (9441): 1215–1216; author reply 1216–1217.

Cohen-Mansfield, J., and Libin, A. 2004. Assessment of agitation in elderly patients with dementia: Correlations between informant rating and direct observation. *Int J Geriatr Psychiatry* 19: 881–891.

Connor, D. J., and Sabbagh, M. N. 2008. Administration and scoring variance on the ADAS-Cog. *J Alzheimers Dis* 15 (3): 461–464.

Coon, K. D., Myers, A. J., Craig, D. W., Webster, J. A., Pearson, J. V., Lince, D. H., Zismann, V. L., Beach, T. G., Leung, D., Bryden, L., Halperin, R. F., Marlowe, L., Kaleem, M., Walker, D. G., Ravid, R., Heward, C. B., Rogers, J., Papassotiropoulos, A., Reiman, E. M., Hardy, J., and Stephan, D. A. 2007. A high-density whole-genome association study reveals that APOE is the major susceptibility gene for sporadic late-onset Alzheimer's disease. *J Clin Psychiatry* 68 (4): 613–618.

Courtney, C., Farrell, D., Gray, R., Hills, R., Lynch, L., Sellwood, E., Edwards, S., Hardyman, W., Raftery, J., Crome, P., Lendon, C., Shaw, H., Bentham, P., and Group. AD2000 Collaborative. 2004. Long-term donepezil treatment in 565 patients with Alzheimer's disease (AD2000): Randomised double-blind trial. *Lancet Neurol* 363 (9427): 2105–2115.

Craft, S. 2007. Insulin resistance and Alzheimer's disease pathogenesis: Potential mechanisms and implications for treatment. *Curr Alzheimer Res* 4 (2): 147–152.

Crawford, J. G. 1998. Alzheimer's disease risk factors as related to cerebral blood flow: Additional evidence. *Med Hypotheses* 50 (1): 25–36.

Cummings, J. L. 1997. The Neuropsychiatric Inventory: Assessing psychopathology in dementia patients. *Neurology* 48 (5 Suppl 6): S10–6.

Cummings, J. L., Mega, M., Gray, K., Rosenberg-Thompson, S., Carusi, D. A., and Gornbein, J. 1994. The Neuropsychiatric Inventory: Comprehensive assessment of psychopathology in dementia. *Neurology* 44 (12): 2308–2314.

David, R., Mulin, E., Mallea, P., and Robert, P. H. 2010. Measurement of neuropsychiatric symptoms in clinical trials targeting Alzheimer's disease and related disorders. *Pharmaceuticals* 3: 2387–2397.

de Jong, D., Jansen, R., Hoefnagels, W., Jellesma-Eggenkamp, M., Verbeek, M., Borm, G., and Kremer, B. 2008. No effect of one-year treatment with indomethacin on Alzheimer's disease progression: A randomized controlled trial. 2008. *PLoS One* 3 (1): e1475, doi:10.1371/journal.pone.0001475.

de Jonghe, J. F., Wetzels, R. B., Mulders, A., Zuidema, S. U., and Koopmans, R. T. 2009. Validity of the Severe Impairment Battery Short Version. *J Neurol Neurosurg Psychiatry* 80 (9): 954–959.

de Medeiros, K., Robert, P., Gauthier, S., Stella, F., Politis, A., Leoutsakos, J., Taragano, F., Kremer, J., Brugnolo, A., Porsteinsson, A. P., Geda, Y. E., Brodaty, H., Gazdag, G., Cummings, J., and Lyketsos, C. 2010. The Neuropsychiatric Inventory-Clinician rating scale (NPI-C): Reliability and validity of a revised assessment of neuropsychiatric symptoms in dementia. *Int Psychogeriatr* 22 (6): 984–994.

DeKosky, S. T., Carrillo, M. C., Phelps, C., Knopman, D., Petersen, R. C., Frank, R., Schenk, D., Masterman, D., Siemers, E. R., Cedarbaum, J. M., Gold, M., Miller, D. S., Morimoto, B. H., Khachaturian, A. S., and Mohs, R. C. 2011. Revision of the criteria for Alzheimer's disease: A symposium. *Alzheimers Dement* 7 (1): e1–12.

DeMattos, R. B., Bales, K. R., Cummins, D. J., Dodart, J. C., Paul, S. M., and Holtzman, D. M. 2001. Peripheral anti-A beta antibody alters CNS and plasma A beta clearance and decreases brain A beta burden in a mouse model of Alzheimer's disease. *Proc Natl Acad Sci USA* 98 (15): 8850–8855.

Dickerson, B. C., Stoub, T. R., Shah, R. C., Sperling, R. A., Killiany, R. J., Albert, M. S., Hyman, B. T., Blacker, D., and Detoledo-Morrell, L. 2011. Alzheimer-signature MRI biomarker predicts AD dementia in cognitively normal adults. *Neurology* 76 (16): 1395–1402.

Dodart, J. C., Bales, K. R., Gannon, K. S., Greene, S. J., DeMattos, R. B., Mathis, C., DeLong, C. A., Wu, S., Wu, X., Holtzman, D. M., and Paul, S. M. 2002. Immunization reverses memory deficits without reducing brain Abeta burden in Alzheimer's disease model. *Nat Neurosci* 5 (5): 452–457.

Dodel, R. C., Du, Y., Depboylu, C., Hampel, H., Frolich, L., Haag, A., Hemmeter, U., Paulsen, S., Teipel, S. J., Brettschneider, S., Spottke, A., Nolker, C., Moller, H. J., Wei, X., Farlow, M., Sommer, N., and Oertel, W. H. 2004. Intravenous immunoglobulins containing antibodies against beta-amyloid for the treatment of Alzheimer's disease. *J Neurol Neurosurg Psychiatry* 75 (10): 1472–1474.

Doody, R. S., Gavrilova, S. I., Sano, M., Thomas, R. G., Aisen, P. S., Bachurin, S. O., Seely, L., and Hung, D. 2008. Effect of dimebon on cognition, activities of daily living, behaviour, and global function in patients with mild-to-moderate Alzheimer's disease: a randomised, double-blind, placebo-controlled study. *Lancet* 372 (9634): 207–215.

Doody, R. S., Tariot, P. N., Pfeiffer, E., Olin, JT., and Graham, S. M. 2007. Meta-analysis of six-month memantine trials in Alzheimer's disease. *Alzheimers Dement* 3 (1): 7–17.

Doraiswamy, P. M., Krishen, A., Stallone, F., Martin, W. L., Potts, N. L., Metz, A., and DeVeaugh-Geiss, J. 1995. Cognitive performance on the Alzheimer's Disease Assessment Scale: Effect of education. *Neurology* 45 (11): 1980–1984.

Duara, R., Loewenstein, D. A., Potter, E., Appel, J., Greig, M. T., Urs, R., Shen, Q., Raj, A., Small, B., Barker, W., Schofield, E., Wu, Y., and Potter, H. 2008. Medial temporal lobe atrophy on MRI scans and the diagnosis of Alzheimer disease. *Neurology* 71 (24): 1986–1992.

Eli Lilly and Company. 2010. Lilly halts development of semagacestat for Alzheimer's disease based on preliminary results of phase III clinical trials, http://newsroom.lilly.com/releasedetail.cfm?releaseid=499794 (accessed August 17, 2010).

Emre, M., Bernabei, R., Blesa, R., Bullock, R., Cunha, L., Daniëls, H., Dziadulewicz, E., Förstl, H., Frölich, L., Gabryelewicz, T., Levin, O., Lindesay, J., Martínez-Lage, P., Monsch, A., Tsolaki, M., and van Laar, T. 2010. Drug profile: Transdermal rivastigmine patch in the treatment of Alzheimer disease. *CNS Neurosci Ther* 16 (4): 246–253.

Engler, H., Forsberg, A., Almkvist, O., Blomquist, G., Larsson, E., Savitcheva, I., Wall, A., Ringheim, A., Langstrom, B., and Nordberg, A. 2006. Two-year follow-up of amyloid deposition in patients with Alzheimer's disease. *Brain* 129 (Pt 11): 2856–2866.

Eriksen, J. L., Sagi, S. A., Smith, T. E., Weggen, S., Das, P., McLendon, D. C., Ozols, V. V., Jessing, K. W., Zavitz, K. H., Koo, E. H., and Golde, T. E. 2003. NSAIDs and enantiomers of flurbiprofen target gamma-secretase and lower Abeta 42 in vivo. *J Clin Invest* 112 (3): 440–449.

Espinoza, R. 2001. Limitations of MMSE when screening for dementia. *Geriatrics* 56 (9): 14.

Etcheberrigaray, R., Tan, M., Dewachter, I., Kuiperi, C., Van der Auwera, I., Wera, S., Qiao, L., Bank, B., Nelson, T. J., Kozikowski, A. P., Van Leuven, F., and Alkon, D. L. 2004. Therapeutic effects of PKC activators in Alzheimer's disease transgenic mice. *Proc Natl Acad Sci USA* 101 (30): 11141–11146.

European Medicines Agency. 2008. Guideline on medicinal products for the treatment of Alzheimer's disease and other dementias. 2008, http://www.ema.europa.eu/docs/en_GB/document_library/Scientific_guideline/2009/09/WC500003562.pdf (accessed May 10, 2011).

Fagan, A. M., Roe, C. M., Xiong, C., Mintun, M. A., Morris, J. C., and Holtzman, D. M. 2007. Cerebrospinal fluid tau/beta-amyloid(42) ratio as a prediction of cognitive decline in nondemented older adults. *Arch Neurol* 64 (3): 343–349.

Farlow, M. R., Salloway, S., Tariot, P. N., Yardley, J., Moline, M. L., Wang, Q., Brand-Schieber, E., Zou, H., Hsu, T., and Satlin, A. 2010. Effectiveness and tolerability of high-dose (23 mg/d) versus standard-dose (10 mg/d) donepezil in moderate to severe Alzheimer's disease: A 24-week, randomized, double-blind study. *Clin Ther* 32 (7): 1234–1251.

Farlow, M. R., Small, G. W., Quarg, P., and Krause, A. 2005. Efficacy of rivastigmine in Alzheimer's disease patients with rapid disease progression: Results of a meta-analysis. *Dement Geriatr Cogn Disord* 20 (2–3): 192–197.

Fassbender, K., Simons, M., Bergmann, C., Stroick, M., Lutjohann, D., Keller, P., Runz, H., Kuhl, S., Bertsch, T., von Bergmann, K., Hennerici, M., Beyreuther, K., and Hartmann, T. 2001. Simvastatin strongly reduces levels of Alzheimer's disease beta-amyloid peptides Abeta 42 and Abeta 40 in vitro and in vivo. *Proc Natl Acad Sci USA* 98 (10): 5856–5861.

Feldman, H. H., Doody, R. S., Kivipelto, M., Sparks, D. L., Waters, D. D., Jones, R. W., Schwam, E., Schindler, R., Hey-Hadavi, J., DeMicco, D. A., and Breazna, A. 2010. Randomized controlled trial of atorvastatin in mild to moderate Alzheimer disease: LEADe. *Neurology* 74 (12): 956–964.

Festuccia, W. T., Oztezcan, S., Laplante, M., Berthiaume, M., Michel, C., Dohgu, S., Denis, R. G., Brito, M. N., Brito, N. A., Miller, D. S., Banks, W. A., Bartness, T. J., Richard, D., and Deshaies, Y. 2008. Peroxisome proliferator-activated receptor-gamma-mediated positive energy balance in the rat is associated with reduced sympathetic drive to adipose tissues and thyroid status. *Endocrinology* 149 (5): 2121–2130.

First, M. B. 2010. Paradigm shifts and the development of the diagnostic and statistical manual of mental disorders: Past experiences and future aspirations. *Can J Psychiatry* 55 (11): 692–700.

Fleisher, A. S., Raman, R., Siemers, E. R., Becerra, L., Clark, C. M., Dean, R. A., Farlow, M. R., Galvin, J. E., et al. 2008. Phase 2 safety trial targeting amyloid beta production with a gamma-secretase inhibitor in Alzheimer disease. *Arch Neurol* 65(8): 1031–1038.

Fleischman, D. A., Wilson, R. S., Gabrieli, J. D., Schneider, J. A., Bienias, J. L., and Bennett, D. A. 2005. Implicit memory and Alzheimer's disease neuropathology. *Brain* 128 (Pt 9): 2006–2015.

Floyd, R. A. 1999. Neuroinflammatory processes are important in neurodegenerative diseases: An hypothesis to explain the increased formation of reactive oxygen and nitrogen species as major factors involved in neurodegenerative disease development. *Free Radic Biol Med* 26 (9–10): 1346–1355.

Folstein, M. F., Folstein, S. E., and McHugh, P. R. 1975. "Mini-mental state." A practical method for grading the cognitive state of patients for the clinician. *J Psychiatr Res* 12 (3): 189–198.

Food and Drug Administration. 1991. An interim report from the FDA. *N Engl J Med* 324 (5): 349–352.

Forti, P., Pisacane, N., Rietti, E., Lucicesare, A., Olivelli, V., Mariani, E., Mecocci, P., and Ravaglia, G. 2010. Metabolic syndrome and risk of dementia in older adults. *J Am Geriatr Soc* 58 (3): 487–492.

Fox, N. C., Cousens, S., Scahill, R., Harvey, R. J., and Rossor, M. N. 2000. Using serial registered brain magnetic resonance imaging to measure disease progression in Alzheimer disease: Power calculations and estimates of sample size to detect treatment effects. *Arch Neurol* 57 (3): 339–344.

Frenkel, D., Solomon, B., and Benhar, I. 2000. Modulation of Alzheimer's beta-amyloid neurotoxicity by site-directed single-chain antibody. *J Neuroimmunol* 106 (1–2): 23–31.

Freund-Levi, Y., Eriksdotter-Jonhagen, M., Cederholm, T., Basun, H., Faxen-Irving, G., Garlind, A., Vedin, I., Vessby, B., Wahlund, L. O., and Palmblad, J. 2006. Omega-3 fatty acid treatment in 174 patients with mild to moderate Alzheimer disease: OmegAD study: A randomized double-blind trial. *Arch Neurol* 63 (10): 1402–1408.

Furukawa, K., Sopher, B. L., Rydel, R. E., Begley, J. G., Pham, D. G., Martin, G. M., Fox, M., and Mattson, M. P. 1996. Increased activity-regulating and neuroprotective efficacy of alpha-secretase-derived secreted amyloid precursor protein conferred by a C-terminal heparin-binding domain. *J Neurochem* 67 (5): 1882–1896.

Fuschillo, C., Ascoli, E., Franzese, G., Campana, F., Cello, C., Galdi, M., La Pia, S., and Cetrangolo, C. 2004. Alzheimer's disease and acetylcholinesterase inhibitor agents: A two-year longitudinal study. *Arch Gerontol Geriatr Suppl* (9): 187–194.

Galasko, D., Schmitt, F., Thomas, R., Jin, S., and Bennett, D. 2005. Detailed assessment of activities of daily living in moderate to severe Alzheimer's disease. *J Int Neuropsychol Soc* 11 (4): 446–453.

Galasko, D. R., Graff-Radford, N., May, S., Hendrix, S., Cottrell, B. A., Sagi, S. A., Mather, G., Laughlin, M., Zavitz, K. H., Swabb, E., Golde, T. E., Murphy, M. P., and Koo, E. H. 2007. Safety, tolerability, pharmacokinetics, and Abeta levels after short-term administration of R-flurbiprofen in healthy elderly individuals. *Alzheimer Dis Assoc Disord* 21 (4): 292–299.

Garzone, P., Koller, M. , Pastrak, A., Jhee, S. S., Ereshefsky, L., Moran, S., Cedarbaum, J. M., Xu, V., and Ross, B. 2009. Oral amyloid anti-aggregating agent ELND005 is measurable in CSF and brain of healthy adult men. Paper presented at the Alzheimer's Association International Conference on Alzheimer's Disease, Vienna, July 11–16.

Gauthier, S., Cummings, J., Ballard, C., Brodaty, H., Grossberg, G., Robert, P., and Lyketsos, C. 2010. Management of behavioral problems in Alzheimer's disease. *Int Psychogeriatr* 22 (3): 346–372.

Gauthier, S., Wirth, Y., and Möbius, H. J. 2005. Effects of memantine on behavioural symptoms in Alzheimer's disease patients: An analysis of the Neuropsychiatric Inventory (NPI) data of two randomised, controlled studies. *Int J Geriatr Psychiatry* 20 (5): 459–464.

Geldmacher, D. S., Fritsch, T., McClendon, M. J., and Landreth, G. 2011. A randomized pilot clinical trial of the safety of pioglitazone in treatment of patients with Alzheimer disease. *Arch Neurol* 68 (1): 45–50.

Gelinas, I., Gautheir, L., McIntyre, M., and Gauthier, S. 1998. Development of a functional measure for persons with Alzheimer's Disease: The Disability Assessment for Dementia. *Am J Occup Ther* 53: 471–481.

Gervais, F., Paquette, J., Morissette, C., Krzywkowski, P., Yu, M., Azzi, M., Lacombe, D., Kong, X., Aman, A., Laurin, J., Szarek, W. A., and Tremblay, P. 2007. Targeting soluble Abeta peptide with Tramiprosate for the treatment of brain amyloidosis. *Neurobiol Aging* 28 (4): 537–547.

Gill, S. S., Anderson, G. M., Fischer, H. D., Bell, C. M., Li, P., Normand, S. L., and Rochon, P. A. 2009. Syncope and its consequences in patients with dementia receiving cholinesterase inhibitors: A population-based cohort study. *Arch Intern Med* 169 (9): 867–873.

Gilman, S., Koller, M., Black, R. S., Jenkins, L., Griffith, S. G., Fox, N. C., Eisner, L., Kirby, L., Rovira, M. B., Forette, F., and Orgogozo, J. M. 2005. Clinical effects of Abeta immunization (AN1792) in patients with AD in an interrupted trial. *Neurology* 64 (9): 1553–1562.

Glenner, G. G., and Wong, C. W. 1984a. Alzheimer's disease and Down's syndrome: Sharing of a unique cerebrovascular amyloid fibril protein. *Biochem Biophys Res Commun* 122 (3): 1131–1135.

Glenner, G. G., and Wong, C. W. 1984b. Alzheimer's disease: Initial report of the purification and characterization of a novel cerebrovascular amyloid protein. *Biochem Biophys Res Commun* 120 (3): 885–890.

Goedert, M., Klug, A., and Crowther, R. A. 2006. Tau protein, the paired helical filament and Alzheimer's disease. *J Alzheimers Dis* 9 (3 Supplement): 195–207.

Goekoop, R., Scheltens, P., Barkhof, F., and Rombouts, S. A. 2006. Cholinergic challenge in Alzheimer patients and mild cognitive impairment differentially affects hippocampal activation: A pharmacological fMRI study. *Brain* 129 (Pt 1): 141–157.

Gold, M., Alderton, C., Zvartau-Hind, M., Egginton, S., Saunders, A. M., Irizarry, M., Craft, S., Landreth, G., Linnamagi, U., and Sawchak, S. 2010. Rosiglitazone monotherapy in mild-to-moderate Alzheimer's disease: Results from a randomized, double-blind, placebo-controlled phase III study. *Dement Geriatr Cogn Disord* 30 (2) :131–146.

Gong, Y., Chang, L., Viola, K. L., Lacor, P. N., Lambert, M. P., Finch, C. E., Krafft, G. A., and Klein, W. L. 2003. Alzheimer's disease-affected brain: Presence of oligomeric A beta ligands (ADDLs) suggests a molecular basis for reversible memory loss. *Proc Natl Acad Sci USA* 100 (18): 10417–10422.

Goto, T., Fujikoshi, S., Uenaka, K., Nishiuma, S., Siemers, E. R., Dean, R. A., and Takahashi, M. 2010. Solanezumab was safe and well-tolerated for Asian patients with mild-to-moderate Alzheimer's disease in a multicenter, randomized, open-label, multidose study. Paper presented at the Alzheimer's Association International Conference on Alzheimer's Disease, Honolulu, Hawaii, July 10–15.

Graham, D. P., Cully, J. A., Snow, A. L., Massman, P., and Doody, R. 2004. The Alzheimer's Disease Assessment Scale-Cognitive subscale: Normative data for older adult controls. *Alzheimer Dis Assoc Disord* 18 (4): 236–240.

Green, R. C., Schneider, L. S., Amato, D. A., Beelen, A. P., Wilcock, G., Swabb, E. A., and Zavitz, K. H. 2009. Effect of tarenflurbil on cognitive decline and activities of daily living in patients with mild Alzheimer disease: A randomized controlled trial. *JAMA* 302 (23): 2557–2564.

Griffiths, H. H., Morten, I. J., and Hooper, N. M. 2008. Emerging and potential therapies for Alzheimer's disease. *Expert Opin Ther Targets* 12 (6): 693–704.

Grossman, H., Marzloff, G., Luo, X., LeRoith, D., and Sano, M. 2009. NIC5-15 as a treatment for Alzheimer's: Safety, pharmacokinetics and clinical variables. Paper presented at the Alzheimer's Association International Conference on Alzheimer's Disease, Vienna, July 11–16.

Guo, J. P., Yu, S., and McGeer, P. L. 2010. Simple in vitro assays to identify amyloid-beta aggregation blockers for Alzheimer's disease therapy. *J Alzheimers Dis* 19 (4): 1359–1370.

Haass, C., and Selkoe, D. J. 2007. Soluble protein oligomers in neurodegeneration: Lessons from the Alzheimer's amyloid beta-peptide. *Nat Rev Mol Cell Biol* 8 (2): 101–112.

Hampel, H., Burger, K., Teipel, S. J., Bokde, A. L., Zetterberg, H., and Blennow, K. 2008. Core candidate neurochemical and imaging biomarkers of Alzheimer's disease. *Alzheimers Dement* 4 (1): 38–48.

Hampel, H., Ewers, M., Burger, K., Annas, P., Mortberg, A., Bogstedt, A., Frolich, L., Schroder, J., Schonknecht, P., Riepe, M. W., Kraft, I., Gasser, T., Leyhe, T., Moller, H. J., Kurz, A., and Basun, H. 2009. Lithium trial in Alzheimer's disease: A randomized, single-blind, placebo-controlled, multicenter 10-week study. *J Clin Psychiatry* 70 (6): 922–931.

Hansen, R. A., Gartlehner, G., Lohr, K. N., and Kaufer, D. I. 2007. Functional outcomes of drug treatment in Alzheimer's disease: A systematic review and meta-analysis. *Drugs Aging* 24 (2): 155–167.

Hansen, R. A., Gartlehner, G., Webb, A. P., Morgan, L. C., Moore, C. G., and Jonas, D. E. 2008. Efficacy and safety of donepezil, galantamine, and rivastigmine for the treatment of Alzheimer's disease: A systematic review and meta-analysis. *Clin Interv Aging* 3 (2): 211–225.

Hansson Petersen, C. A., Alikhani, N., Behbahani, H., Wiehager, B., Pavlov, P. F., Alafuzoff, I., Leinonen, V., Ito, A., Winblad, B., Glaser, E., and Ankarcrona, M. 2008. The amyloid beta-peptide is imported into mitochondria via the TOM import machinery and localized to mitochondrial cristae. *Proc Natl Acad Sci USA* 105 (35): 13145–13150.

Hardy, J. A., and Higgins, G. A. 1992. Alzheimer's disease: The amyloid cascade hypothesis. *Science* 256 (5054): 184–185.

Harry, R. D., and Zakzanis, K. K. 2005. A comparison of donepezil and galantamine in the treatment of cognitive symptoms of Alzheimer's disease: A meta-analysis. 2005. *Hum Psychopharmacol* 20 (3): 183–187.

Hartmann, D., Tournoy, J., Saftig, P., Annaert, W., and De Strooper, B. 2001. Implication of APP secretases in notch signaling. *J Mol Neurosci* 17 (2): 171–181.

Herrmann, N. 2007. Trials and tribulations of evidence-based medicine: The case of Alzheimer disease therapeutics. *Can J Psychiatry* 52 (10): 617–619.

Herrmann, N., Lanctôt, K. L., Sambrook, R., Lesnikova, N., Hebert, R., McCracken, P., Robillard, A., and Nguyen, E. 2006. The contribution of neuropsychiatric symptoms to the cost of dementia care. *Int J Geriatr Psychiatry* 21 (10): 972–976.

Hoglund, K., and Blennow, K. 2007. Effect of HMG-CoA reductase inhibitors on beta-amyloid peptide levels: Implications for Alzheimer's disease. *CNS Drugs* 21 (6): 449–462.

Holmes, C., Boche, D., Wilkinson, D., Yadegarfar, G., Hopkins, V., Bayer, A., Jones, R. W., Bullock, R., Love, S., Neal, J. W., Zotova, E., and Nicoll, J. A. 2008. Long-term effects of Abeta42 immunisation in Alzheimer's disease: Follow-up of a randomised, placebo-controlled phase I trial. *Lancet* 372 (9634): 216–223.

Holmes, C., Burns, A., Passmore, P., Forsyth, D., and Wilkinson, D. 2004a. AD2000: Design and conclusions. *Lancet* 364 (9441): 1213–1214; author reply 1216–1217.

Holmes, C., Wilkinson, D., Dean, C., Vethanayagam, S., Olivieri, S., Langley, A., Pandita-Gunawardena, N. D., Hogg, F., Clare, C., and Damms, J. 2004b. The efficacy of done-pezil in the treatment of neuropsychiatric symptoms in Alzheimer disease. *Neurology* 63 (2): 214–219.

Howard, R. J., Juszczak, E., Ballard, C. G., Bentham, P., Brown, R. G., Bullock, R., Burns, A. S., Holmes, C., Jacoby, R., Johnson, T., Knapp, M., Lindesay, J., O'Brien, J. T., Wilcock, G., Katona, C., Jones, R. W., DeCesare, J., Rodger, M., et al., 2007. CALM-AD Trial. Donepezil for the treatment of agitation in Alzheimer's disease. *N Engl J Med* 357 (14): 1382–1392.

Howe, I. 2004. AD2000: Design and conclusions. *Lancet* 364 (9441): 1214–1215; author reply 1216–1217.

Jack, C. R., Jr., Lowe, V. J., Weigand, S. D., Wiste, H. J., Senjem, M. L., Knopman, D. S., Shiung, M. M., Gunter, J. L., Boeve, B. F., Kemp, B. J., Weiner, M., and Petersen, R. C. 2009. Serial PIB and MRI in normal, mild cognitive impairment and Alzheimer's disease: Implications for sequence of pathological events in Alzheimer's disease. *Brain* 132 (Pt 5): 1355–1365.

Jack, C. R., Jr., Petersen, R. C., Xu, Y., O'Brien, P. C., Smith, G. E., Ivnik, R. J., Boeve, B. F., Tangalos, E. G., and Kokmen, E. 2000. Rates of hippocampal atrophy correlate with change in clinical status in aging and AD. *Neurology* 55 (4): 484–489.

Jacobsen, S., Comery, T., Kreft, A., Mayer, S., Zaleska, M., Riddell, D., Bard, J., Gonzales, C., Frick, G., Raje, S., Forlow, S., Balliet, C., Burczynski, M., Wan, H., Harrison, B., Reinhart, P., Pangalos, M., and Martone, R. 2009. GSI-953 is a potent APP-selective gamma-secretase inhibitor for the treatment of Alzheimer's disease. In *Alzheimer's Association International Conference on Alzheimer's Disease*. Vienna: Alzheimers Dement.

Jessen, F., Traeber, F., Freymann, K., Maier, W., Schild, H. H., and Block, W. 2006. Treatment monitoring and response prediction with proton MR spectroscopy in AD. *Neurology* 67 (3): 528–530.

Jiang, Q., Heneka, M., and Landreth, G. E. 2008. The role of peroxisome proliferator-activated receptor-gamma (PPARgamma) in Alzheimer's disease: Therapeutic implications. *CNS Drugs* 22 (1): 1–14.

Jick, H., Zornberg, G. L., Jick, S. S., Seshadri, S., and Drachman, D. A. 2000. Statins and the risk of dementia. *Lancet* 356 (9242): 1627–1631.

Joffres, C., Graham, J., and Rockwood, K. 2000. Qualitative analysis of the clinician inter-view-based impression of change (Plus): Methodological issues and implications for clinical research. *Int Psychogeriatr* 12 (3): 403–413.

Jones, R. W., Soininen, H., Hager, K., Aarsland, D., Passmore, P., Murthy, A., Zhang, R., and Bahra, R. 2004. A multinational, randomised, 12-week study comparing the effects of donepezil and galantamine in patients with mild to moderate Alzheimer's disease. *Int J Geriatr Psychiatry* 19 (1): 58–67.

Kadir, A., Andreasen, N., Almkvist, O., Wall, A., Forsberg, A., Engler, H., Hagman, G., Larksater, M., Winblad, B., Zetterberg, H., Blennow, K., Langstrom, B., and Nordberg, A. 2008. Effect of phenserine treatment on brain functional activity and amyloid in Alzheimer's disease. *Ann Neurol* 63 (5): 621–631.

Kaduszkiewicz, H., Zimmermann, T., Beck-Bornholdt, H. P., and van den Bussche, H. 2005. Cholinesterase inhibitors for patients with Alzheimer's disease: Systematic review of randomised clinical trials. *BMJ* 331 (7512): 321–327.

Kalmijn, S., Launer, L. J., Ott, A., Witteman, J. C., Hofman, A., and Breteler, M. M. 1997. Dietary fat intake and the risk of incident dementia in the Rotterdam Study. *Ann Neurol* 42 (5): 776–782.

Kauwe, J. S., Wang, J., Mayo, K., Morris, J. C., Fagan, A. M., Holtzman, D. M., and Goate, A. M. 2009. Alzheimer's disease risk variants show association with cerebrospinal fluid amyloid beta. *Neurogenetics* 10 (1): 13–17.

Kircher, T. T., Erb, M., Grodd, W., and Leube, D. T. 2005. Cortical activation during cholinesterase-inhibitor treatment in Alzheimer disease: Preliminary findings from a pharmaco-fMRI study. *Am J Geriatr Psychiatry* 13 (11): 1006–1013.

Klunk, W. E., Engler, H., Nordberg, A., Wang, Y., Blomqvist, G., Holt, D. P., Bergstrom, M., Savitcheva, I., Huang, G. F., Estrada, S., Ausen, B., Debnath, M. L., Barletta, J., Price, J. C., Sandell, J., Lopresti, B. J., Wall, A., Koivisto, P., Antoni, G., Mathis, C. A., and Langstrom, B. 2004. Imaging brain amyloid in Alzheimer's disease with Pittsburgh Compound-B. *Ann Neurol* 55 (3): 306–319.

Knapp, M. J., Knopman, D. S., Solomon, P. R., Pendlebury, W. W., Davis, C. S., and Gracon, S. I. 1994. A 30-week randomized controlled trial of high-dose tacrine in patients with Alzheimer's disease. The Tacrine Study Group. *JAMA* 271 (13): 985–991.

Knopman, D. S. 2007. Commentary on "Meta-analysis of six-month memantine trials in Alzheimer's disease." Memantine has negligible benefits in mild to moderate Alzheimer's disease. *Alzheimers Dement* 3 (1): 21–22.

Kosaka, T., Imagawa, M., Seki, K., Arai, H., Sasaki, H., Tsuji, S., Asami-Odaka, A., Fukushima, T., Imai, K., and Iwatsubo, T. 1997. The beta APP717 Alzheimer mutation increases the percentage of plasma amyloid-beta protein ending at A beta42(43). *Neurology* 48 (3): 741–745.

Kosasa, T., Kuriya, Y., Matsui, K. , and Yamanishi, Y. 2000. Inhibitory effect of orally administered donepezil hydrochloride (E2020), a novel treatment for Alzheimer's disease, on cholinesterase activity in rats. *Eur J Pharmacol* 389 (2–3): 173–179.

Kumar-Singh, S., Theuns, J., Van Broeck, B., Pirici, D., Vennekens, K., Corsmit, E., Cruts, M., Dermaut, B., Wang, R., and Van Broeckhoven, C. 2006. Mean age-of-onset of familial Alzheimer disease caused by presenilin mutations correlates with both increased Abeta42 and decreased Abeta40. *Hum Mutat* 27 (7): 686–695.

Laakso, M. P., Soininen, H., Partanen, K., Lehtovirta, M., Hallikainen, M., Hanninen, T., Helkala, E. L., Vainio, P., and Riekkinen, P. J., Sr. 1998. MRI of the hippocampus in Alzheimer's disease: Sensitivity, specificity, and analysis of the incorrectly classified subjects. *Neurobiol Aging* 19 (1): 23–31.

Lanctôt, K. L. Herrmann, N., Yau, K. K., Khan, LR., Liu, B. A., LouLou, M. M., and Einarson, T. R. 2003. Efficacy and safety of cholinesterase inhibitors in Alzheimer's disease: A meta-analysis. *CMAJ* 169 (6): 557–564.

Lannfelt, L., Blennow, K., Zetterberg, H., Batsman, S., Ames, D., Harrison, J., Masters, C. L., Targum, S., Bush, A. I., Murdoch, R., Wilson, J., and Ritchie, C. W. 2008. Safety, efficacy, and biomarker findings of PBT2 in targeting Abeta as a modifying therapy for Alzheimer's disease: A phase IIa, double-blind, randomised, placebo-controlled trial. *Lancet Neurol* 7 (9): 779–786.

Lee, V. M., and Trojanowski, J. Q. 2006. Progress from Alzheimer's tangles to pathological tau points towards more effective therapies now. *J Alzheimers Dis* 9 (3 Supplement): 257–262.

Lerch, J. P., Pruessner, J., Zijdenbos, A. P., Collins, D. L., Teipel, S. J., Hampel, H., and Evans, A. C. 2008. Automated cortical thickness measurements from MRI can accurately separate Alzheimer's patients from normal elderly controls. *Neurobiol Aging* 29 (1): 23–30.

Levites, Y., Amit, T., Mandel, S., and Youdim, M. B. 2003. Neuroprotection and neurorescue against Abeta toxicity and PKC-dependent release of nonamyloidogenic soluble precursor protein by green tea polyphenol (-)-epigallocatechin-3-gallate. *FASEB J* 17 (8): 952–954.

Lewis, H. D., Perez Revuelta, B. I., Nadin, A., Neduvelil, J. G., Harrison, T., Pollack, S. J., and Shearman, M. S. 2003. Catalytic site-directed gamma-secretase complex inhibitors do not discriminate pharmacologically between Notch S3 and beta-APP cleavages. *Biochemistry* 42 (24): 7580–7586.

Li, J., Wu, H. M., Zhou, R. L., Liu, G. J., and Dong, B. R. 2008. Huperzine A for Alzheimer's disease. *Cochrane Database Syst Rev* 16 (2): CD005592.

Livingston, G., Katona, C., Roch, B., Guilhaume, C., and Rive, B. 2004. A dependency model for patients with Alzheimer's disease: Its validation and relationship to the costs of care—the LASER-AD Study. *Curr Med Res Opin* 20 (7): 1007–1016.

Llinas Regla, J., Lozano Gallego, M., Lopez, O. L., Gudayol Portabella, M., Lopez-Pousa, S., Vilalta Franch, J., and J., Saxton. 1995. Validacion de la adaptacion espanola de la Severe Impairment Battery (SIB). *Neurologia* 10 (1): 14–18.

Lockhart, A., Lamb, J. R., Osredkar, T., Sue, L. I., Joyce, J. N., Ye, L., Libri, V., Leppert, D., and Beach, T. G. 2007. PIB is a non-specific imaging marker of amyloid-beta (Abeta) peptide-related cerebral amyloidosis. *Brain* 130 (Pt 10): 2607–2615.

Lockhart, I. A., Mitchell, S. A., and Kelly, S. 2009. Safety and tolerability of donepezil, rivastigmine and galantamine for patients with Alzheimer's disease: Systematic review of the "real-world" evidence. *Dement Geriatr Cogn Disord* 28 (5): 389–403.

Logothetis, N. K. 2002. The neural basis of the blood-oxygen-level-dependent functional magnetic resonance imaging signal. *Philos Trans R Soc Lond B Biol Sci* 357 (1424): 1003–1037.

Lopez-Pousa, S., Turon-Estrada, A., Garre-Olmo, J., Pericot-Nierga, I., Lozano-Gallego, M., Vilalta-Franch, M., Hernandez-Ferrandiz, M., Morante-Munoz, V., Isern-Vila, A., Gelada-Batlle, E., and Majo-Llopart, J. 2005. Differential efficacy of treatment with acetylcholinesterase inhibitors in patients with mild and moderate Alzheimer's disease over a 6-month period. *Dement Geriatr Cogn Disord* 19 (4): 189–195.

Loy, C., and Schneider, L. 2006. Galantamine for Alzheimer's disease and mild cognitive impairment. *Cochrane Database Syst Rev* 25 (1): CD001747.

Luckmann, R. 2006. Review: Cholinesterase inhibitors may be effective in Alzheimer's disease. *Evid Based Med* 11 (1): 23.

Maidment, I. D., Fox, C. G., Boustani, M., Rodriguez, J., Brown, R. C., and Katona, C. L. 2008. Efficacy of memantine on behavioral and psychological symptoms related to dementia: A systematic meta-analysis. *Ann Pharmacother* 42 (1): 32–38.

Mangialasche, F., Solomon, A., Winblad, B., Mecocci, P., and Kivipelto, M. 2010. Alzheimer's disease: Clinical trials and drug development. *Lancet Neurol* 9 (7): 702–716.

Marcade, M., Bourdin, J., Loiseau, N., Peillon, H., Rayer, A., Drouin, D., Schweighoffer, F., and Desire, L. 2008. Etazolate, a neuroprotective drug linking GABA(A) receptor pharmacology to amyloid precursor protein processing. *J Neurochem* 106 (1): 392–404.

Mayeux, R., and Sano, M. 1999. Treatment of Alzheimer's disease. *N Engl J Med* 341 (22): 1670–1679.

McGeer, P. L., and McGeer, E. G. 2007. NSAIDs and Alzheimer disease: Epidemiological, animal model and clinical studies. *Neurobiol Aging* 28 (5): 639–647.

McGeer, P. L., Schulzer, M., and McGeer, E. G. 1996. Arthritis and anti-inflammatory agents as possible protective factors for Alzheimer's disease: A review of 17 epidemiologic studies. *Neurology* 47 (2): 425–432.

McGuinness, B., O'Hare, J., Craig, D., Bullock, R., Malouf, R., and Passmore, P. 2010. Statins for the treatment of dementia. In *Cochrane Database Syst Rev* (8): CD007514.

McKhann, G., Drachman, D., Folstein, M., Katzman, R., Price, D., and Stadlan, E. M. 1984. Clinical diagnosis of Alzheimer's disease: Report of the NINCDS-ADRDA Work Group under the auspices of Department of Health and Human Services Task Force on Alzheimer's Disease. *Neurology* 34 (7): 939–944.

McKhann, G. M., Knopman, D. S., Chertkow, H., Hyman, B. T., Jack C. R, Jr., Kawas, C. H., Klunk, W. E., Koroshetz, W. J., Manly, J. J., Mayeux, R., Mohs, R. C., Morris, J. C., Rossor, M. N., Scheltens, P., Carrillo, M. C., Thies, B., Weintraub, S., and Phelps, C. H. 2011. The diagnosis of dementia due to Alzheimer's disease: Recommendations from the National Institute on Aging-Alzheimer's Association workgroups on diagnostic guidelines for Alzheimer's disease. *Alzheimers Dement* 7 (3): 263–269.

McShane, R., Areosa Sastre, A., and Minakaran, N. 2006. Memantine for dementia. *Cochrane Database Syst Rev* 19 (2): CD003154.

Medivation. 2010. Pfizer and Medivation announce results from two phase 3 studies In dimebon (latrepirdine*) Alzheimer's disease clinical development program, http://investors. medivation.com/releasedetail.cfm?ReleaseID=448818 (accessed March 3, 2010).

Mega, M. S., Dinov, I. D., Porter, V., Chow, G., Reback, E., Davoodi, P., O'Connor, S. M., Carter, M. F., Amezcua, H., and Cummings, J. L. 2005. Metabolic patterns associated with the clinical response to galantamine therapy: A fludeoxyglucose f 18 positron emission tomographic study. *Arch Neurol* 62 (5): 721–728.

Meziane, H., Dodart, J. C., Mathis, C., Little, S., Clemens, J., Paul, S. M., and Ungerer, A. 1998. Memory-enhancing effects of secreted forms of the beta-amyloid precursor protein in normal and amnestic mice. *Proc Natl Acad Sci USA* 95 (21): 12683–12688.

Moffett, J. R., Ross, B., Arun, P., Madhavarao, C. N., and Namboodiri, A. M. 2007. N-Acetylaspartate in the CNS: From neurodiagnostics to neurobiology. *Prog Neurobiol* 81 (2): 89–131.

Mohs, R. C., and Cohen, L. 1988. Alzheimer's Disease Assessment Scale (ADAS). *Psychopharmacol Bull* 24 (4): 627–628.

Mohs, R. C., Knopman, D., Petersen, R. C., Ferris, S. H., Ernesto, C., Grundman, M., Sano, M., Bieliauskas, L., Geldmacher, D., Clark, C., and Thal, L. J. 1997. Development of cognitive instruments for use in clinical trials of antidementia drugs: Additions to the Alzheimer's Disease Assessment Scale that broaden its scope. The Alzheimer's Disease Cooperative Study. *Alzheimer Dis Assoc Disord* 11 Suppl 2: S13–21.

Morihara, T., Chu, T., Ubeda, O., Beech, W., and Cole, G. M. 2002. Selective inhibition of Abeta42 production by NSAID R-enantiomers. *J Neurochem* 83 (4): 1009–1012.

Morinaga, A., Ono, K., Ikeda, T., Ikeda, Y., Shima, K., Noguchi-Shinohara, M., Samuraki, M., Yanase, D., Yoshita, M., Iwasa, K., Mastunari, I., and Yamada, M. 2010. A comparison of the diagnostic sensitivity of MRI, CBF-SPECT, FDG-PET and cerebrospinal fluid biomarkers for detecting Alzheimer's disease in a memory clinic. *Dement Geriatr Cogn Disord* 30 (4): 285–292.

Morris, M. C., Evans, D. A., Bienias, J. L., Tangney, C. C., Bennett, D. A., Wilson, R. S., Aggarwal, N., and Schneider, J. 2003. Consumption of fish and n-3 fatty acids and risk of incident Alzheimer disease. *Arch Neurol* 60 (7): 940–946.

Mosconi, L. 2005. Brain glucose metabolism in the early and specific diagnosis of Alzheimer's disease. FDG-PET studies in MCI and AD. *Eur J Nucl Med Mol Imaging* 32 (4): 486–510.

Mossello, E., Tonon, E., Caleri, V., Tilli, S., Cantini, C., Cavallini, M. C., Bencini, F., Mecacci, R., Marini, M., Bardelli, F., Sarcone, E., Razzi, E., Biagini, C. A., and Masotti, G. 2004. Effectiveness and safety of cholinesterase inhibitors in elderly subjects with Alzheimer's disease: A "real world" study. *Arch Gerontol Geriatr Suppl* (9): 297–307.

Mungas, D. 1991. In-office mental status testing: a practical guide. *Geriatrics* 46 (7): 54–58, 63, 66.

Nordberg, A. 2006. Mechanisms behind the neuroprotective actions of cholinesterase inhibitors in Alzheimer disease. *Alzheimer Dis Assoc Disord* 20 (2 Suppl 1): S12–18.

Okamura, N., and Yanai, K. 2010. Florbetapir (18F), a PET imaging agent that binds to amyloid plaques for the potential detection of Alzheimer's disease. *IDrugs* 13 (12): 890–899.

Olsson, A., Vanderstichele, H., Andreasen, N., De Meyer, G., Wallin, A., Holmberg, B., Rosengren, L., Vanmechelen, E., and Blennow, K. 2005. Simultaneous measurement of beta-amyloid(1-42), total tau, and phosphorylated tau (Thr181) in cerebrospinal fluid by the xMAP technology. *Clin Chem* 51 (2): 336–345.

Oz, M., Lorke, D. E., and Petroianu, G. A. 2009. Methylene blue and Alzheimer's disease. *Biochem Pharmacol* 78 (8): 927–932.

Pakrasi, S., Mukaetova-Ladinska, E. B., McKeith, I. G., and O'Brien, J. T. 2003. Clinical predictors of response to Acetyl Cholinesterase Inhibitors: Experience from routine clinical use in Newcastle. *Int J Geriatr Psychiatry* 18 (10): 879–886.

Pakrasi, S., and O'Brien, J. T. 2005. Emission tomography in dementia. *Nucl Med Commun* 26 (3): 189–196.

Panisset, M., Roudier, M., Saxton, J., and Boller, F. 1992. Batterie d'evaluation neuropsychologique pour la demence grave. *Presse Me Âdicale* 21: 1271–1274.

Park-Wyllie, L. Y., Mamdani, M. M., Li, P., Gill, S. S., Laupacis, A., and Juurlink, D. N. 2009. Cholinesterase inhibitors and hospitalization for bradycardia: A population-based study. *PLoS Med 6* (9): e1000157, doi:10.1371/journal.pmed.1000157.

Perry, E. K., Tomlinson, B. E., Blessed, G., Bergmann, K., Gibson, P. H., and Perry, R. H. 1978. Correlation of cholinergic abnormalities with senile plaques and mental test scores in senile dementia. *Br Med J* 2 (6150): 1457–1459.

Pimplikar, S. W. 2009. Reassessing the amyloid cascade hypothesis of Alzheimer's disease. *Int J Biochem Cell Biol* 41 (6): 1261–1268.

Pippi, M., Mecocci, P., Saxton, J., Bartorelli, L., Pettenati, C., Bonaiuto, S., Cucinotta, D., Masaraki, G., Neri, M., Tammaro, A. E., Vergani, C., Chionne, F., and Senin, U. 1999. Neuropsychological assessment of the severely impaired elderly patient: Validation of the Italian short version of the Severe Impairment Battery (SIB). Gruppo di Studio sull'Invecchiamento Cerebrale della Societa Italiana di Gerontologia e Geriatria. *Aging* (Milano) 11 (4): 221–226.

Poirier, J., Delisle, M. C., Quirion, R., Aubert, I., Farlow, M., Lahiri, D., Hui, S., Bertrand, P., Nalbantoglu, J., Gilfix, B. M., and Gauthier, S. 1995. Apolipoprotein E4 allele as a predictor of cholinergic deficits and treatment outcome in Alzheimer disease. *Proc Natl Acad Sci USA* 92 (26): 12260–12264.

Polinsky, R. J. 1998. Clinical pharmacology of rivastigmine: A new-generation acetylcholinesterase inhibitor for the treatment of Alzheimer's disease. *Clin Ther* 20 (4): 634–647.

Profenno, L. A., Porsteinsson, A. P., and Faraone, S. V. 2010. Meta-analysis of Alzheimer's disease risk with obesity, diabetes, and related disorders. *Biol Psychiatry* 67 (6): 505–512.

Quinn, J. F., Raman, R., Thomas, R. G., Yurko-Mauro, K., Nelson, E. B., Van Dyck, C., Galvin, J. E., Emond, J., Jack, C. R., Jr., Weiner, M., Shinto, L., and Aisen, P. S. 2010. Docosahexaenoic acid supplementation and cognitive decline in Alzheimer disease: A randomized trial. *JAMA* 304 (17): 1903–1911.

Rafii, M. S., Walsh, S., Little, J. T., Behan, K., Reynolds, B., Ward, C., Jin, S., Thomas, R., and Aisen, P. S. 2011. A phase II trial of huperzine A in mild to moderate Alzheimer disease. *Neurology* 76 (16): 1389–1394.

Raina, P. Santaguida, P., Ismaila, A., Patterson, C., Cowan, D., Levine, M., Booker, L., and Oremus, M. 2008. Effectiveness of cholinesterase inhibitors and memantine for treating dementia: Evidence review for a clinical practice guideline. *Ann Intern Med* 148 (5): 379–397.

Razay, G., and Wilcock, G. K. 2008. Galantamine in Alzheimer's disease. *Expert Rev Neurother* 8 (1): 9–17.

Refolo, L. M., Pappolla, M. A., LaFrancois, J., Malester, B., Schmidt, S. D., Thomas-Bryant, T., Tint, G. S., Wang, R., Mercken, M., Petanceska, S. S., and Duff, K. E. 2001. A cholesterol-lowering drug reduces beta-amyloid pathology in a transgenic mouse model of Alzheimer's disease. *Neurobiol Dis* 8 (5): 890–899.

Reines, S. A., Block, G. A., Morris, J. C., Liu, G., Nessly, M. L., Lines, C. R., Norman, B. A., and Baranak, C. C. 2004. Rofecoxib: No effect on Alzheimer's disease in a 1-year, randomized, blinded, controlled study. *Neurology* 62 (1): 66–71.

Reisberg, B., Borenstein, J., Salob, S. P., Ferris, S. H., Franssen, E., and Georgotas, A. 1987. Behavioral symptoms in Alzheimer's disease: Phenomenology and treatment. *J Clin Psychiatry* 48 Suppl: 9–15.

Reisberg, B., Doody, R., Stoffler, A., Schmitt, F., Ferris, S., and Mobius, H. J. 2003. Memantine in moderate-to-severe Alzheimer's disease. *N Engl J Med* 348 (14): 1333–1341.

Relkin, N. R., Szabo, P., Adamiak, B., Burgut, T., Monthe, C., Lent, R. W., Younkin, S., Younkin, L., Schiff, R., and Weksler, M. E. 2009. 18-Month study of intravenous immunoglobulin for treatment of mild Alzheimer disease. *Neurobiol Aging* 30 (11): 1728–1736.

Risner, M. E., Saunders, A. M., Altman, J. F., Ormandy, G. C., Craft, S., Foley, I. M., Zvartau-Hind, M. E., Hosford, D. A., and Roses, A. D. 2006. Efficacy of rosiglitazone in a genetically defined population with mild-to-moderate Alzheimer's disease. *Pharmacogenomics* J 6 (4): 246–254.

Ritchie, C. W., Ames, D., Clayton, T., and Lai, R. 2004. Metaanalysis of randomized trials of the efficacy and safety of donepezil, galantamine, and rivastigmine for the treatment of Alzheimer disease. *Am J Geriatr Psychiatry* 12 (4):358–369.

Rockwood, K., Kirkland, S., Hogan, D. B., MacKnight, C., Merry, H., Verreault, R., Wolfson, C., and McDowell, I. 2002. Use of lipid-lowering agents, indication bias, and the risk of dementia in community-dwelling elderly people. *Arch Neurol* 59 (2): 223–227.

Rogers, J., Kirby, L. C., Hempelman, S. R., Berry, D. L., McGeer, P. L., Kaszniak, A. W., Zalinski, J., Cofield, M., Mansukhani, L., Willson, P., et al. 1993. Clinical trial of indomethacin in Alzheimer's disease. *Neurology* 43 (8): 1609–1611.

Rosen, W. G., Mohs, R. C., and Davis, K. L. 1984. A new rating scale for Alzheimer's disease. *Am J Psychiatry* 141: 1356–1364.

Rothwell, P. M. 2005. External validity of randomised controlled trials: "To whom do the results of this trial apply?" *Lancet* 365 (9453): 82–93.

Salloway, S., Sperling, R., Gilman, S., Fox, N. C., Blennow, K., Raskind, M., Sabbagh, M., Honig, L. S., Doody, R., van Dyck, C. H., Mulnard, R., Barakos, J., Gregg, K. M., Liu, E., Lieberburg, I., Schenk, D., Black, R., and Grundman, M. 2009. A phase 2 multiple ascending dose trial of bapineuzumab in mild to moderate Alzheimer disease. *Neurology* 73 (24): 2061–2070.

Saumier, D., Duong, A., Haine, D., Garceau, D., and Sampalis, J. 2009. Domain-specific cognitive effects of tramiprosate in patients with mild to moderate Alzheimer's disease: ADAS-cog subscale results from the Alphase Study. *J Nutr Health Aging* 13 (9): 808–812.

Saxton, J., Kastango, K. B., Hugonot-Diener, L., Boller, F., Verny, M., Sarles, C. E., Girgis, R. R., Devouche, E., Mecocci, P., Pollock, B. G., and DeKosky, S. T. 2005. Development of a short form of the Severe Impairment Battery. *Am J Geriatr Psychiatry* 13 (11): 999–1005.

Saxton, J., McGonigle-Gibson, K. L., Swihart, A. A., Miller, V. J., and Boller, F. 1990. Assessment of the severely impaired patient: description and validation of a new neuropsychological test battery. *Psychological Assessment* 2 (3): 298–303.

Schaefer, E. J., Bongard, V., Beiser, A. S., Lamon-Fava, S., Robins, S. J., Au, R., Tucker, K. L., Kyle, D. J., Wilson, P. W., and Wolf, P. A. 2006. Plasma phosphatidylcholine docosa-hexaenoic acid content and risk of dementia and Alzheimer disease: The Framingham Heart Study. *Arch Neurol* 63 (11): 1545–1550.

Schenk, D., Barbour, R., Dunn, W., Gordon, G., Grajeda, H., Guido, T., Hu, K., Huang, J., Johnson-Wood, K., Khan, K., Kholodenko, D., Lee, M., Liao, Z., Lieberburg, I., Motter, R., Mutter, L., Soriano, F., Shopp, G., Vasquez, N., Vandevert, C., Walker, S., Wogulis, M., Yednock, T., Games, D., and Seubert, P. 1999. Immunization with amyloid-beta attenuates Alzheimer-disease-like pathology in the PDAPP mouse. *Nature* 400 (6740): 173–177.

Schmitt, F. A., and Wichems, C. H. 2006. A systematic review of assessment and treatment of moderate to severe Alzheimer's disease. *Prim Care Companion J Clin Psychiatry* 8 (3): 158–159.

Schneeberger, A., Mandler, M., Otawa, O., Zauner, W., Mattner, F., and Schmidt, W. 2009. Development of AFFITOPE vaccines for Alzheimer's disease (AD): From concept to clinical testing. *J Nutr Health Aging* 13 (3): 264–267.

Schneider, A., and Mandelkow, E. 2008. Tau-based treatment strategies in neurodegenerative diseases. *Neurotherapeutics* 5 (3): 443–457.

Schneider, L. S. 2004. AD2000: Donepezil in Alzheimer's disease. *Lancet* 363 (9427): 2100–2101.

Schneider, L. S. 2007. Commentary on "Meta-analysis of six-month memantine trials in Alzheimer's disease." Wuthering forest plots: Distinguishing the forest from the plots. *Alzheimers Dement* 3 (1): 18–20.

Schneider, L. S., Dagerman, K. S., Higgins, J. P., and McShane, R. 2011. Lack of evidence for the efficacy of memantine in mild Alzheimer disease. *Arch Neurol* 68(8): 991–998.

Schneider, L. S., Olin, J. T., Doody, R. S., Clark, C. M., Morris, J. C., Reisberg, B., Schmitt, F. A., Grundman, M., Thomas, R. G., and Ferris, S. H. 1997. Validity and reliability of the Alzheimer's Disease Cooperative Study-Clinical Global Impression of Change. The Alzheimer's Disease Cooperative Study. *Alzheimer Dis Assoc Disord* 11 Suppl 2: S22–32.

Selkoe, D. J. 1991. The molecular pathology of Alzheimer's disease. *Neuron* 6 (4): 487–498.

Selkoe, D. J. 1996. Amyloid beta-protein and the genetics of Alzheimer's disease. *J Biol Chem* 271 (31): 18295–18298.

Sevigny, J. J., Peng, Y., Liu, L., and Lines, C. R. 2010. Item analysis of ADAS-Cog: Effect of baseline cognitive impairment in a clinical AD trial. *Am J Alzheimers Dis Other Demen* 25 (2): 119–124.

Shankar, G. M., Li, S., Mehta, T. H., Garcia-Munoz, A., Shepardson, N. E., Smith, I., Brett, F. M., Farrell, M. A., Rowan, M. J., Lemere, C. A., Regan, C. M., Walsh, D. M., Sabatini, B. L., and Selkoe, D. J. 2008. Amyloid-beta protein dimers isolated directly from Alzheimer's brains impair synaptic plasticity and memory. *Nat Med* 14 (8): 837–842.

Shaw, L. M., Vanderstichele, H., Knapik-Czajka, M., Clark, C. M., Aisen, P. S., Petersen, R. C., Blennow, K., Soares, H., Simon, A., Lewczuk, P., Dean, R., Siemers, E., Potter, W., Lee, V. M., and Trojanowski, J. Q. 2009. Cerebrospinal fluid biomarker signature in Alzheimer's disease neuroimaging initiative subjects. *Ann Neurol* 65 (4): 403–413.

Shimohama, S. 2009. Nicotinic receptor-mediated neuroprotection in neurodegenerative dis-ease models. *Biol Pharm Bull* 32 (3): 332–336.

Siemers, E. R., Friedrich, S., Dean, R. A., Sethuraman, G., DeMattos, R., Jennings, D., Tamagnan, G., Marek, K., and Seibyl, J. 2008. Safety, tolerability and biomarker effects of an Abeta monoclonal antibody administered to patients with Alzheimer's disease. Paper presented at the Alzheimer's Association International Conference on Alzheimer's Disease, Chicago, Illinois, July 26–31.

Siemers, E. R., Friedrich, S., Dean, R. A., Gonzales, C. R., Farlow, M. R., Paul, S. M., and Demattos, R. B. 2010. Safety and changes in plasma and cerebrospinal fluid amyloid beta after a single administration of an amyloid beta monoclonal antibody in subjects with Alzheimer disease. *Clin Neuropharmacol* 33 (2): 67–73.

Siemers, E. R., Quinn, J. F., Kaye, J., Farlow, M. R., Porsteinsson, A., Tariot, P., Zoulnouni, P., et al. 2006. Effects of a gamma-secretase inhibitor in a randomized study of patients with Alzheimer disease. *Neurology* 66(4): 602–604.

Silverman, D. H., Geist, C. L., Kenna, H. A., Williams, K., Wroolie, T., Powers, B., Brooks, J., and Rasgon, N. L. 2011. Differences in regional brain metabolism associated with specific formulations of hormone therapy in postmenopausal women at risk for AD. *Psychoneuroendocrinology* 36 (4): 502–513.

Sims, N. R., Bowen, D. M., Allen, S. J., Smith, C. C., Neary, D., Thomas, D. J., and Davison, A. N. 1983. Presynaptic cholinergic dysfunction in patients with dementia. *J Neurochem* 40 (2): 503–509.

Small, G. W., Bookheimer, S. Y., Thompson, P. M., Cole, G. M., Huang, S. C., Kepe, V., and Barrio, J. R. 2008. Current and future uses of neuroimaging for cognitively impaired patients. *Lancet Neurol* 7(2): 161–172.

Soares, H., Raha, N., Sikpi, M., Liston, D., Brodney, M., Coffman, K., Tate, B., Qiu, R., Wang, E. Q., Li, X., Hidi, R., Banerjee, S., Jhee, S., Ereshefsky, L., and Fullerton, T. 2009. β variability and effect of gamma secretase inhibition on cerebrospinal fluid levels of Aβ in healthy volunteers. Paper presented at the Alzheimer's Association International Conference on Alzheimer's Disease, Vienna, July 11–16.

Sparks, D. L., Connor, D. J., Browne, P. J., Lopez, J. E., and Sabbagh, M. N. 2002. HMG-CoA reductase inhibitors (statins) in the treatment of Alzheimer's disease and why it would be ill-advised to use one that crosses the blood-brain barrier. *J Nutr Health Aging* 6 (5): 324–331.

Sparks, D. L., Connor, D. J., Sabbagh, M. N., Petersen, R. B., Lopez, J., and Browne, P. 2006. Circulating cholesterol levels, apolipoprotein E genotype and dementia severity influence the benefit of atorvastatin treatment in Alzheimer's disease: Results of the Alzheimer's Disease Cholesterol-Lowering Treatment (ADCLT) trial. *Acta Neurol Scand Suppl* 185: 3–7.

Standridge, J. B. 2004. Donepezil did not reduce the rate of institutionalisation or disability in people with mild to moderate Alzheimer's disease. *Evid Based Ment Health* 7 (4): 112.

Stefani, A., Martorana, A., Bernardini, S., Panella, M., Mercati, F., Orlacchio, A., and Pierantozzi, M. 2006. CSF markers in Alzheimer disease patients are not related to the different degree of cognitive impairment. *J Neurol Sci* 251 (1–2): 124–128.

Stefanova, E., Wall, A., Almkvist, O., Nilsson, A., Forsberg, A., Langstrom, B., and Nordberg, A. 2006. Longitudinal PET evaluation of cerebral glucose metabolism in rivastigmine treated patients with mild Alzheimer's disease. *J Neural Transm* 113 (2): 205–218.

Suzuki, N., Cheung, T. T., Cai, X. D., Odaka, A., Otvos, L., Jr., Eckman, C., Golde, T. E., and Younkin, S. G. 1994. An increased percentage of long amyloid beta protein secreted by familial amyloid beta protein precursor (beta APP717) mutants. *Science* 264 (5163): 1336–1340.

Swardfager, W., Lanctôt, K., Rothenburg, L., Wong, A., Cappell, J., and Herrmann, N. 2010. A meta-analysis of cytokines in Alzheimer's disease. *Biol Psychiatry* 68 (10): 930–941.

Szekely, C. A., Thorne, J. E., Zandi, P. P., Ek, M., Messias, E., Breitner, J. C., and Goodman, S. N. 2004. Nonsteroidal anti-inflammatory drugs for the prevention of Alzheimer's disease: A systematic review. *Neuroepidemiology* 23 (4): 159–169.

Tabet, N., and Feldman, H. 2002. Indomethacin for Alzheimer's disease. In *Cochrane Database Syst Rev* (2): CD003673, doi: 10.1002/14651858.CD003673.

Takada, Y., Yonezawa, A., Kume, T., Katsuki, H., Kaneko, S., Sugimoto, H., and Akaike, A. 2003. Nicotinic acetylcholine receptor-mediated neuroprotection by donepezil against glutamate neurotoxicity in rat cortical neurons. *J Pharmacol Exp Ther* 306(2): 772–777.

Tariot, P. N., and Aisen, P. S. 2009. Can lithium or valproate untie tangles in Alzheimer's disease? *J Clin Psychiatry* 70 (6): 919–921.

Tariot, P. N., Aisen, P., Cummings, J., Jakimovich, L., Schneider, L., Thomas, R., Becerra, L., and Loy, R. 2009. The ADCS valproate neuroprotection trial: Primary efficacy and safety results. In *Alzheimer's Association International Conference on Alzheimer's Disease*. Vienna: Alzheimers Dement.

Tariot, P. N., Farlow, M. R., Grossberg, G. T., Graham, S. M., McDonald, S., and Gergel, I. 2004. Memantine treatment in patients with moderate to severe Alzheimer disease already receiving donepezil: A randomized controlled trial. *JAMA* 291 (3): 317–324.

Terry, R. D., Masliah, E., Salmon, D. P., Butters, N., DeTeresa, R., Hill, R., Hansen, L. A., and Katzman, R. 1991. Physical basis of cognitive alterations in Alzheimer's disease: Synapse loss is the major correlate of cognitive impairment. *Ann Neurol* 30 (4): 572–580.

Thal, D. R., Holzer, M., Rub, U., Waldmann, G., Gunzel, S., Zedlick, D., and Schober, R. 2000. Alzheimer-related tau-pathology in the perforant path target zone and in the hippocampal stratum oriens and radiatum correlates with onset and degree of dementia. *Exp Neurol* 163 (1): 98–110.

Tokuda, T., Tamaoka, A., Matsuno, S., Sakurai, S., Shimada, H., Morita, H., and Ikeda, S. 2001. Plasma levels of amyloid beta proteins did not differ between subjects taking statins and those not taking statins. *Ann Neurol* 49 (4): 546–547.

Tombaugh, T. N., and McIntyre, N. J. 1992. The mini-mental state examination: A comprehensive review. *J Am Geriatr Soc* 40 (9): 922–935.

Tsuji, A., Saheki, A., Tamai, I., and Terasaki, T. 1993. Transport mechanism of 3-hydroxy- 3-methylglutaryl coenzyme A reductase inhibitors at the blood-brain barrier. *J Pharmacol Exp Ther* 267 (3): 1085–1090.

Turner, P. R., O'Connor, K., Tate, W. P., and Abraham, W. C. 2003. Roles of amyloid precursor protein and its fragments in regulating neural activity, plasticity and memory. *Prog Neurobiol* 70 (1): 1–32.

Turon-Estrada, A., Lopez-Pousa, S., Gelada-Batlle, E., Garre-Olmo, J., Lozano-Gallego, M., Hernandez-Ferrandiz, M., Fajardo-Tibau, C., Morante-Munoz, V., and Vilalta-Franch, J. 2003. Tolerance and adverse events of treatment with acetylcholinesterase inhibitors in a clinical sample of patients with very slight and mild Alzheimer s disease over a six-month period. *Rev Neurol* 36 (5): 421–424.

United Nations. 2002. *World Population Ageing: 1950–2050*, http://www.un.org/esa/population/publications/worldageing19502050/ (accessed May 10, 2011).

Van Gool, W. A., Weinstein, H. C., Scheltens, P., and Walstra, G. J. 2001. Effect of hydroxychloroquine on progression of dementia in early Alzheimer's disease: An 18-month randomised, double-blind, placebo-controlled study. *Lancet* 358 (9280): 455–460.

Verny, M., Hugonot-Diener, L., Saillon, A., Caputo, L., Dobigny-Roman, N., Dieudonne, B., Geoffre, C., Guard, O., Jachan, T., Meridjen, G., Ousset, P. J., and Boller, F. 1999. Evaluation de la demence severe: Echelles cognitives et comportementales (groupe de travail du GRECO). *L Anne Âege Ârontologique* 13: 156–168.

Wang, C. Y., Finstad, C. L., Walfield, A. M., Sia, C., Sokoll, K. K., Chang, T. Y., Fang, X. D., Hung, C. H., Hutter-Paier, B., and Windisch, M. 2007. Site-specific UBITh amyloid-beta vaccine for immunotherapy of Alzheimer's disease. *Vaccine* 25 (16): 3041–3052.

Watkins, P. B., Zimmerman, H. J., Knapp, M. J., Gracon, S. I., and Lewis, K. W. 1994. Hepatotoxic effects of tacrine administration in patients with Alzheimer's disease. *JAMA* 271 (13): 992–998.

Watson, G. S., and Craft, S. 2003. The role of insulin resistance in the pathogenesis of Alzheimer's disease: Implications for treatment. *CNS Drugs* 17 (1): 27–45.

Wenk, G. L., Parsons, C. G., and Danysz, W. 2006. Potential role of N-methyl-D-aspartate receptors as executors of neurodegeneration resulting from diverse insults: focus on memantine. *Behav Pharmacol* 17 (5–6): 411–424.

Weyer, G., Erzigkeit, H. , Kanowski, S., Ihl, R., and Hadler, D. 1997. Alzheimer's Disease Assessment Scale: Reliability and validity in a multicenter clinical trial. *Int Psychogeriatr* 9 (2): 123–138.

Wilcock, G., Howe, I., Coles, H., Lilienfeld, S., Truyen, L., Zhu, Y., Bullock, R., Kershaw, P., and Group., GAL-GBR-2 Study. 2003. A long-term comparison of galantamine and donepezil in the treatment of Alzheimer's disease. *Drugs Aging* 20 (10): 777–789.

Wilcock, G. K., Black, S. E., Hendrix, S. B., Zavitz, K. H., Swabb, E. A., and Laughlin, M. A. 2008. Efficacy and safety of tarenflurbil in mild to moderate Alzheimer's disease: A randomised phase II trial. *Lancet Neurol* 7 (6): 483–493.

Wilkinson, D. G., Passmore, A. P., Bullock, R., Hopker, S. W., Smith, R., Potocnik, F. C., Maud, C. M., Engelbrecht, I., Hock, C., Ieni, J. R., and Bahra, R. S. 2002. A multinational, randomised, 12-week, comparative study of donepezil and rivastigmine in patients with mild to moderate Alzheimer's disease. *Int J Clin Pract* 56 (6): 441–446.

Winblad, B. 2009. Donepezil in severe Alzheimer's disease. *Am J Alzheimers Dis Other Demen* 24 (3): 185–192.

Winblad, B., Jones, R. W., Wirth, Y., Stöffler, A., and Möbius, H. J. 2007a. Memantine in moderate to severe Alzheimer's disease: A meta-analysis of randomised clinical trials. *Dement Geriatr Cogn Disord* 24 (1): 20–27 [Epub 2007 May 2010].

Winblad, B., Cummings, J., Andreasen, N., Grossberg, G., Onofrj, M., Sadowsky, C., Zechner, S., Nagel, J., and Lane, R. 2007b. A six-month double-blind, randomized, placebo-controlled study of a transdermal patch in Alzheimer's disease: Rivastigmine patch versus capsule. *Int J Geriatr Psychiatry* 22 (5): 456–467.

Winblad, B., Kilander, L. , Eriksson, S., Minthon, L., Båtsman, S., Wetterholm, A. L., Jansson-Blixt, C., and Haglund, A. 2006. Donepezil in patients with severe Alzheimer's disease: Double-blind, parallel-group, placebo-controlled study. *Lancet* 367: 1057–1065.

Wischik, C. M., Bentham, P., Wischik, D. J., and Seng, K. M. 2008. Tau aggregation inhibitor (TAI) therapy with rember™ arrests disease progression in mild and moderate Alzheimer's disease over 50 weeks. *Alzheimers Dement* 4(4): T167.

Wischik, C. M., Edwards, P. C., Lai, R. Y., Roth, M., and Harrington, C. R. 1996. Selective inhibition of Alzheimer disease-like tau aggregation by phenothiazines. *Proc Natl Acad Sci USA* 93 (20): 11213–11218.

Witt, A., Macdonald, N., and Kirkpatrick, P. 2004. Memantine hydrochloride. *Nat Rev Drug Discov* 3 (2): 109–110.

World Health Organization. 1992. *The Tenth Revision of the International Classification of Diseases and Relative Health Problems (ICD-10)*. Geneva: World Health Organization.

Wu, J., Li, Q., and Bezprozvanny, I. 2008. Evaluation of Dimebon in cellular model of Huntington's disease. *Mol Neurodegener* 3: 15.

Younkin, S. G. 1995. Evidence that A beta 42 is the real culprit in Alzheimer's disease. *Ann Neurol* 37 (3): 287–288.

Yuan, X., Shan, B., Ma, Y., Tian, J., Jiang, K., Cao, Q., and Wang, R. 2010. Multi-center study on Alzheimer's disease using FDG PET: Group and individual analyses. *J Alzheimers Dis* 19 (3): 927–935.

Zhang, S., Hedskog, L., Petersen, C. A., Winblad, B., and Ankarcrona, M. 2010. Dimebon (latrepirdine) enhances mitochondrial function and protects neuronal cells from death. *J Alzheimers Dis* 21 (2): 389–402.

5 New Small Molecule Drug Discovery for Alzheimer's Disease

Kangning Liu, Minhua Zhang,
and Guhan Nagappan

CONTENTS

5.1   INTRODUCTION

Among the many progressive neurodegenerative diseases causing dementia, Alzheimer's disease (AD) is the most common, for which aging remains the most significant risk factor. Current Food and Drug Administration (FDA)-approved medications, donepezil (Aricept), galantamine (Razadyne), rivastigmine (Exelon), and memantine (Namenda) only provide limited symptomatic relief of cognitive manifestation, yet none alters disease progression. As the aged population rapidly increases around the globe, AD is projected by some to affect 1 in every 85 people by the year 2050 (Brookmeyer et al., 2007). Therefore, it is of urgent need to develop more potent symptomatic agents to manage cognitive impairment and other clinical manifestations of AD; and to develop *disease-modifying* agents that can either prevent or delay the onset of the disease, slow down disease progression once it starts, and more optimistically, reverse disease pathology and cognitive decline.

Pathologically, AD is defined by extracellular amyloid plaques, of which amyloid beta (Abeta) peptide is the primary component, and intraneuronal neurofibrillary tangles, which contain hyperphosphorylated tau, a neuronal microtubule-associated protein (Hyman and Trojanowski, 1997). All genetic mutations that cause familial AD (fAD) are linked to the generation of Abeta, while tau mutations are associated with AD and several other forms of neurodegenerative diseases including frontotemporal dementia (Bertram et al., 2010; Brouwers et al., 2008). Based on genetic and molecular evidences, the amyloid hypothesis was proposed (Glenner and Wong, 1984; Hardy and Higgins, 1992; Selkoe, 2002). It states that Abeta aggregation triggers downstream cascades to cause synaptic dysfunction, tau pathology, gliosis and inflammation, neurotransmitter loss, and ultimately neurodegeneration (Hardy and Selkoe, 2002; Harkany et al., 2000; Selkoe, 2001, 2002; Verdier et al., 2004). Over time, the identity of the primary toxic Abeta species has evolved from fibrillar Abeta to more soluble oligomeric Abeta (Haass and Selkoe, 2007; Klein, 2002; Selkoe, 2008). Guided by the amyloid hypothesis, historically, efforts and strategies to treat AD have largely been centered on Abeta. This includes inhibitors to reduce Abeta generation, disaggregators to disrupt or prevent Abeta aggregation, vaccine or immunotherapy to promote Abeta clearance, and approaches to ameliorate Abeta-induced toxicity. However, disappointing results from recent clinical trials targeting Abeta have instigated a reassessment of the amyloid hypothesis and further highlight the need for a better understanding of the disease biology (Haass, 2010).

In this chapter, we will review recent progress made in small-molecule disease-modifier drug discovery efforts for AD, specifically focusing on new targets and efforts in the area of: (1) Abeta; (2) tau; and (3) the emerging neuroprotective/neuro-repair approaches, which may provide therapeutic benefits not only to AD but also to other neurodegenerative diseases.

5.2 APPROACHES TARGETING ABETA

A primary component of amyloid plaques, Abeta is generated from amyloid precursor protein (APP) by sequential proteolytic cleavages by the beta- and gamma-secretase enzymes (Hardy and Selkoe, 2002; Selkoe, 2002). fAD mutations are mostly associated with increased Abeta production or increased Abeta 42-to-40 ratio. These include mutations in genes encoding APP, presenilin 1 and 2 (Brouwers et al., 2008). APP gene duplication and triplication (in Down syndrome) have also been reported. Correspondingly, Abeta-targeting approaches can be classified into the following categories as illustrated in Figure 5.1:

1. Reducing generation of pathogenic Abeta
   a. Inhibiting beta- and gamma-secretases, the two rate-limiting enzymes involved in the generation of amyloidogenic Abeta
   b. Activating alpha-secretase to generate nonamyloidogenic Abeta fragments thereby indirectly reducing the level of amyloidogenic Abeta. sAPPalpha, a co-product of alpha cleavage, was also shown to provide neuroprotection and promote neurogenesis (Caille et al., 2004; Goodman and Mattson, 1994; Ohsawa et al., 1999)
2. Reducing Abeta accumulation
   a. Active vaccinations against Abeta or passive immunization with anti-Abeta antibodies to promote Abeta clearance
   b. Enhance degradation of amyloidogenic peptides by activating enzymes such as neprilysin and insulin-degradation enzyme (IDE)
   c. Interfering with Abeta oligomerization and aggregation. Small soluble oligomeric Abeta has emerged as the culprit for early synaptic deterioration (Haass and Selkoe, 2007; Klein, 2002; Selkoe, 2008), although the precise form(s) of toxic Abeta species in vivo is yet to be determined.

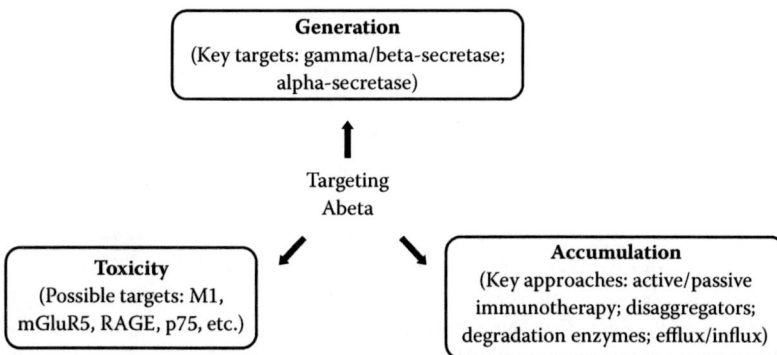

FIGURE 5.1 Diagrams showing various approaches targeting Abeta. Current drug discovery efforts targeting Abeta can be categorized into three classes: (A) inhibiting generation of pathogenic Abeta, (B) removing/preventing Abeta accumulation, and (C) blocking Abeta-induced toxicity.

The therapeutic approach to interrupt Abeta aggregation is reviewed in detail elsewhere in this book and will not be discussed here.

   d. Activation of Abeta efflux or inhibition of Abeta influx to reduce the Abeta load in the brain

3. Reducing Abeta-induced toxicity by blocking Abeta binding to molecules/ receptors

In the following section, we will discuss some of these strategies in detail citing specific examples.

5.2.1 Reducing Pathogenic Abeta Generation

5.2.1.1 Gamma-Secretase: Recent Advances in Developing Selective Gamma-Secretase Modulators

As one of the key rate-limiting enzymes responsible for Abeta production, gamma-secretase has been the target of intense drug discovery efforts. Four components, presenilin, nicastrin, anterior pharynx-defective 1 (APH-1), and presenilin enhancer 2 (PEN-2), reconstitute the full gamma-secretase activity in vitro and in model systems such as fruit fly and yeast (Edbauer et al., 2003; Kimberly et al., 2003; Takasugi et al., 2003; Wolfe, 2008). Additional supportive evidences include the following: Deletion of *presenilin-1* and *presenilin-2* genes completely eliminates gamma-secretase activity (Herreman et al., 2000). Mutations in *presenilin* genes cause familial AD (Brouwers et al., 2008). Up-regulation of presenilin messenger RNA (mRNA) and protein was also reported in postmortem brains of sporadic AD patients (Ikeda et al., 2000; Smith et al., 2004).

Historically, initial efforts targeting gamma-secretase activity led to the identification of nonselective gamma-secretase inhibitors (GSIs). However, the community quickly recognized that the lack of substrate selectivity could lead to mechanism-associated adverse effects: Gamma-secretase processes >40 other substrates (Hemming et al., 2008; Rochette and Murphy, 2002) including Notch, a transmembrane receptor critical in development and cell fate determination (Jorissen and De Strooper, 2010). Not surprisingly, inhibition of Notch cleavage results in abnormalities in the gastrointestinal tract (Milano et al., 2004; Stanger et al., 2005) and the immune system (Maillard et al., 2003). In addition, in some preclinical studies, inhibition of gamma-secretase impaired learning and memory (Saura et al., 2004) and caused skin cancer (Kang et al., 2002; Xia et al., 2001). In 2010, Eli Lilly and Company announced termination of Semagacestat (LY-450139) (Figure 5.2A), the most advanced GSI program. Preliminary results from two phase III trials (the IDENTITY and IDENTITY-2 trials) revealed lack of improvement in cognitive functions in patients with mild to moderate AD. Instead, it worsened cognitive decline and increased the risk for developing skin cancer (Eli Lilly News Release, "Lilly Halts Development of Semagacestat for AD Based on Preliminary Results of Phase III Clinical Trials," http://newsroom.lilly.com/releasedetail.cfm?releaseid=499794).

Subsequently, the strategy was modified to discover and develop APP-selective GSIs. While it remains challenging to establish selectivity among >40 substrates

I. GSI/GSM:

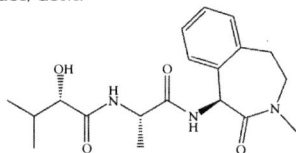

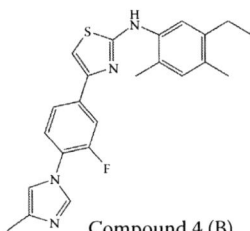

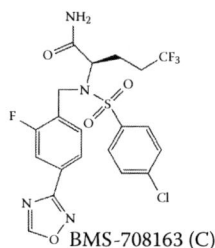

Semagacestat (A)   Compound 4 (B)   BMS-708163 (C)

II. Beta-secretase inhibitors:

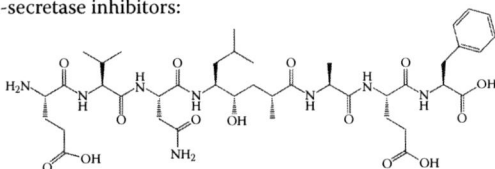

OM99-2 (D)

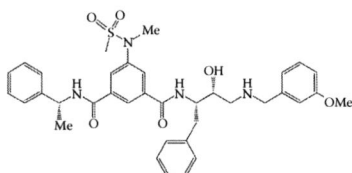

GRL-8234 (E)

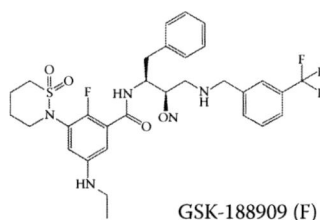

GSK-188909 (F)

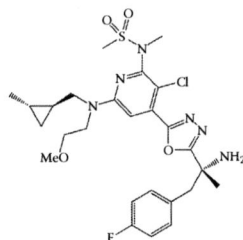

Merck compound 10 (G)

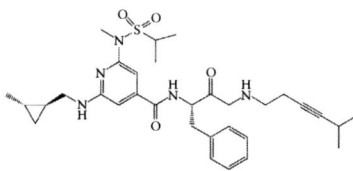

Medivir compound (H)
(WO 2010107384)

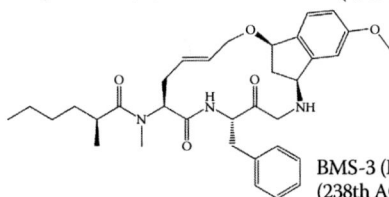

BMS-3 (I)
(238th ACS (Washington, DC), 2009, MEDI 212)

FIGURE 5.2 Representative structures discussed in the Abeta session. I. Gamma-secretase inhibitors/modulators: (A) Semagacestat (LY-450139); (B) Compound 4, an aminothiazole-containing GSM; (C) BMS-708163; II. Beta-secretase inhibitors; (D) OM99-2, one of the earliest reported BACE1 inhibitors; (E) GRL-8234, one of the earliest drug-like BACE1 inhibitors; (F) GSK-188909, one of the first reported orally available BACE1 inhibitors; (G–I) recently reported potent BACE1 inhibitors;

III. M1 agonists:

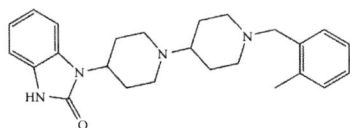

TBPB (J)

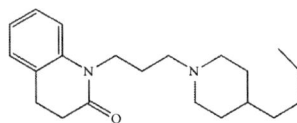

77-LH-28-1 (K)

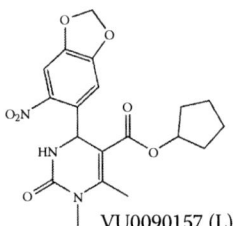

VU0090157 (L)

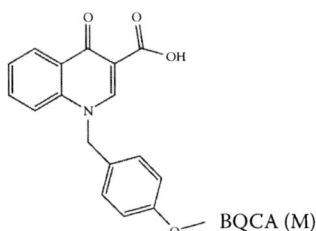

BQCA (M)

IV. mGluR5 antagonists/NAM:

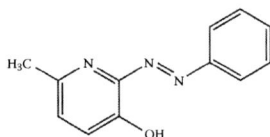

SIB-1757 (N)

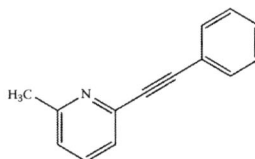

MPEP (O)

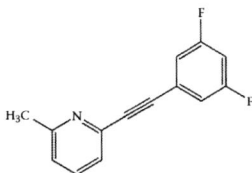

Structure from the
Addex10059 series (P)

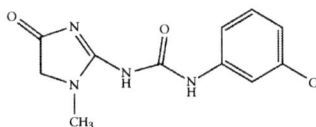

Fenobam (Q)

FIGURE 5.2 (CONTINUED) III. M1 agonists: selective allosteric M1 agonists TBPB (J) and 77-LH-28-1 (K) activate M1 via different mechanisms; VU0090197 (L) and BQCA (M) are positive allosteric modulators of M1; IV. mGluR5 antagonists: SIB-1757 (N) and more potent derivative MPEP (O) are both negative allosteric modulators of mGluR5. Addex10059 (structure from the series shown in P) and Fenobam (Q) are currently in clinical trials.

and profile their potential biological impact in vivo, it may be possible to achieve selectivity against APP. However, GSIs induce accumulation of beta-C terminal fragment (CTF), which may cause paradoxical increase of Abeta in plasma, as observed with LY-450139 in humans (Imbimbo, 2008) and in preclinical animal species (Lanz et al., 2004; Lanz et al., 2006). This potential GSI-induced rebound may not be removed by APP-selective GSIs.

More recently, the field has evolved to develop gamma-secretase modulators (GSMs). By shifting the gamma-cleavage site to generate shorter and thus less amyloidogenic fragments of Abeta, GSMs aim to preserve the function of non-APP substrates, which may be less affected by such shifted cleavage.

For example, in a recent study, Kounnas and colleagues reported a class of "potent, selective and brain permeable" aminothiazole-containing small-molecule GSMs (AGSM) (Kounnas et al., 2010). These AGSMs differentiate from GSI (conventional or allosteric) as well as previously reported GSMs including some NSAIDs (Kukar et al., 2008; Weggen et al., 2001) in several aspects. Specifically, first, they selectively inhibit Abeta 42 and 40 production, and increase nonamyloidogenic Abeta species, such as Abeta 37/38/39, without changing the total level of Abeta. Second, they do not affect APP or Notch epsilon cleavage, and therefore do not impact generation of the APP intracellular domain (AICD) or Notch intracellular domain (NICD). However, comprehensive profiling against other known substrates of gamma-secretase is needed to further confirm its selectivity.

In vivo, single-dosing or short-term repeated dosing treatment with Compound 4 of AGSM (Figure 5.2B) lowered Abeta 42 and 40 in a dose-dependent fashion in the Tg2576 APP overexpressing transgenic mouse model, more so against plasma Abeta. Chronic dosing at 50 mg/kg/day up to 29 weeks (on chow) appeared to be well tolerated with no detectable GI abnormalities, although a comprehensive long-term toxicology study with careful monitoring of dosing variability is needed. Given the unexpected reduction in Abeta 38 upon chronic dosing, it is important to understand the biology of chronic GSM-mediated Abeta reduction in more detail.

In the clinic, several potential APP-selective GSIs or GSMs are being tested, including BMS-708163 (from BMS, Figure 5.2C) and NIC5-15 (from Humanetics) in phase II (clinical trial: NCT00810147, NCT00470418, ClinicalTrials.gov), CHF 5074 (from Chlesl) and ELND006/007 (from Elan) in phase I (clinical trial: NCT00954252, ClinicalTrials.gov). As more data become available, it is of great interest to see whether the improved selectivity could provide a wider therapeutic window and achieve higher efficacy.

Additionally, the recent reports of Abeta-selective gamma-secretase regulators such as gamma-secretase activating protein (GSAP) (He et al., 2010) may offer an alternative mechanism for selective inhibition of Abeta generation. Identified as a small protein that binds to the anticancer drug Gleevec (also known as Imatinib or STI571), GSAP was shown to selectively activate Abeta generation with no apparent effect on Notch processing (He et al., 2010). Using Gleevec as a tool molecule, the primary assays are in place for a structure activity relationship (SAR) study to identify a brain-permeable small molecule that may selectively decrease Abeta generation. Better understanding of how GSAP itself is regulated may offer additional intervening opportunities. Given other previously reported gamma-secretase regulators selective for Abeta generation, such as CD147 (Zhou et al., 2005), TMP21 (Chen et al., 2006), and GPCR3 (Thathiah et al., 2009), it remains to be seen whether targeting GSAP alone will provide sufficient inhibition of Abeta production.

5.2.1.2 Beta-Secretase Inhibitors

As the other rate-limiting enzyme in Abeta generation, beta-site APP-cleaving enzyme 1 (BACE1) is the primary beta-secretase (Hong et al., 2000; Lin et al., 2000; Sinha et al., 1999; Vassar et al., 1999; Yan et al., 1999) that initiates Abeta production and plays an essential role in AD pathogenesis. Deletion of BACE1 significantly reduced Abeta production (Cai et al., 2001; Luo et al., 2003; Luo et al., 2001; Nishitomi et al., 2006; Roberds et al., 2001). Conversely, double-transgenic mice overexpressing BACE1 and APP showed enhanced Abeta generation and exacerbated Abeta pathology (Mohajeri et al., 2004; Ozmen et al., 2005; Willem et al., 2004). Furthermore, an association has been suggested between Abeta load and BACE1 elevation, based on the observation of increase in BACE1 protein and activity in postmortem AD brain tissue and AD transgenic mouse lines (Li et al., 2004; Zhao et al., 2007). Although initial reports suggested a rather benign phenotype, later studies reported deficits in synaptic function, neuronal activity, and myelination in BACE1 knockout mice (Hu et al., 2006; Hu et al., 2010; Laird et al., 2005; Wang et al., 2008). These potential mechanism-associated issues need to be taken into consideration when developing BACE1 inhibitors for therapy.

As a membrane-bound aspartic protease, BACE protein possesses two aspartic residues at the site of peptide bond hydrolysis, while the substrate recognition site shapes like a long cleft (Ghosh et al., 2008). The crystal structure of BACE1 has been instructive in structure-guided inhibitor design (Hong et al., 2000; Hong et al., 2002). To address the selectivity issue, BACE2 and Cathepsin D, two major aspartic proteases, have been routinely used in counter assays (Ghosh et al., 2008). Some of the inhibitors developed in both industry and academia have been reviewed previously, including OM99-2 (Figure 5.2D), GRL-8234 (Figure 5.2E), KNI-1027, GSK-188909 (Figure 5.2F), and compounds from Wyeth (now Pfizer) and Johnson & Johnson (Ghosh et al., 2008; Tomita, 2009). Other potent inhibitors reported recently include the tertiary carbinamine-derived Merck Compound 10 (Figure 5.2G) (Zhu et al., 2010), Medivir compound (Figure 5.2H) (WO 2010107384), and BMS compounds (Figure 5.2I), which demonstrate single-digit nanomolar potency against BACE1 in vitro.

A greater part of reported BACE1 inhibitors (e.g., hydroxyethylene, statin, and hydroxymethylcarbonyl isostere) are peptidomimetic compounds that inhibit the enzyme in its transition state (Tomita, 2009). It is suggested that aspartic acid protease inhibitor drugs that are in clinical use against HIV protease and renin arrest the enzymes in their transition state, which may also be the case for BACE1 inhibitors (Ghosh et al., 2008).

Several BACE1 inhibitors are in clinical development. CoMentis (previously Athenagen) is developing CTS-21166 (ASP-1702), an orally available lead compound in the ZPQ-1 series of BACE1 inhibitors, for the treatment of AD (clinical trial: NCT00621010, ClinicalTrials.gov). In a dose-escalation phase I trial in 48 healthy volunteers, a single intravenous injection of CTS-21166 reduced plasma levels of Abeta by more than 60%. A sustained reduction (>70%) was observed at higher doses over a 72-hour period (press releases, CoMentis, June 18, 2007[*], January 7, 2008[†], and July 28, 2008[‡]). Additional small-molecule BACE1 inhibitors that are being currently tested in the clinic include ACI-91 from AC Immune, LY2886721 from Lilly (clinical trial: NCT01133405, ClinicalTrials.gov) and an orally available iminohydantoin BACE1 inhibitor from Merck & Co (Schering-Plough before the merger).

5.2.2　Targeting Abeta-Mediated Toxicity

Abeta aggregation is a complicated process, starting with monomeric Abeta, and oligomeric Abeta being largely considered an intermediate species. Preclinical data suggest that diffusible oligomeric aggregates are responsible for early synaptic dysfunction that both precedes neuronal degeneration and better correlates with disease progression (Dahlgren et al., 2002; Hartley et al., 1999; Kayed et al., 2003; Lambert et al., 1998; Podlisny et al., 1998; Selkoe, 2002; Walsh et al., 2002), although it awaits further proof in the clinic. Additionally, fibrillar Abeta induces cytotoxicity and contributes to AD pathogenesis, partially through gliocytosis (El Khoury et al., 2003; Fassbender et al., 2001; Muehlhauser et al., 2001; Selkoe, 2002). We will next examine some of the targets and strategies that block Abeta-induced toxicity.

5.2.2.1　Symptomatic Treatment with Potential Disease-Modifying Benefit

5.2.2.1.1　Abeta and Muscarinic Acetylcholine Receptor M1 (M1)

Based on the cholinergic hypothesis (Thathiah and De Strooper, 2009), muscarinic acetylcholine receptors (mAChRs) are considered as viable drug targets for AD therapy. Among the many subtypes, M1 is suggested to most likely modulate cognition, attention, and sensory processing (Conn et al., 2009), therefore offering symptomatic relief to AD patients. Earlier observations of altered APP processing, and decreased tau and Abeta pathology upon agonizing M1 also suggest that this may be potentially disease modifying (Fisher, 2008). For example, treatment of 3xTg-AD mice (APPswe, PS1M146V, TauP301L) with AF267B, an M1 agonist with limited selectivity decreased amyloidogenic processing of APP, reduced both amyloid and tau pathologies, and rescued cognitive impairments (Caccamo et al., 2006). Upon chronic AF267B treatment, both cerebrospinal fluid (CSF) and brain Abeta levels decreased in the rabbit hypercholesterolemia model of cholinergic dysfunction and Abeta pathology (Beach et al., 2001; Fisher, 2008).

The major challenge in targeting mAChRs has been to develop subtype selective agonists (for M1 and M4) to minimize adverse effects associated with activation of peripheral mAChRs, especially M2 and M3. AF267B, for example, although suggested as a selective M1 agonist, has similar profiles as the previous orthosteric agonists and activates multiple mAChR subtypes including M3 and M5 (Conn et al., 2009; Jones et al., 2008). Encouragingly, in recent years, major advances were

---

[*] http://www.marketwire.com/press-release/comentis-receives-fda-clearance-begin-human-clinical-trials-its-disease-modifying-alzheimers-743079.htm

[†] http://www.marketwire.com/press-release/comentis-announces-proof-activity-data-from-its-phase-i-study-disease-modifying-alzheimers-808028.htm

[‡] http://www.marketwire.com/press-release/comentis-astellas-present-alzheimers-disease-research-international-conference-on-alzheimers-883083.htm

made in generating selective allosteric agonists and potentiators for M1 mAChR. Discovery of brucine, AC-42, and other early mAChR allosteric agonists paved the way for the identification of selective and systemically active M1 allosteric agonists such as [1-(1'-2-methylbenzyl)-1,4'-bipiperidin-4-yl)-1H-benzo[d]imidazol-2(3H)-one] (TBPB) (Figure 5.2J) (Bridges et al., 2008; Jones et al., 2008) and 77-LH-28-1 (Figure 5.2K) (Langmead et al., 2008; Thomas et al., 2008). TBPB is highly selective and brain permeable without major peripheral side effects in rats (Jones et al., 2008). Consistent with an earlier observation, in vitro, TBPB shifts APP processing toward nonamyloidogenic alpha cleavage. It is therefore interesting to see whether chronic treatment with TBPB in AD transgenic rodent models can achieve similar effect on Abeta and tau pathology, in addition to the expected cognitive benefit. Apparently, TBPB and 77-LH-28-1 activate M1 via different mechanisms: while TBPB exclusively binds to allosteric site on M1, 77-LH-28-1 is *bi-topic*; its binding site overlaps both the orthosteric and allosteric site that modulates *orthosteric-site* affinity (Conn et al., 2009; Lebon et al., 2009).

Additionally, novel positive allosteric modulators (PAM) of M1 have recently been reported, including VU0090157 (Figure 5.2L), VU0029767 (Marlo et al., 2009), and highly selective and potent benzyl quinolone carboxylic acid (BQCA) (Figure 5.2M) (Conn et al., 2009; Ma et al., 2009). As in the example of TBPB and 77-LH-28-1, VU0090157 and VU0029767 differentially regulate coupling of the receptor to different signaling pathways. On the other hand, BQCA was reported to reverse scopolamine-induced memory deficits in contextual fear conditioning, increase blood flow to the cerebral cortex, and increase wakefulness while reducing delta sleep, supporting the hypothesis that allosteric modulation of M1 could enhance memory without directly agonizing the receptor itself (Conn et al., 2009; Ma et al., 2009). At the molecular level, however, the mechanism of selectivity exhibited by these allosteric activators/modulators have not been fully understood (Conn et al., 2009).

A few M1 agonists have been tested in the clinic for AD, such as PD-151832 (or CI-1017) sponsored by Pfizer; talsaclidine fumarate, sponsored by Boehringer Ingelheim (Hock et al., 2003); NGX-267, sponsored by Raptor Pharmaceutical (formerly TorreyPines Therapeutics); MCD-386 by Mithridion (http://www.mithridion. com); Sabcomeline by Braincells; and GSK-1034702 by GSK (clinical trial: NCT00937846, ClinicalTrials.gov). However, for many of these compounds, subtype selectivity is limited. It remains to be tested whether the newly developed selective M1 agonists and positive potentiators could offer superior therapeutic benefit, and halt disease progression, in addition to offering a better safety profile.

5.2.2.1.2 *Abeta and Metabotropic Glutamate Receptor 5 (mGluR5)*

Abeta binds to the lipid membranes, which facilitate Abeta aggregation. In turn, this alters and disturbs the membrane structure and function. Specifically, binding of Abeta to membrane lipids was suggested to affect membrane fluidity (Kremer et al., 2000; Mason et al., 1999), perturb structure of the plasma membrane (Eckert et al., 2000), discharge lipids from the neuronal plasma membrane (Michikawa et al., 2001), and assemble functional ion channels (Arispe et al., 1993; Kagan et al., 2002; Kourie et al., 2001; Tran et al., 2002; Verdier et al., 2004). Using single-particle tracking of quantum dot–labeled oligomers and synaptic proteins in hippocampal neurons, Renner and colleagues have shown that diffusion of membrane-attached oligomers was strikingly hampered upon deposit at synapses, aberrantly clustering mGluR5 (Renner et al., 2010). This clustering of mGluR5 increases intracellular Ca^{2+} and causes synaptic N-methyl-D-aspartate (NMDA) receptor NR1 subunit loss. In vitro, such a loss could be abolished by antagonizing mGluR5 genetically or pharmacologically using SIB1757 ([6-methyl-2-(phenylazo)-3-pyridinol]), a selective antagonist for mGluR5 discovered by Novartis AG (Figure 5.2N) (Renner et al., 2010; Varney et al., 1999). Interestingly, the clustering caused by the Abeta oligomer seems to be selective for mGluR5, sparing gamma-aminobutyric acid receptor (GABAR) or alpha-amino-3-hydroxy-5-methyl-4-isoxazolepropinonic acid receptor (AMPAR); the latter has also been suggested to mediate Abeta oligomer-induced synaptic toxicity (Hsieh et al., 2006). 2-methyl-6-(phenylethynyl)pyridine (MPEP) (Figure 5.2O), the more potent derivative of SIB-1757 that has been widely studied as a mGluR5 antagonizing tool compound, protected against NMDA- and Abeta-induced toxicity in vitro (Bruno et al., 2000).

In the clinic, several small-molecule negative allosteric modulators (NAM) of mGluR5 are being developed for various indications such as migraine, Parkinson's disease, anxiety, Fragile X syndrome, and gastroesophageal reflux disease (GERD). These mGluR5 NAMs include Addex10059 (Figure 5.2P for this structural series) and 48621, AFQ056 from Novartis (clinical trial: NCT00582673, ClinicalTrials. gov), AZD2066 from AstraZenica (clinical trial: NCT00684502, ClinicalTrials. gov), RG-7090 from Hoffmann-La Roche (NCT01437657), STX-107 from Merck (NCT01325740), and Fenobam by Roche/Neuropharm (Figure 5.2Q) (Berry-Kravis et al., 2009). Inhibiting a well-investigated drug target that fine-tunes synaptic function and controls the accuracy and sharpness of transmission, mGluR5 antagonists have demonstrated a broad anxiolytic-like profile and other beneficial effects in a variety of preclinical animal models (Breysse et al., 2002; Gasparini et al., 2008; Spooren et al., 2000). In contrast to targeting the ionotropic glutamate receptors (iGluRs) including NMDA, AMPA, and kainate receptors, allosteric modulation of mGluR5 may achieve a wide therapeutic window with a much-desired safety profile (Gasparini et al., 2008; Lindsley and Emmitte, 2009). As proof of principle, it is of great interest whether any of these potent and selective mGluR5 NAMs improve the behavior abnormality and synaptic impairment in APP or APP/PS1 transgenic mouse models, where the cognitive deficits were induced at least partially by oligomeric Abeta aggregates (Lesne et al., 2006). If the results are indeed positive, then this could raise an intriguing possibility of antagonizing mGluR5 as a potential disease-modifying therapy for AD.

5.2.2.2 Inhibition of Abeta-Induced Signaling

Abeta 40 and 42 are prone to nonspecific protein binding. Many membrane proteins have been shown to directly bind to Abeta (monomer or aggregated), and be involved in Abeta-induced cytotoxicity. These include the insulin receptor, serpin complex receptor, alpha7 nicotinic acetylcholine receptor (alpha7nAchR), Integrin beta1, receptor for advanced glycosylation end products (RAGE), NMDA receptor, APP and p75 neurotrophin receptor (p75NTR), to name a few (Verdier et al., 2004). Among these, several are worth discussing given the recent progress.

5.2.2.2.1   Abeta and Alpha7nAChR

Both monomeric and oligomeric Abeta have been shown to bind alpha7nAChR, an integral membrane protein modulating Ca^{2+} homeostasis and acetylcholine release (Dineley et al., 2002; Lee and Wang, 2003; Wang et al., 2000a; Wang et al., 2000b). The selective and nanomolar affinity binding of Abeta 42 to alpha7nAChR was suggested to block receptor function (Lee and Wang, 2003; Li and Buccafusco, 2003; Liu et al., 2001), mediate Abeta 1-42-induced tau phosphorylation (Wang et al., 2003), and facilitate internalization of Abeta 1-42 itself (Nagele et al., 2002). However, in a different experimental system, binding of nonaggregated Abeta to the receptor activated alpha7nAChR instead (Dineley et al., 2002). Adding to this complexity, it has been reported that Tg2576 transgenic mouse, when crossed with an alpha7nAChR knockout mouse line (A7KO), demonstrated unexpected increase in Abeta oligomer accumulation, with severe deficits in learning and memory, and septohippocampal pathology at young age (5 months) (Hernandez et al., 2010). The data actually suggest a neuroprotective role for alpha7nAChR in the early stage of disease development in this model. More detailed studies are needed to reconcile these differences.

In a recently published detailed postmortem study on the first AD patient that was ever imaged by Pittsburgh Compound B (PIB), Kadir and colleagues performed binding assays on the brain homogenates to look at synaptic changes (Kadir et al., 2011). While the density of the alpha4beta2 nicotinic receptor subunit was lower in brain regions with high amyloid load, consistent with an interaction, there was no correlation between amyloid load and the density of the alpha7 subunit.

Current alpha7 receptor agonists that are in clinical trials include EVP-6124 from Envivo (clinical trial: NCT01073228, ClinicalTrials.gov) and RG3487/RO-5313534/MEM3534 from Roche (clinical trial: NCT00884507, ClinicalTrials.gov), both in phase II for AD.

5.2.2.2.2   Abeta and RAGE

RAGE is a multiligand receptor in the immunoglobulin superfamily expressed on neurons, glia (Yan et al., 1996), and endothelial cells in vasculature (Ueno et al., 2010). Binding to neuronal RAGE, although suggested not to directly mediate Abeta neurotoxicity (Liu et al., 1997), generates oxidative stress and enhances expression of macrophage colony-stimulating factor (M-CSF) via activating the transcription factor nuclear factor kappa B (NFkB), which in turn stimulates microglia cell proliferation and migration (Du Yan et al., 1997; Lue et al., 2001; Yan et al., 1996). Abeta-RAGE-mediated microglial activation further augments RAGE and M-CSF expression, thus providing a positive-feedback loop (Lue et al., 2001). Immunohistochemical studies also support a role for RAGE in uptake and lysosomal degradation of Abeta in astrocytes (Sasaki et al., 2001). It is interesting, in this context, to note the recent report of an association between a single nucleotide polymorphism (SNP) G82S (rs2070600) in the RAGE-encoding gene AGER and the risk for AD (Daborg et al., 2010; Li et al., 2010). Finally, RAGE up-regulation in cerebral vasculature has been reported in AD patients and in the Tg2576 AD transgenic mouse model (Deane et al., 2003). RAGE expressed along the vessel wall has been shown to function as a major influx receptor for Abeta across the blood–brain barrier (BBB) and induce neurovascular stress. Inhibition of RAGE–ligand interaction via systemic administration of a recombinant truncated form of RAGE or RAGE-blocking antibody suppressed brain parenchymal accumulation of Abeta and restored endothelial function in two different APP transgenic mouse models, respectively (Deane et al., 2003; Ueno et al., 2010).

In the clinic, Pfizer (TransTech Pharma) has recently completed a double-blind, placebo-controlled, randomized, phase II multicenter study to evaluate the efficacy and safety of an orally active small-molecule RAGE antagonist PF04494700 (TTP488) in patients with mild to moderate AD, which was initiated in December 2007 (clinical trial: NCT00566397, ClinicalTrials.gov). Preclinically, in a systemic amyloidosis mouse model, TTP-488 effectively reduced the amyloid load and the expression of IL-6 and M-CSF in the spleen. In a model of AD, it effectively reduced brain amyloid burden after 90 days treatment, and rescued spatial memory (TransTech, August 22, 2006, http://www.ttpharma.com/TherapeuticAreas/AlzheimersDisease/TTP488/tabid/123/Default.aspx).

5.2.2.2.3   Abeta and p75NTR

p75NTR is another receptor that has been shown to bind to aggregated Abeta in vitro. As a member of the death receptor family, p75NTR is a pan-neurotrophin receptor that can bind nerve growth factor (NGF), brain-derived neurotrophin factor (BDNF), neurotrophin-3 (NT-3), and neurotrophin-4 (NT-4). Binding of p75NTR with fibrillar Abeta has been shown to both cause and protect against apoptosis (Tsukamoto et al., 2003; Yaar et al., 2002; Yaar et al., 1997; Zhang et al., 2003), likely suggesting a cell-type, tissue-context, or species-specific difference. Recently, it was reported that p75NTR binds to oligomeric Abeta, and blocking such an interaction with a peptidomimetic small molecule can abolish Abeta oligomer-induced toxicity (Yaar et al., 2007). Further studies are needed to validate p75NTR as a receptor mediating Abeta-induced toxicity (Bengoechea et al., 2009; Coulson, 2006; Knowles et al., 2009; Kuner et al., 1998). We will revisit this target in detail in the neuroprotection session.

Finally, prion protein has recently been reported to selectively bind to Abeta oligomers (Lauren et al., 2009). But it is still under investigation whether prion is a functional receptor mediating Abeta oligomer-induced toxicity in vivo (Balducci et al., 2010; Benilova and De Strooper, 2010; Calella et al., 2010; Kessels et al., 2010).

5.2.3   SUMMARY AND FUTURE DIRECTION FOR ABETA-CENTERED APPROACHES

In the current section, we have briefly reviewed small-molecule drug discovery efforts targeting Abeta, but it is far from comprehensive. Significant progress has been made in the area of metal chelation (Duce and Bush, 2010; Duce et al., 2010; Faux et al., 2010), for example, which we have not discussed here due to space limitations. As the field continues to advance, novel mechanisms will emerge and mature, hopefully strengthening the pipeline for AD drug discovery.

On the other hand, it is the authors' opinion that there are multiple challenges that the field has to conquer first, such as inconsistency in Abeta oligomer preparation and uncertainty over the disease-relevant toxic species in vivo. Furthermore, preclinical animal models overexpressing fAD APP mutations have significant limitations and have yet to provide robust and consistent disease-relevant phenotypes.

The amyloid hypothesis has been instrumental in advancing our understanding of Abeta generation, aggregation, and toxicity. It still requires ultimate testing with an appropriate agent and an optimal trial design, possibly through guidance with biomarkers. As we continue to improve our understanding in Abeta biology, other pathways have also emerged that could play an equally important role in AD pathogenesis.

5.3 TAU-BASED THERAPEUTIC APPROACHES

Neurofibrillary degeneration, including intraneuronal tangles, neurophil threads, and dystrophic neurites surrounding neuritic plaques, is one of the hallmarks of AD pathology. The microtubule-associated protein (MAP), tau, is the major component of neurofibrillary degeneration pathology. It is expressed mainly in neurons, in particular, axons to regulate microtubule assembly and stability (Cleveland et al., 1977; Weingarten et al., 1975). In the diseased brain, tau is hyperphosphorylated and aggregated to form intraneuronal tau tangle.

Given its critical role in AD pathogenesis, targeting tau using small molecules may provide an effective treatment for AD. However, unlike Abeta-targeting approaches, where significant research and drug discovery efforts were invested in the last two decades, only a handful of clinical trials are targeting tau for AD (Table 5.1). In this section, we will first briefly introduce the current understanding of tau biology and its role in AD pathogenesis. We will then discuss in detail the status of drug discovery efforts targeting tau (Figure 5.3), focusing on (1) reducing tau hyperphosphorylation, (2) disassembling tau aggregates, and (3) enhancing tau clearance.

5.3.1 PHYSIOLOGICAL FUNCTIONS AND PATHOLOGICAL ROLES OF TAU

In humans there are six isoforms of tau produced by alternative splicing of exons 2, 3, and 10 of the single MAPT gene (alias tau) on chromosome 17q21.3 (Goedert et al., 1989; Neve et al., 1986). Tau isoforms differ by the presence or absence of

TABLE 5.1
Summary of Clinical Trials Targeting Tau

Drug Name	Overview	Global Status	Originator	Reference
Methylthioninium chloride, TauRx Rember Trx0014	An orally available tau aggregation inhibitor	Phase II	TauRx Pharmaceuticals	NCT00515333, ClinicalTrial.gov
Davunetide	Microtubule stabilizer; neuroprotectant	Phase II	Allon Therapeutics	NCT00422981, ClinicalTrial.gov
Tideglusib	GSK3beta inhibitor	Phase II	Zeltia/Noscira {Zeltia/ NeuroPharma}	NCT01350362, ClinicalTrial.gov
Lithium	GSK3beta inhibitor	Phase II	NINDS	NCT00088387, ClinicalTrial.gov

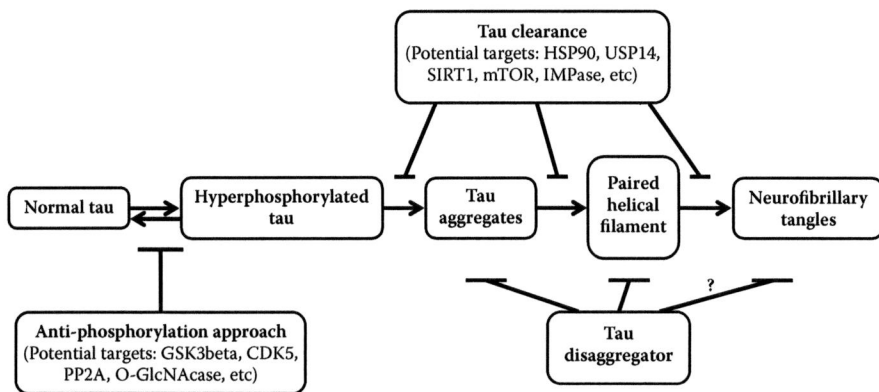

FIGURE 5.3 Tau-targeting approaches for small molecule drug discovery: Drug discovery efforts and potential novel targets are discussed along the possible mechanisms of tau toxicity.

one or two N-terminal inserts (N1, N2) and the presence of three or four pseudo-repeats (3R, 4R) in the microtubule binding domain. Binding to the microtubule is regulated by both the N- and C-terminus of tau (Preuss et al., 1997). The number of repeats in the microtubule binding domain affects the binding affinity and dynamics of tau, with less affinity for the 3R isoform (Panda et al., 2003). Physiologically, tau is phosphorylated by many kinases and phosphorylation regulates its binding affinity to the microtubule (Alonso et al., 1994; Lindwall and Cole, 1984). In addition, tau could interact with other cytoskeletal proteins such as actin (He et al., 2009), or with proteins involved in signal transduction (Ittner et al., 2010; Lee et al., 1998), and plays a critical role in regulating axonal transport (Stoothoff et al., 2009).

In AD brain, the neurofibrillary tangles (NFT) are composed of hyperphosphory-lated tau that forms filamentous amyloid aggregates. The NFT pathology starts from the entorhinal cortex and gradually progresses to hippocampus and other cortical regions (the so-called Braak staging of AD) (Braak and Braak, 1991). The occurrence and number of NFTs correlate with cognitive function in AD patients (Grober et al., 1999). The neurodegenerative processes occurring in the AD brain are also reflected in the CSF, where the levels of hyperphosphorylated tau and total tau are elevated (Buerger et al., 2006; Tapiola et al., 1997). In addition to AD, tau pathologies also occur in a set of neurodegenerative diseases (tauopathies) including frontotemporal dementia and Parkinsonism linked to chromosome 17 (FTDP-17), Pick's disease, progressive supranuclear palsy (PSP), etc. (Braak and Braak, 1991; Goedert and Jakes, 2005; Mimuro et al., 2010). Though the regional pattern of tau tangles and the vulnerable neuronal network differ among tauopathies, it does suggest that abnormality of tau is sufficient to cause neurodegeneration and functional impairments in human brain.

Multiple direct and indirect mechanisms have been proposed to explain how tau dysfunction perturbs neuronal function and eventually triggers neurodegeneration. Here tau hyperphosphorylation and tau aggregation will be discussed in detail along with the drug discovery efforts targeting them.

5.3.2 Targeting Tau Hyperphosphorylation

The largest human brain tau isoform contains 45 serine, 35 threonine, and 5 tyrosine residues. At least half of them have been demonstrated to be phosphorylated both in vitro and in vivo. Among the serines and threonines, 17 sites are serine/proline or threonine/proline sites, which are phosphorylated by proline-directed kinases, such as glycogen synthase kinase 3 beta (GSK3beta) (Buee et al., 2000; Gong et al., 2005). In the paired helical filament (PHF) isolated from AD brains, tau is hyperphosphorylated at nearly all phosphorylation sites (Morishima-Kawashima et al., 1995).

Tau hyperphosphorylation induces neuronal toxicity. Overexpression of a pseudohyperphosphorylated tau in PC12 cells induces cytotoxicity and cell apoptosis, while overexpression of wild-type tau has no effect on cell viability (Fath et al., 2002). Tau hyperphosphorylation also promotes tau aggregation (Haase et al., 2004), which then dissociates tau from the microtubule and disrupts microtubule integrity. Hyperphosphorylated tau could further sequester normal tau and induce dissociation of tau from the microtubule (Alonso et al., 1996). The unbound hyperphosphorylated tau can be missorted to dendritic spine and disrupt synaptic function by impairing glutamate receptor trafficking (Hoover et al., 2010). Interestingly, hyperphosphorylated tau has higher binding affinity to kinesin-1 than normal tau. Therefore, in the diseased condition, the unbound hyperphosphorylated tau could potentially affect axonal transport of kinesin cargos such as neurofilament to create toxicity (Cuchillo-Ibanez et al., 2008; Dubey et al., 2008). Thus, inhibiting tau hyperphosphorylation could potentially reduce tau aggregation, restore microtubule stability, and eliminate cytotoxicity.

Next we will discuss various approaches targeting tau hyperphosphorylation. These include inhibiting tau kinases, activating tau phosphatases, and modulating tau glycosylation.

5.3.2.1 Inhibiting Tau Kinases

Among many kinases involved in tau phosphorylation, GSK3beta is considered the major one (Hanger et al., 1992; Mandelkow et al., 1992). An increased activity of GSK3beta was detected in AD brains (Pei et al., 1997), while inhibition of GSK3beta, by both pharmacological and genetic approaches, reduced tau phosphorylation and rescued tau-related pathology in preclinical models (Bhat et al., 2003; Engel et al., 2006; Hong et al., 1997). Interestingly, GSK3beta is also involved in Abeta production by modulating APP processing, yet the mechanism is unclear (Phiel et al., 2003; Ryder et al., 2003). NP-12 (Tideglusib) is a GSK3beta inhibitor that is currently in a phase II clinical trial for AD. It is structurally related to thiadiazolidinone (TDZD) (Figure 5.4A) and is a non-ATP-competitive GSK3beta inhibitor (Martinez et al., 2005; Medina and Castro, 2008). In 2009, the European Commission and the US FDA granted the Noscira company the orphan drug status to Nypta® (NP-12 or Tideglusib) for treating PSP, a form of tauopathy. Lithium, a mood stabilizer, also inhibits GSK3beta and it has been evaluated in AD patients (Macdonald et al., 2008) (clinical trial: NCT00088387, ClinicalTrials.gov). However, GSK3beta not only phosphorylates tau, but is also critically involved in glucose metabolism and

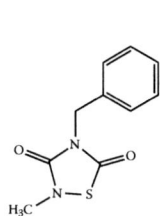

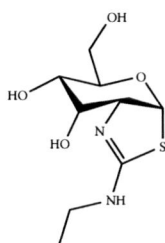

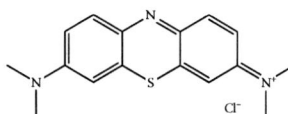

TDZD-8, a compound in TDZD series (A)   Thiamet-G (B)   Rember (C)

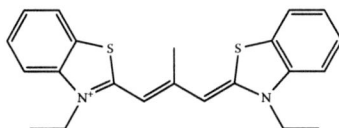

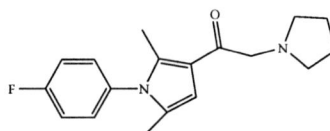

Cyanine dye C11 (D)   USP14 inhibitor IU1 (E)

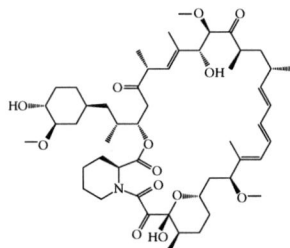

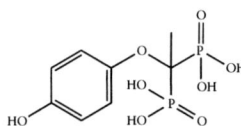

Rapamycin (F)   L-690330 (G)

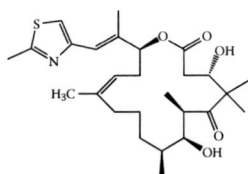

Epothilone D (H)

FIGURE 5.4 Representative structures discussed in the tau session. (A) GSK3beta inhibitor TDZD-8, a compound in thiadiazolidinone (TDZD) series; (B) O-GlcNAcase inhibitor Thiamet-G; (C) tau disaggregator Rember; (D) tau disaggregator cyanine dye C11; (E) USP14 inhibitor IU1; (F) mTOR inhibitor Rapamycin; (G) IMPase inhibitor L-690330; (H) microtubule stabilizer Epothilone D.

oncogenesis (Rayasam et al., 2009). Substrate-selective modulation of GSK3beta-mediated phosphorylation may be a challenge.

Development of inhibitors targeting other tau kinases is still at preclinical stage. Cyclin-dependent kinase 5 (CDK5) is a proline-directed tau kinase. Together with postmortem brain analysis, in vitro and in vivo studies have established the link between CDK5 activation and tau pathogenesis in AD (Cruz et al., 2003; Patrick et al., 1999; Pei et al., 1998). Suppression of the *cdk5* gene via virus-delivered RNA interference decreased tau phosphorylation and the number of NFTs in 3xTg AD mouse model (Piedrahita et al., 2010). Conversely, activation of CDK5 by its activator p25 enhanced tau phosphorylation and aggregation in vivo (Cruz et al., 2003; Noble et al., 2003). Furthermore, administration of roscovitine, a purine CDK5 inhibitor with an IC50 of 0.16 micromolar reduced tau hyperphosphorylation in transgenic AD animal model (Kitazawa et al., 2005). Unfortunately, CDK5 inhibitor development has been hampered by lack of selectivity against other kinases. The inhibitors developed so far (purine olomoncine, flavopiridol, aloisines, and indirubins) also inhibit other CDKs and GSK3beta. Preclinical studies further suggest that inhibition of CDK5 could enhance GSK3beta activity (Plattner et al., 2006). Thus, the therapeutic potential of CDK5 inhibitor remains uncertain.

5.3.2.2 Activating Tau Phosphatases

The kinase-phosphatase cycle maintains the steady-state level of phosphorylated tau and this regulation is disrupted under diseased conditions. Activation of phosphatases is therefore an alternative approach to reduce tau hyperphosphorylation. Protein phosphatase 2A (PP2A) is the major tau phosphatase. Intriguingly, the activity of PP2A is significantly decreased in postmortem AD brains (Sontag et al., 2004). Sodium selenate was recently shown to activate PP2A in a cell-free system (selectivity and other profiles of this compound are not yet reported). As proof of principle, when given to tau transgenic mice (TAU441), selenate significantly reduced tau phosphorylation and improved spatial learning and memory (Corcoran et al., 2010).

PP2A is an abundant protein whose catalytic subunit makes up to 0.1% of total cell protein (Virshup and Shenolikar, 2009). It has a broad spectrum of substrates. Thus, directly activating PP2A could generate undesired side effects. Instead, selectively modulating PP2A activity responsible for tau dephosphorylation may be a better alternative, as discussed in the following text.

First, PP2A is a multimeric enzyme with three subunits (A, B-alpha, and C). It partially achieves tissue or substrate specificity by interacting with different isoforms of regulatory B subunit, which has tissue- and cell-specific distribution (Virshup and Shenolikar, 2009). The B-alpha subunit selectively and markedly facilitates dephosphorylation of the phosphorylated tau (Sontag et al., 1996). In human AD brain, the levels of PP2A complex A-B-alpha-C is reduced in cortex, and consequently the total PP2A activity is decreased (Sontag et al., 2004). The interaction between B-alpha and A (scaffold subunit)-C (catalytic subunit) dimer is regulated by the methylation of leucine 309 (L309) in the catalytic subunit of PP2A. Mutation of L309 into alanine reduces B-alpha subunit association with the AC holoenzyme, and thereby increases tau phosphorylation (Schild et al., 2006). Therefore, targeting PP2A methylation enzymes may offer intervening opportunities.

Secondly, PP2A activity is regulated by two endogenous inhibitory proteins, I_1^{PP2A} and I_2^{PP2A} (Li et al., 1995; Li et al., 1996), which are up-regulated in AD brain (Tanimukai et al., 2005). In animal models, overexpression of the C-terminal fragment of I_2^{PP2A} reduced PP2A activity and induced AD like pathology including tau hyperphosphorylation and neurodegeneration (Wang, Blanchard et al., 2010). Inhibiting these proteins may therefore provide another mechanism for augmenting PP2A activity responsible for tau dephosphorylation, although more research is required to better elucidate the biology.

5.3.2.3 Modulating Tau Glycosylation

Since the majority of phosphorylation in tau occurs at serine and threonine sites, posttranslational modifications such as O-linked glycosylation can significantly alter the availability of hydroxyl groups for phosphorylation. In fact, in healthy adult brain, tau is extensively glycosylated by O-linked beta-N-acetylglucosamine (O-GlcNAc) at multiple serine and threonine sites (Arnold et al., 1996; Liu et al., 2004), and in AD patient brain the level of O-GlcNAc on tau is significantly reduced (Liu et al., 2004). Therefore targeting mechanisms responsible for O-linked glycosylation may be another approach to reduce tau phosphorylation.

O-linked glycosylation is catalyzed by O-GlcNAc transferases (O-GlcNAcase). Based on enzyme crystal structure, a specific O-GlcNAcase inhibitor (Thiamet-G) (Figure 5.4B) was designed and tested both in vitro and in vivo (Yuzwa et al., 2008). Administration of Thiamet-G significantly increased O-GlcNAc levels and reduced tau phosphorylation at several serine and threonine sites (Yuzwa et al., 2008). Recently, Merck partnered with Alectos Therapeutics to develop the O-GlcNAcase inhibitor (http://www.merck.com/licensing/our-partnership/Alectos-partnership.html). It is worth noting, however, that O-GlcNAcase glycosylates many nuclear and cytoplasmic proteins (Hart et al., 2007) and inhibition of O-GlcNAcase could affect glycosylation levels of various proteins in the cells.

5.3.3 Tau Disaggregators

Tau is a highly soluble protein with a poorly defined secondary structure. Hyperphosphorylation or truncation of tau is thought to dissociate tau from microtubules, which then adopts a conformation that has a higher propensity to form aggregates. The hexapeptide motifs (VQIINK and VQIVYK) in the repeat region of microtubule binding domain help tau to switch its conformation and form a beta-sheet structure (von Bergen et al., 2000). Tau polymerizes, both in vitro and in vivo, into higher-order structures such as PHF and straight filaments, and eventually develops into tangles.

Accumulating evidence suggests that tau aggregates are neurotoxic. For example, FTDP-17 ΔK280 mutation promotes tau aggregation and tangle formation (proaggregation), while another tau mutation (ΔK280 /I277P/I308P) inhibits tau aggregation and tangle formation (anti-aggregation). Transgenic mice overexpressing the *pro-aggregation* tau mutation displayed significant neuronal loss and gliosis, whereas no neuronal loss was observed in mice overexpressing the *anti-aggregation* tau mutation (Mocanu et al., 2008). In humans it is clear that the pattern/stage of NFT pathology (Braak and Braak, 1991) and the number of NFTs, but not senile plaques, correlate with the disease progression and severity of AD (Arriagada et al., 1992). These findings strongly support the notion that tau aggregation is cytotoxic and suggest disaggregating tau as a potential therapeutic strategy.

Indeed, the concept is currently being tested in a phase II clinical trial using methylthioninium chloride (Rember) (Figure 5.4C) developed by TauRx pharmaceuticals. However, its clinical development could prove challenging. The compound may hit multiple targets, in addition to its reported tau disaggregation property (Oz et al., 2011; Wischik et al., 1996). Moreover, the blue color of the compound confounds clinical trial design. Thus, efforts are in progress to identify more potent, selective, and brain-penetrable tau disaggregators.

In fact, utilizing a cell-free tau aggregation system and in silico virtual screening, many compounds have been identified with the ability to disaggregate tau (e.g., rhodamines, phenylthiazolylhydrazides, N-phenylamines, anthraquinones, benzothiazoles, phenothiazines) (Bulic et al., 2009). These compounds have been subsequently tested in cell-based assays and in ex vivo brain slice culture from tau transgenic mice (Chang et al., 2009; Duff et al., 2010; Larbig et al., 2007).

Tau disaggregator approach does carry intrinsic challenges. First, many of these compounds are of a dye-like structure, and self-aggregate at higher concentrations. For instance, the cyanine dye C11 (Figure 5.4D) at 1 nanomolar disaggregates about 50% of tau aggregates in brain slices, but at 1 micromolar, it induces tau aggregation to 200% compared to control (Duff et al., 2010). Second, many identified tau disaggregators are charged, thus limiting their ability to be developed. Third, for effective disaggregation, large numbers of disaggregators must be present in the brain to counter abundant tau. Finally, special attention has to be paid to ensure compound selectivity so that it can spare normal cellular protein–protein interaction.

Conversely, many protein aggregates form a beta-sheet-like structure. It will be interesting to see whether potent tau disaggregators could also disaggregate other pathological protein aggregates, such as huntingtin aggregation in Huntington's disease, alpha-synuclein aggregation in Parkinson's disease, and even Abeta aggregates in AD.

5.3.4 TAU CLEARANCE

In cells, tau aggregates are cleared by both proteasomal and autophagy pathways. Enhancing these mechanisms to remove abnormal tau, while maintaining normal tau functions, may be another therapeutic approach for AD and tauopathies. In this category, several targets are of special interest.

First, heat shock proteins (HSPs) play a critical role in directing tau for proteasomal degradation. Inhibiting HSP90 by small molecules directly promotes clearance of phosphorylated tau or tau aggregates (Dickey et al., 2005; Dickey et al., 2007; Luo et al., 2007). Inhibition of HSP90 also activates heat shock factor 1 (HSF1), a transcription factor that up-regulates expression of heat shock proteins and enhances degradation of aggregated proteins (Kimura et al., 2010).

Next, USP14 is a proteasome-associated deubiquitinating enzyme that modulates proteasome function. A USP14 inhibitor has been shown to enhance proteasomal degradation of tau and other proteins involved in neurodegeneration in vitro (Figure 5.4E) (Lee et al., 2010).

Thirdly, tau was recently reported to be acetylated and acetylation inhibits tau degradation. In patients with mild to moderate tau pathology, the acetylation level of tau is increased. As tau acetylation is regulated by p300 (for acetylation) and SIRT1 (for deacetylation) (Min et al., 2010), it is interesting to test whether small-molecule SIRT1 activators could reduce tau acetylation and promote tau degradation.

Finally, there are several approaches to enhance autophagy function and small molecules that could enhance cellular autophagy activity have been identified (Sarkar and Rubinsztein, 2008). Rapamycin (Figure 5.4F), for example, specifically inhibits mTOR, a key regulator of autophagy (Ravikumar et al., 2004). It was shown to reduce cellular tau aggregates and protect cells against apoptotic insults in vitro (Berger et al., 2006; Ravikumar et al., 2006). Lithium and L-690330 (Atack et al., 1993) (Figure 5.4G), interestingly, could enhance autophagy activity by inhibiting inositol monophosphatase (IMPase), a key enzyme catalyzing the hydrolysis of inositol monophosphate into free inositol (Sarkar et al., 2005; Sarkar and Rubinsztein, 2006).

For these approaches to augment proteasome and autophagy degradation, the challenge lies in selective manipulation of pathological proteins to maintain normal cellular function.

5.3.5 OTHER MECHANISMS

As discussed earlier, tau is a microtubule binding protein, and tau aggregates are thought to dissociate from microtubules resulting in microtubule disassembly and disruption of axonal transport. Hence, microtubule stabilizers may compensate for the dysfunction. Davunetide (AL-108) is an intranasal formulation of NAP (a peptide of eight amino acids, NAPVSIPQ) that is currently in phase II trials for AD. It was reported to stabilize microtubules and reduce tau hyperphosphorylation (Gozes et al., 2009). In 2010, the FDA granted orphan drug designation to davunetide for treating PSP.

Small-molecule microtubule stabilizers are commonly used in cancer therapy (Altmann, 2001) and multiple FDA-approved drugs are available. Interestingly, some of the compounds also showed beneficial effects in preclinical AD animal models. For example, Epothilone D (Figure 5.4H), a CNS-penetrable microtubule stabilizer, has been shown to improve microtubule density and cognition in the PS19 tau transgenic mouse model (Brunden et al., 2011; Brunden et al., 2010). Unexpectedly, the dose used in the animal study is much less compared to that used for cancer (Beer et al., 2007; Brunden et al., 2010), suggesting a possibility to dissociate toxicity from microtubule stabilizing effect. Currently, Bristol-Myers Squibb is developing small-molecule microtubule stabilizers for AD (http://www.bms.com/Documents/investors/ICM_Cuss.pdf).

As exciting new mechanisms for tau toxicity are emerging, elucidating the underlying biology may help to formulate novel strategies targeting tau. For example, the tau propagation hypothesis (Clavaguera et al., 2009; Frost et al., 2009) and how extracellular tau triggers the intracellular tau aggregation is an exciting area for research. tau oligomers have been identified in early AD brains (Maeda et al., 2006) and are reportedly more toxic than monomers in SH-SY5Y cells (Lasagna-Reeves et al., 2010). Tau missorting and the mechanism of tau-induced synaptic toxicity is another research area that is unfolding (Hoover et al., 2010; Thies and Mandelkow, 2007). Finally, it is important to understand how tau influences Abeta-mediated cytotoxicity (Gotz et al., 2001; Ittner et al., 2010; Rapoport et al., 2002; Roberson et al., 2007).

5.3.6 CHALLENGES

Besides the specific challenges associated with the mechanisms discussed above, one general challenge in tau drug discovery is the limited understanding of tau biology. For example, tau has many phosphorylation sites, yet the contribution of each phosphorylation site to disease pathogenesis is not completely understood. It is unknown whether a specific tau kinase inhibitor will be sufficient to achieve overall biological efficacy. The identity of toxic tau species (hyperphosphorylated tau, tau oligomers, or tau fibrils) and how they each contribute to AD pathogenesis are other key questions that may impact tau drug discovery strategy. As the role of tau in AD pathogenesis being increasingly appreciated, scientific research and drug discovery efforts on tau will likely further intensify over the next few years. This will hopefully further enhance our understanding of tau biology to fill these gaps.

5.4 NEUROPROTECTION, NEUROREPAIR, AND NEUROREGENERATION

As discussed earlier, AD is a progressive disease with synaptic dysfunction and loss preceding neuronal degeneration. The majority of the current approaches in AD drug discovery aim at inhibiting disease pathologies like Abeta and tau, which may halt or delay disease progression depending on the degree of toxin reduction. Neuroprotection and neurorepair, on the other hand, could not only counteract the deleterious effects generated by the pathological neurotoxins but also protect or promote synapse formation and neuronal survival, thereby enhancing cognitive function. In this section, we will discuss three major approaches: (a) *neuroprotection,* which prevents neuronal death by regulating mechanisms that alter neuronal homeostasis; (b) *neurorepair,* which targets the endogenous growth factor pathway to promote neuronal survival; and (c) *neuroregeneration,* which promotes adult neurogenesis or survival of newborn neurons to compensate for the neuronal loss in diseases. These approaches may provide therapeutic benefits not only for AD but also for other neurodegenerative diseases.

5.4.1 NEUROPROTECTIVE APPROACH

5.4.1.1 L-Type Calcium Channel Blockers

Cognitive decline in AD patients has been linked to neuronal damage caused by calcium influx-mediated excitotoxicity driven by persistent hyperactivation of NMDA receptors and voltage-gated and voltage-sensitive calcium channels induced by the excitatory neurotransmitter glutamate. Multiple mechanisms (including Abeta) have been proposed to disturb cytosolic calcium homeostasis, which mediates downstream signaling events resulting in neurodegeneration (Supnet and Bezprozvanny, 2010a). Since calcium is a key cellular second messenger, a high degree of selectivity would be required to gain a sufficient safety margin. From a drug development perspective, identifying targets that specifically restore calcium homeostasis in the diseased condition will be desirable, although identification of such a target is highly challenging.

Different types of receptors and ion channels, including voltage-gated calcium channels (VGCC), sarco/endoplasmic reticulum Ca^{2+}-ATPase (SERCA), ryanodine receptors (RyRs), and inositol 1,4,5-trisphosphate (IP3) receptors regulate intracellular calcium and have been considered as targets for treating AD (Buxbaum et al., 1994; Cheung et al., 2008; Supnet and Bezprozvanny, 2010a; Supnet et al., 2010). All three classes of conventional calcium channel inhibitors (dihydropyridine or DHP, phenyl-alkylamine or PAA, benzothiazepine or BTZ) inhibit the long-lasting calcium current mediated by the L-type VGCCs (Elmslie, 2004; Kochegarov, 2003), which have prolonged channel opening properties and whose expression level is elevated under the diseased condition (Coon et al., 1999). AD clinical trials using nimodipine (a DHP derivative and L-VGCC antagonist) have been largely variable with the undesirable side effect of reducing blood pressure, although meta-analysis suggests the drug was well tolerated in dementia patients (Lopez-Arrieta and Birks, 2002). MEM-1003 (developed by Memory Pharmaceuticals), another L-VGCC-specific antagonist with better brain permeability, did not meet the primary endpoint in a 12-week phase II AD clinical trial (clinical trial: NCT00257673, ClinicalTrials.gov). A similar class of L-VGCC antagonist, isradipine (Dynacirc CR) is currently in a phase II STEADY-PD trial for Parkinson's disease (clinical trial: NCT00909545, ClinicalTrials.gov).

5.4.1.2 Mitochondrial Stabilizers

In addition to their function as the energy-producing organelle in cells, mitochondria also act as a sink to buffer excessive cytosolic calcium. Above a certain threshold, mitochondria lose their buffering capacity and open mitochondrial permeability transition pores (mPTPs) resulting in mitochondrial permeability transition and dysfunction, which is conserved across different species (Azzolin et al., 2010; Supnet and Bezprozvanny, 2010a; Supnet and Bezprozvanny, 2010b). Cyclophilin D is a mitochondrial isoform of cyclophilins (a family of peptidylprolyl cis-trans isomerases) that facilitates formation of mPTP in the mitochondrial inner membrane. Inhibiting cyclophilin D via a genetic or pharmacological approach stabilized mitochondria and rescued cell viability in vitro and in vivo (Malouitre et al., 2009; Millay et al., 2008). However, available cyclophilin D inhibitors are not brain permeable. Dimebon (latrepirdine) (Figure 5.5A) is another potential mitochondrial stabilizer that has been used as an antihistamine drug in Russia for more than two decades (Bachurin et al., 2001). In addition to evidence suggesting Dimebon as a blocker of mPTP (Bachurin et al., 2004), this molecule has also been reported to inhibit NMDA receptors (Grigorev et al., 2003) and VGCCs (Lermontova et al., 2001), albeit at very high concentrations (IC50 = 10–50 micromolar). Although Dimebon demonstrated significant therapeutic effects in a six-month randomized, double-blind, placebo-controlled phase II study (Doody et al., 2008), it failed in the large phase III AD CONNECTION trial sponsored by Pfizer and Medivation, in both primary (ADAS-Cog) and secondary efficacy measures (clinical trial: NCT00675623, ClinicalTrials.gov). Potent, selective, and brain-permeable mitochondrial stabilizers are needed to further test whether targeting mitochondria will provide therapeutic benefits to AD patients.

5.4.1.3 Antagonizing p75NTR

The pan-neurotrophin receptor p75NTR (NGFR or CD271) belongs to the tumor necrosis factor (TNF) superfamily of cell death receptors. In a normal brain, p75NTR is highly expressed during development, but its expression in adult neurons is largely limited to basal forebrain cholinergic neurons (Allen et al., 1989; Hefti and Mash, 1989;

I. Neuroprotection:

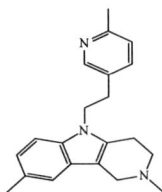 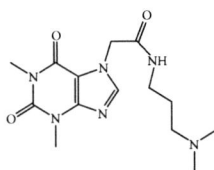 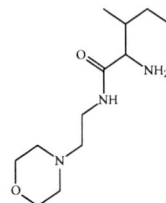

Dimebon (A)   LM11A-24 (B)   LM11A-31 (C)

II. Neurorepair:

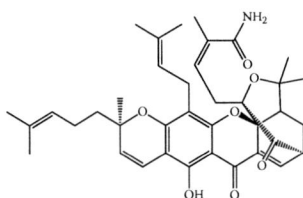 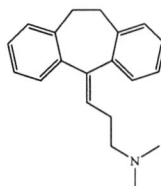

Gambogic amide (D)   Amitriptyline (E)

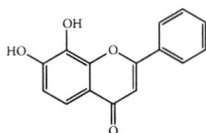 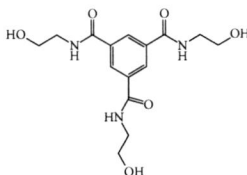 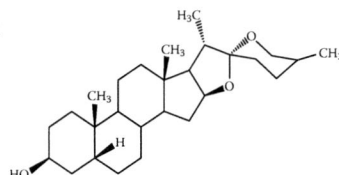

7,8 – dihydroxyflavone (F)   LM22A-4 (G)   PYM50028 (H)

III. Neuroregeneration:

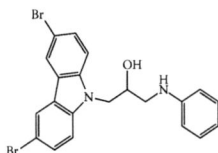 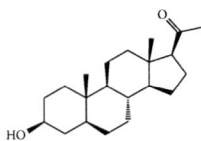 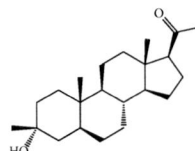

P7C3 (I)   Allopregnanolone (J)   Ganaxolone (K)

FIGURE 5.5 Representative structures discussed in the Neuroprotection/Neurorepair-Neuroregeneration session. I. Neuroprotection: (A) Dimebon is a multifunctional molecule with mitochondrial stabilizing property; (B–C) LM11A-24 and 31 antagonizing p75NTR in vitro; II. Neurorepair: Gambogic amide (D) and Amitriptyline (E) activate NGF-TrkA pathway; 7,8-dihydroxyflavone (F) and LM22A-4 (G) activate BDNF-TrkB pathway; PYM50028 (H) is suggested to increase BDNF level among other functions; III. Neuroregeneration: P7C3 (I) and Allopregnanolone (J) may have neuroregeneration potential. Ganaxolone (K) is a structural analogue of (J).

Kordower et al., 1989; Mufson et al., 1989a). Remarkably, p75NTR level is dramatically increased in neurons that are damaged in AD (Mufson et al., 1989b), amyotrophic lateral sclerosis (ALS) (Lowry et al., 2001; Seeburger et al., 1993), and in oligodendrocytes in multiple sclerosis (Dowling et al., 1999). Thus, inhibiting p75NTR could potentially rescue the dying neurons specifically without affecting surrounding normal cells.

In adult brain, p75NTR promotes survival of cholinergic neurons in conjunction with the tropomyosin-related kinase A (TrkA) (Chen et al., 1996; Naumann et al., 2002). Nerve growth factor (NGF) binds TrkA and promotes the survival of cholinergic neurons. In disease conditions, the TrkA level reduces, while p75NTR is up-regulated and/or remains unaffected (Counts et al., 2004; Ginsberg et al., 2006; Hu et al., 2002), shifting the balance from promoting cholinergic neuron survival to apoptosis. In addition, p75NTR has been reported to (a) increase processing of APP by beta-secretase (Costantini et al., 2005); (b) function as a potential signaling receptor for Abeta to induce cell death (Knowles et al., 2009; Sotthibundhu et al., 2008; Yaar et al., 1997); and (c) act as a signaling receptor for proneurotrophins like proNGF (Pedraza et al., 2005; Podlesniy et al., 2006).

High-throughput screening (HTS) for small molecules that inhibit p75NTR-mediated cell death identified molecules that interfere with NGF binding rather than those that directly antagonize p75NTR (Colquhoun et al., 2004; Jaen et al., 1995; Niederhauser et al., 2000). Peptidomimetic antagonists against p75NTR appeared cell-protective in vitro, yet attempts to demonstrate efficacy in vivo upon systemic administration failed (Turner et al., 2004; Yaar et al., 2007). However, pharmacokinetic profile and brain exposure of the peptidomimetics are unknown. In silico virtual screening identified small molecules against p75NTR with a more favorable drug-like profile such as LM11A-24 (Figure 5.5B) and LM11A-31 (Figure 5.5C) (Massa et al., 2006). These molecules promoted hippocampal neuronal survival with no cross activation of tropomyosin-related kinase B (TrkB). These compounds displaced NGF and p75NTR extracellular domain binding antibodies from p75NTR. But they showed cytotoxicity at higher concentrations, and failed to prevent NGF-TrkA binding and their survival effect. In vitro, binding of LM11A compounds to p75NTR selectively promoted early components of the NFκB pathway stimulated by neurotrophins, blocked Abeta-induced cytotoxicity (Yang et al., 2008), and protected oligodendrocytes against cell death induced by proNGF (Massa et al., 2006). In vivo proof-of-principle tests would require better tool compounds.

Finally, anti-inflammation and antioxidant approaches could also be categorized as neuroprotection. The subject of neuroinflammation and AD has been reviewed extensively (Agostinho et al., 2010; Eikelenboom et al., 2010; El Khoury, 2010; Glass et al., 2010; Hensley, 2010). While the involvement of microglia and astrocyte in the onset and progress of the neurodegenerative process in AD has been increasingly recognized, neuroinflammation (with oxidative stress) is often referred to as a "double-edged sword" as it can have both detrimental and beneficial effects on the neural tissue (Agostinho et al., 2010). Therefore, a better strategy to modulate neuroinflammation to achieve therapeutic benefit still awaits further elucidation. So far, clinical trials using monotreatment of antioxidants (Vitamin E, Vitamin C, etc.) or in combination with other drugs have yielded inconclusive results as brain penetration may be limited in some cases. A simple scavenger approach requires a high concentration of scavenging agents in the brain to quench a high level of reactive oxygen species (ROS), and therefore may not be efficient. Alternatively, active inhibition of ROS production may be a better approach.

5.4.2 Neurorepair: Growth Factor Approach

Neurotrophins are endogenous trophic factors that promote neuronal survival and differentiation during development, and regulate synapse plasticity and cognition in the adult. Two of the neurotrophic factors, NGF and BDNF, and their cognate receptors, TrkA and TrkB, respectively, are expressed in adult brain and have been considered as targets for AD therapy. While growth factors per se as a treatment face a huge hurdle as they cannot enter the brain, recent advances in the field may pave the way for alternative strategies to target growth factors using small molecules.

5.4.2.1 Agonizing NGF-TrkA Pathway

The *cholinergic hypothesis* stipulates that agents promoting the survival and/or function of cholinergic neurons should provide a disease-modifying benefit (Thathiah and De Strooper, 2009). NGF and its receptor TrkA have long been demonstrated to promote survival of cholinergic neurons in vivo (Fagan et al., 1997). For example, AD patients or nonhuman primates surgically implanted with heterologous cells secreting NGF in the medial septal region showed significant improvement in cognitive functions as well as in activities of daily life (Kordower et al., 1994; Tuszynski et al., 2005). Based on these promising findings, significant efforts have been made to identify small molecules that can directly activate TrkA, potentiate NGF action, and/or enhance NGF secretion.

Intuitively, molecules that either potentiate the effects of NGF or increase NGF expression may only provide temporary therapeutic benefits as the level of NGF will significantly decrease in AD patients as disease progresses (Counts and Mufson, 2005). Increasing the expression of NGF in the diseased condition may instead be counterproductive because it could result in the accumulation of precursor proNGF, which has pro-apoptotic properties (Fahnestock et al., 2001). Therefore, molecules that can directly activate or modulate TrkA function may be more desirable.

Toward this end, two different approaches have been adopted. The first uses an agonistic TrkA monoclonal antibody to generate a class of small peptidomimetics to activate TrkA and promote cell survival (LeSauteur et al., 1996; Maliartchouk et al., 2000). Given that these molecules bind to sites on TrkA other than the ligand-binding domain, it will be important to determine whether they could achieve similar efficacy as NGFs in vivo.

Second, screening of small molecules that either promote survival or provide resistance to staurosporine-induced cell death identified gambogic amide (GA) (Figure 5.5D) as a selective activator of TrkA. Activation of downstream signaling events (pAkt, pMAPK) results in neuronal protection against glutamate and kainic acid insults in vitro. In vivo, GA decreased infarct volume in the transient middle cerebral artery occlusion model of stroke in rodents (Jang et al., 2007). A tricyclic antidepressant, amitriptyline (Figure 5.5E), was recently reported to bind and activate TrkA in vitro and promote cell survival against oxygen-glucose deprivation and kainic acid insults (Jang et al., 2009). However, this neuroprotective effect was not observed with the structurally related drugs imipramine or clomipramine.

5.4.2.2 Agonizing BDNF-TrkB Pathway

TrkB is ubiquitously expressed in the central neurons, and plays a critical role in learning and memory, in addition to promoting neuronal survival and preventing synapse loss. As proof of principle, when delivered bilaterally using lentivirus to the entorhinal cortex of J20-APP mice (overexpressing Swedish and Indiana APP mutations) six months after the disease onset, within one month of treatment, BDNF significantly rescued both spatial and associative memory deficits as well as synapse loss without affecting number of neurons or Abeta plaque load (Nagahara et al., 2009). These results indicate that the behavioral benefits were achieved without affecting Abeta, suggesting that BDNF effects are primarily mediated by synaptic protection/repair.

A few nonpeptidyl small molecules have been claimed so far as TrkB agonists. One group identified 7,8-dihydroxyflavone (7,8-DHF) (Figure 5.5F) and deoxygedunin as TrkB-specific agonists through a cell-based survival assay and/or an in silico screening approach based on a BDNF loop-domain pharmacophore (Jang et al., 2010a; Jang et al., 2010b; Massa et al., 2010). 7,8-DHF, for example, specifically protected neurons against glutamate and oxygen-glucose deprivation in vitro. In vivo, the compound protected against neuronal degeneration in an kainic acid–induced epileptic model, in an ischemic model of stroke, and in an MPTP mouse model of Parkinson's disease (Jang et al., 2010b; Liu et al., 2010). Using structure-based drug design, a second group identified LM22A-4 (Figure 5.5G) as a TrkB agonist. In vivo, LM22A-4 progressively restored deficits in rotarod performance after 2–3 weeks of parietal controlled cortical impact injury in rats (Massa et al., 2010). Although these compounds possess a broad neuroprotectant potential, the efficacy of these compounds in preclinical AD models remains to be tested. Given the long history of failures to identify TrkB agonists, it is essential to validate these compounds for more direct TrkB receptor binding and activation in vitro, and target engagement in vivo.

In addition, several molecules have been reported to promote neuronal survival by stimulating neurotrophin synthesis and secretion directly or indirectly. For example, PYM50028 (or sapogenin from Phytopharm) (Figure 5.5H) isolated from a Chinese medicinal herb has been shown to not only increase the level of BDNF, but also increase glial celline–derived neurotrophic factor (GDNF) and M1 muscarinic acetylcholine receptor levels (Hu et al., 2008; Hu et al., 2005). It was taken into phase II study for AD (clinical trials: NCT00130429, ClinicalTrials.gov), but did not meet the primary endpoints after 12-week treatment. It is unclear whether lack of target engagement could partially explain the lack of efficacy. Similarly, Sirt1 (Gao et al., 2010) and magnesium- L- threonate (Slutsky et al., 2010) have been reported to increase BDNF expression, although in the former case, the challenge has been to selectively activate the deacetylating enzyme via a small-molecule approach given its broad range of substrates (Beher et al., 2009; Donmez et al., 2010; Kim et al., 2007; Min et al., 2010; Pacholec et al., 2010).

5.4.3 EMERGING NEUROREGENERATIVE APPROACH

In humans, adult neurogenesis predominantly exists in two regions: the subgranular zone (SGZ) in the dentate gyrus of hippocampus, and the subventricular zone (SVZ) lining the lateral ventricles. Only a fraction of the newborn neurons survive and integrate into the neuronal network while the majority die. With age there is a significant reduction in neurogenesis (Bhardwaj et al., 2006; Knoth et al., 2010; Siwak-Tapp et al., 2007). Efforts are being made to develop/identify small molecules that can either promote proliferation and differentiation of neural stem cells or promote survival of newborn neurons, to potentially compensate for some of the neuronal loss during neurodegeneration.

A recent in vivo screen for such small molecules with an ability to promote neuroregeneration identified aminopropyl carbazole (designated P7C3) (Figure 5.5I) as a possible candidate (Pieper et al., 2010). Two months treatment with P7C3 at 10 mg/kg significantly improved spatial memory in the Morris water maze test in aged rats. Another study demonstrated that allopregnanolone (APα) (Figure 5.5J), a small lipophilic and naturally produced molecule in humans, could increase the proliferation of neural precursor cells in both SVZ and SGZ regions in rodents (Wang, Singh et al., 2010). Interestingly, a single subcutaneous injection (10 mg/kg) of APα not only elevated the level of neurogenesis but also rescued the memory deficit in trace eye-blink conditioning in the 3xTg AD mouse model after 7 or 22 days of chronic treatment. Moreover, there was a clear association between the dose of APα, amount of neurogenesis, and improvement in memory function. With these recent findings it would be interesting to see whether Epalon 1000 (ganaxolone, a 3α-methylated synthetic analog of 3α-hydroxy-5α-pregnan-20-one) (Figure 5.5K), developed as an anti-epileptic/anti-anxiolytic medication by Purdue Pharma/Marinus Pharmaceuticals with a good safety profile, would provide desired cognitive benefits in preclinical AD animal models.

5.4.4 CHALLENGES

While neuroprotective, neurorepair, and neuroregenerative mechanisms may offer additional advantages, major challenges are expected. First, the majority of the growth factor receptors require dimerization for their activation, which involves complex protein–protein interactions. Whether small molecules can efficiently induce dimerization to activate the receptors is a key question. Second, activating growth factor pathways is intrinsically associated with tumorogenic potential. Since Trk receptors are also expressed in peripheral tissues, activation using small molecules may lead to undesired pleiotrophic side effects (myalgia and other pain) due to activation of nociceptive neurons, which was observed in NGF clinical trials (Petty et al., 1994). Finally, it is worth noting that from a neuroprotection perspective, to achieve substantial disease modification, the therapy may be most efficacious during the early stages of disease and long-term treatment may be required to observe clinical benefits.

5.5 FUTURE PERSPECTIVES

In this chapter, we briefly reviewed small-molecule disease-modifying drug discovery efforts in AD, mainly focusing on the most recent advances in targeting Abeta, tau, and emerging neuroprotection and neurorepair mechanisms. Strategy-specific challenges were discussed in each section. In addition, there are common hurdles that the whole community working in neurodegenerative diseases, including AD, is facing. These include heterogeneity of diseases both in biology and clinical symptoms, the complicated nature of pathologies with limited understanding of disease biology, lack of translatable animal models, and limited disease-based biomarkers. Furthermore, many targets at the discovery stage are associated with potential mechanism-associated adverse effects (or an expected limited safety margin). Some mechanisms of action require interference of protein–protein interaction, which is historically proven as being highly challenging for small-molecule drug discovery.

Despite all these major challenges, the discovery community is making steady progress. The Alzheimer's Disease Neuroimaging Initiative (ADNI) sets a good example of how information sharing among the entire research community and cooperatively working together could lead to fruitful progress. As we reflect back on AD drug discovery and look forward to the future, it is our firm belief that exciting science and innovative technologies combined with holding the highest standard at every step of drug discovery will pave the way toward successfully generating medicines for AD and other neurodegenerative diseases.

ACKNOWLEDGMENTS

We would like to thank Drs. Yasuji Matsuoka, Andy Lockhart, and Bai Lu for their critical reading and editing of this book chapter. We'd also like to thank other colleagues for their support during the writing process. We sincerely apologize to colleagues in the field whose important work may have not been cited here.

REFERENCES

Agostinho, P., Cunha, R. A., and Oliveira, C. 2010. Neuroinflammation, oxidative stress and the pathogenesis of Alzheimer's disease. *Curr Pharm Des* 16: 2766–2778.

Allen, S. J., Dawbarn, D., Spillantini, M. G., Goedert, M., Wilcock, G. K., Moss, T. H., and Semenenko, F. M. 1989. Distribution of beta-nerve growth factor receptors in the human basal forebrain. *J Comp Neurol* 289: 626–640.

Alonso, A. C., Grundke-Iqbal, I., and Iqbal, K. 1996. Alzheimer's disease hyperphosphorylated tau sequesters normal tau into tangles of filaments and disassembles microtubules. *Nat Med* 2: 783–787.

Alonso, A. C., Zaidi, T., Grundke-Iqbal, I., and Iqbal, K. 1994. Role of abnormally phosphorylated tau in the breakdown of microtubules in Alzheimer disease. *Proc Natl Acad Sci USA* 91: 5562–5566.

Altmann, K. H. 2001. Microtubule-stabilizing agents: A growing class of important anticancer drugs. *Curr Opin Chem Biol* 5: 424–431.

Arispe, N., Rojas, E., and Pollard, H. B. 1993. Alzheimer disease amyloid beta protein forms calcium channels in bilayer membranes: Blockade by tromethamine and aluminum. *Proc Natl Acad Sci USA* 90: 567–571.

Arnold, C. S., Johnson, G. V., Cole, R. N., Dong, D. L., Lee, M., and Hart, G. W. 1996. The microtubule-associated protein tau is extensively modified with O-linked N-acetylglucosamine. *J Biol Chem* 271: 28741–28744.

Arriagada, P. V., Growdon, J. H., Hedley-Whyte, E. T., and Hyman, B. T. 1992. Neurofibrillary tangles but not senile plaques parallel duration and severity of Alzheimer's disease. *Neurology* 42: 631–639.

Atack, J. R., Cook, S. M., Watt, A. P., Fletcher, S. R., and Ragan, C. I. 1993. In vitro and in vivo inhibition of inositol monophosphatase by the bisphosphonate L-690,330. *J Neurochem* 60: 652–658.

Azzolin, L., von Stockum, S., Basso, E., Petronilli, V., Forte, M. A., and Bernardi, P. 2010. The mitochondrial permeability transition from yeast to mammals. *FEBS Lett* 584: 2504–2509.

Bachurin, S., Bukatina, E., Lermontova, N., Tkachenko, S., Afanasiev, A., Grigoriev, V., Grigorieva, I., Ivanov, Y., Sablin, S., and Zefirov, N. 2001. Antihistamine agent Dimebon as a novel neuroprotector and a cognition enhancer. *Ann N Y Acad Sci* 939: 425–435.

Bachurin, S. O., Shevtsova, E. P., Kireeva, E. G., Oxenkrug, G. F., and Sablin, S. O. 2004. Mitochondria as a target for neurotoxins and neuroprotective agents. *Ann N Y Acad Sci* 993: 334–344; discussion 345–339.

Balducci, C., Beeg, M., Stravalaci, M., Bastone, A., Sclip, A., Biasini, E., Tapella, L., Colombo, L., Manzoni, C., Borsello, T., Chiesa, R., Gobbi, M., Salmona, M., and Forloni, G. 2010. Synthetic amyloid-beta oligomers impair long-term memory independently of cellular prion protein. *Proc Natl Acad Sci USA* 107: 2295–2300.

Beach, T. G., Walker, D. G., Potter, P. E., Sue, L. I., and Fisher, A. 2001. Reduction of cerebrospinal fluid amyloid beta after systemic administration of M1 muscarinic agonists. *Brain Res* 905: 220–223.

Beer, T. M., Higano, C. S., Saleh, M., Dreicer, R., Hudes, G., Picus, J., Rarick, M., Fehrenbacher, L., and Hannah, A. L. 2007. Phase II study of KOS-862 in patients with metastatic androgen independent prostate cancer previously treated with docetaxel. *Invest New Drugs* 25: 565–570.

Beher, D., Wu, J., Cumine, S., Kim, K. W., Lu, S.C., Atangan, L., and Wang, M. 2009. Resveratrol is not a direct activator of SIRT1 enzyme activity. *Chem Biol Drug Des* 74: 619–624.

Bengoechea, T. G., Chen, Z., O'Leary, D. A., Masliah, E., and Lee, K. F. 2009. p75 reduces beta-amyloid-induced sympathetic innervation deficits in an Alzheimer's disease mouse model. *Proc Natl Acad Sci USA* 106: 7870–7875.

Benilova, I., and De Strooper, B. Prion protein in Alzheimer's pathogenesis: A hot and controversial issue. 2010. *EMBO Molecular Medicine* 2: 289–290.

Berger, Z., Ravikumar, B., Menzies, F. M., Oroz, L. G., Underwood, B. R., Pangalos, M. N., Schmitt, I., Wullner, U., Evert, B. O., O'Kane, C. J., and Rubinsztein, D. C. 2006. Rapamycin alleviates toxicity of different aggregate-prone proteins. *Hum Mol Genet* 15: 433–442.

Berry-Kravis, E., Hessl, D., Coffey, S., Hervey, C., Schneider, A., Yuhas, J., Hutchison, J., Snape, M., Tranfaglia, M., Nguyen, D. V., and Hagerman, R. 2009. A pilot open label, single dose trial of fenobam in adults with fragile X syndrome. *J Med Genet* 46: 266–271.

Bertram, L., Lill, C. M., and Tanzi, R. E. 2010. The genetics of Alzheimer disease: Back to the future. *Neuron* 68: 270–281.

Bhardwaj, R. D., Curtis, M. A., Spalding, K. L., Buchholz, B. A., Fink, D., Bjork-Eriksson, T., Nordborg, C., Gage, F. H., Druid, H., Eriksson, P. S., and Frisen, J. 2006. Neocortical neurogenesis in humans is restricted to development. *Proc Natl Acad Sci USA* 103: 12564–12568.

Bhat, R., Xue, Y., Berg, S., Hellberg, S., Ormo, M., Nilsson, Y., Radesater, A. C., Jerning, E., Markgren, P. O., Borgegard, T., Nylof, M., Gimenez-Cassina, A., Hernandez, F., Lucas, J. J., Diaz-Nido, J., and Avila, J. 2003. Structural insights and biological effects of glycogen synthase kinase 3-specific inhibitor AR-A014418. *J Biol Chem* 278: 45937–45945.

Braak, H., and Braak, E. 1991. Neuropathological staging of Alzheimer-related changes. *Acta Neuropathol* 82: 239–259.

Breysse, N., Baunez, C., Spooren, W., Gasparini, F., and Amalric, M. 2002. Chronic but not acute treatment with a metabotropic glutamate 5 receptor antagonist reverses the akinetic deficits in a rat model of parkinsonism. *J Neurosci* 22: 5669–5678.

Bridges, T. M., Brady, A. E., Kennedy, J. P., Daniels, R. N., Miller, N. R., Kim, K., Breininger, M. L., Gentry, P. R., Brogan, J. T., Jones, C. K., Conn, P. J., and Lindsley, C. W. 2008. Synthesis and SAR of analogues of the M1 allosteric agonist TBPB. Part I: Exploration of alternative benzyl and privileged structure moieties. *Bioorg Med Chem Lett* 18: 5439–5442.

Brookmeyer, R., Johnson, E., Ziegler-Graham, K., and Arrighi, H. M. 2007. Forecasting the global burden of Alzheimer's disease. *Alzheimers Dement* 3: 186–191.

Brouwers, N., Sleegers, K., and Van Broeckhoven, C. 2008. Molecular genetics of Alzheimer's disease: An update. *Ann Med* 40: 562–583.

Brunden, K. R., Yao, Y., Potuzak, J. S., Ferrer, N. I., Ballatore, C., James, M. J., Hogan, A. M., Trojanowski, J. Q., Smith, A. B., 3rd, and Lee, V. M. 2011. The characterization of microtubule-stabilizing drugs as possible therapeutic agents for Alzheimer's disease and related tauopathies. *Pharmacol Res* 63: 341–351.

Brunden, K. R., Zhang, B., Carroll, J., Yao, Y., Potuzak, J. S., Hogan, A. M., Iba, M., James, M. J., Xie, S. X., Ballatore, C., Smith, A. B., III, Lee, V. M., and Trojanowski, J. Q. 2010. Epothilone D improves microtubule density, axonal integrity, and cognition in a transgenic mouse model of tauopathy. *J Neurosci* 30: 13861–13866.

Bruno, V., Ksiazek, I., Battaglia, G., Lukic, S., Leonhardt, T., Sauer, D., Gasparini, F., Kuhn, R., Nicoletti, F., and Flor, P. J. 2000. Selective blockade of metabotropic glutamate receptor subtype 5 is neuroprotective. *Neuropharmacology* 39: 2223–2230.

Buee, L., Bussiere, T., Buee-Scherrer, V., Delacourte, A., and Hof, P. R. 2000. Tau protein isoforms, phosphorylation and role in neurodegenerative disorders. *Brain Res Brain Res Rev* 33: 95–130.

Buerger, K., Ewers, M., Pirttila, T., Zinkowski, R., Alafuzoff, I., Teipel, S. J., DeBernardis, J., Kerkman, D., McCulloch, C., Soininen, H., and Hampel, H. 2006. CSF phosphorylated tau protein correlates with neocortical neurofibrillary pathology in Alzheimer's disease. *Brain* 129: 3035–3041.

Bulic, B., Pickhardt, M., Schmidt, B., Mandelkow, E. M., Waldmann, H., and Mandelkow, E. 2009. Development of tau aggregation inhibitors for Alzheimer's disease. *Angew Chem Int Ed Engl* 48: 1740–1752.

Buxbaum, J. D., Ruefli, A. A., Parker, C. A., Cypess, A. M., and Greengard, P. 1994. Calcium regulates processing of the Alzheimer amyloid protein precursor in a protein kinase C-independent manner. *Proc Natl Acad Sci USA* 91: 4489–4493.

Caccamo, A., Oddo, S., Billings, L. M., Green, K. N., Martinez-Coria, H., Fisher, A., and LaFerla, F. M. 2006. M1 receptors play a central role in modulating AD-like pathology in transgenic mice. *Neuron* 49: 671–682.

Cai, H., Wang, Y., McCarthy, D., Wen, H., Borchelt, D.R., Price, D. L., and Wong, P. C. 2001. BACE1 is the major beta-secretase for generation of Abeta peptides by neurons. *Nat Neurosci* 4: 233–234.

Caille, I., Allinquant, B., Dupont, E., Bouillot, C., Langer, A., Muller, U., and Prochiantz, A. 2004. Soluble form of amyloid precursor protein regulates proliferation of progenitors in the adult subventricular zone. *Development* 131: 2173–2181.

Calella, A. M., Farinelli, M., Nuvolone, M., Mirante, O., Moos, R., Falsig, J., Mansuy, I. M., and Aguzzi, A. 2010. Prion protein and Abeta-related synaptic toxicity impairment. *EMBO Molecular Medicine* 2: 306–314.

Chang, E., Congdon, E. E., Honson, N. S., Duff, K. E., and Kuret, J. 2009. Structure-activity relationship of cyanine tau aggregation inhibitors. *J Med Chem* 52: 3539–3547.

Chen, E. Y., Mufson, E. J., and Kordower, J. H. 1996. TRK and p75 neurotrophin receptor systems in the developing human brain. *J Comp Neurol* 369: 591–618.

Chen, F., Hasegawa, H., Schmitt-Ulms, G., Kawarai, T., Bohm, C., Katayama, T., Gu, Y., Sanjo, N., Glista, M., Rogaeva, E., Wakutani, Y., Pardossi-Piquard, R., Ruan, X., Tandon, A., Checler, F., Marambaud, P., Hansen, K., Westaway, D., St George-Hyslop, P., and Fraser, P. 2006. TMP21 is a presenilin complex component that modulates gamma-secretase but not epsilon-secretase activity. *Nature* 440: 1208–1212.

Cheung, K. H., Shineman, D., Muller, M., Cardenas, C., Mei, L., Yang, J., Tomita, T., Iwatsubo, T., Lee, V. M., and Foskett, J. K. 2008. Mechanism of Ca2+ disruption in Alzheimer's disease by presenilin regulation of InsP3 receptor channel gating. *Neuron* 58: 871–883.

Clavaguera, F., Bolmont, T., Crowther, R. A., Abramowski, D., Frank, S., Probst, A., Fraser, G., Stalder, A. K., Beibel, M., Staufenbiel, M., Jucker, M., Goedert, M., and Tolnay, M. 2009. Transmission and spreading of tauopathy in transgenic mouse brain. *Nat Cell Biol* 11: 909–913.

Cleveland, D. W., Hwo, S. Y., and Kirschner, M. W. 1977. Purification of tau, a microtubule-associated protein that induces assembly of microtubules from purified tubulin. *J Mol Biol* 116: 207–225.

Colquhoun, A., Lawrance, G. M., Shamovsky, I. L., Riopelle, R. J., and Ross, G. M. 2004. Differential activity of the nerve growth factor (NGF) antagonist PD90780 [7-(benzolylamino)-4,9-dihydro-4-methyl-9-oxo-pyrazolo[5,1-b]quinazoline-2-carboxylic acid] suggests altered NGF-p75NTR interactions in the presence of TrkA. *J Pharmacol Exp Ther* 310: 505–511.

Conn, P. J., Jones, C. K., and Lindsley, C. W. 2009. Subtype-selective allosteric modulators of muscarinic receptors for the treatment of CNS disorders. *Trends Pharmacol Sci* 30: 148–155.

Coon, A. L., Wallace, D. R., Mactutus, C. F., and Booze, R. M. 1999. L-type calcium channels in the hippocampus and cerebellum of Alzheimer's disease brain tissue. *Neurobiol Aging* 20: 597–603.

Corcoran, N. M., Martin, D., Hutter-Paier, B., Windisch, M., Nguyen, T., Nheu, L., Sundstrom, L. E., Costello, A. J., and Hovens, C. M. 2010. Sodium selenate specifically activates PP2A phosphatase, dephosphorylates tau and reverses memory deficits in an Alzheimer's disease model. *J Clin Neurosci* 17: 1025–1033.

Costantini, C., Weindruch, R., Della Valle, G., and Puglielli, L. 2005. A TrkA-to-p75NTR molecular switch activates amyloid beta-peptide generation during aging. *Biochem J* 391: 59–67.

Coulson, E. J. 2006. Does the p75 neurotrophin receptor mediate Abeta-induced toxicity in Alzheimer's disease? *J Neurochem* 98: 654–660.

Counts, S. E., and Mufson, E. J. 2005. The role of nerve growth factor receptors in cholinergic basal forebrain degeneration in prodromal Alzheimer disease. *J Neuropathol Exp Neurol* 64: 263–272.

Counts, S. E., Nadeem, M., Wuu, J., Ginsberg, S. D., Saragovi, H. U., and Mufson, E. J. 2004. Reduction of cortical TrkA but not p75(NTR) protein in early stage Alzheimer's disease. *Ann Neurol* 56: 520–531.

Cruz, J. C., Tseng, H. C., Goldman, J. A., Shih, H., and Tsai, L. H. 2003. Aberrant Cdk5 activation by p25 triggers pathological events leading to neurodegeneration and neurofibrillary tangles. *Neuron* 40: 471–483.

Cuchillo-Ibanez, I., Seereeram, A., Byers, H. L., Leung, K. Y., Ward, M. A., Anderton, B. H., and Hanger, D. P. 2008. Phosphorylation of tau regulates its axonal transport by controlling its binding to kinesin. *Faseb J* 22: 3186–3195.

Daborg, J., von Otter, M., Sjolander, A., Nilsson, S., Minthon, L., Gustafson, D. R., Skoog, I., Blennow, K., and Zetterberg, H. 2010. Association of the RAGE G82S polymorphism with Alzheimer's disease. *J Neural Transm* 117: 861–867.

Dahlgren, K. N., Manelli, A. M., Stine, W. B., Jr., Baker, L. K., Krafft, G. A., and LaDu, M. J. 2002. Oligomeric and fibrillar species of amyloid-beta peptides differentially affect neuronal viability. *J Biol Chem* 277: 32046–32053.

Deane, R., Du Yan, S., Submamaryan, R. K., LaRue, B., Jovanovic, S., Hogg, E., Welch, D., Manness, L., Lin, C., Yu, J., Zhu, H., Ghiso, J., Frangione, B., Stern, A., Schmidt, A. M., Armstrong, D. L., Arnold, B., Liliensiek, B., Nawroth, P., Hofman, F., Kindy, M., Stern, D., and Zlokovic, B. 2003. RAGE mediates amyloid-beta peptide transport across the blood-brain barrier and accumulation in brain. *Nat Med* 9: 907–913.

Dickey, C. A., Eriksen, J., Kamal, A., Burrows, F., Kasibhatla, S., Eckman, C. B., Hutton, M., and Petrucelli, L. 2005. Development of a high throughput drug screening assay for the detection of changes in tau levels—proof of concept with HSP90 inhibitors. *Curr Alzheimer Res* 2: 231–238.

Dickey, C. A., Kamal, A., Lundgren, K., Klosak, N., Bailey, R. M., Dunmore, J., Ash, P., Shoraka, S., Zlatkovic, J., Eckman, C. B., Patterson, C., Dickson, D. W., Nahman, N. S., Jr., Hutton, M., Burrows, F., and Petrucelli, L. 2007. The high-affinity HSP90-CHIP complex recognizes and selectively degrades phosphorylated tau client proteins. *J Clin Invest* 117: 648–658.

Dineley, K. T., Bell, K. A., Bui, D., and Sweatt, J. D. 2002. Beta-amyloid peptide activates alpha 7 nicotinic acetylcholine receptors expressed in Xenopus oocytes. *J Biol Chem* 277: 25056–25061.

Donmez, G., Wang, D., Cohen, D. E., and Guarente, L. 2010. SIRT1 suppresses beta-amyloid production by activating the alpha-secretase gene ADAM10. *Cell* 142: 320–332.

Doody, R. S., Gavrilova, S. I., Sano, M., Thomas, R. G., Aisen, P. S., Bachurin, S. O., Seely, L., and Hung, D. 2008. Effect of dimebon on cognition, activities of daily living, behaviour, and global function in patients with mild-to-moderate Alzheimer's disease: A randomised, double-blind, placebo-controlled study. *Lancet* 372: 207–215.

Dowling, P., Ming, X., Raval, S., Husar, W., Casaccia-Bonnefil, P., Chao, M., Cook, S., and Blumberg, B. 1999. Up-regulated p75NTR neurotrophin receptor on glial cells in MS plaques. *Neurology* 53: 1676–1682.

Du Yan, S., Zhu, H., Fu, J., Yan, S. F., Roher, A., Tourtellotte, W. W., Rajavashisth, T., Chen, X., Godman, G. C., Stern, D., and Schmidt, A. M. 1997. Amyloid-beta peptide-receptor for advanced glycation end-product interaction elicits neuronal expression of macrophage-colony stimulating factor: A proinflammatory pathway in Alzheimer disease. *Proc Natl Acad Sci USA* 94: 5296–5301.

Dubey, M., Chaudhury, P., Kabiru, H., and Shea, T. B. 2008. Tau inhibits anterograde axonal transport and perturbs stability in growing axonal neurites in part by displacing kinesin cargo: Neurofilaments attenuate tau-mediated neurite instability. *Cell Motil Cytoskeleton* 65: 89–99.

Duce, J. A., and Bush, A. I. 2010. Biological metals and Alzheimer's disease: implications for therapeutics and diagnostics. *Prog Neurobiol* 92: 1–18.

Duce, J. A., Tsatsanis, A., Cater, M. A., James, S. A., Robb, E., Wikhe, K., Leong, S. L., Perez, K., Johanssen, T., Greenough, M. A., Cho, H. H., Galatis, D., Moir, R. D., Masters, C. L., McLean, C., Tanzi, R. E., Cappai, R., Barnham, K. J., Ciccotosto, G. D., Rogers, J. T., and Bush, A. I. 2010. Iron-export ferroxidase activity of beta-amyloid precursor protein is inhibited by zinc in Alzheimer's disease. *Cell* 142: 857–867.

Duff, K., Kuret, J., and Congdon, E. E. 2010. Disaggregation of tau as a therapeutic approach to tauopathies. *Curr Alzheimer Res* 7: 235–240.

Eckert, G. P., Cairns, N. J., Maras, A., Gattaz, W. F., and Muller, W. E. 2000. Cholesterol modulates the membrane-disordering effects of beta-amyloid peptides in the hippocampus: Specific changes in Alzheimer's disease. *Dement Geriatr Cogn Disord* 11: 181–186.

Edbauer, D., Winkler, E., Regula, J. T., Pesold, B., Steiner, H., and Haass, C. 2003. Reconstitution of gamma-secretase activity. *Nat Cell Biol* 5: 486–488.

Eikelenboom, P., van Exel, E., Hoozemans, J. J., Veerhuis, R., Rozemuller, A. J., and van Gool, W. A. 2010. Neuroinflammation—an early event in both the history and pathogenesis of Alzheimer's disease. *Neurodegener Dis* 7: 38–41.

El Khoury, J. 2010. Neurodegeneration and the neuroimmune system. *Nat Med* 16: 1369–1370.

El Khoury, J. B., Moore, K. J., Means, T. K., Leung, J., Terada, K., Toft, M., Freeman, M. W., and Luster, A. D. 2003. CD36 mediates the innate host response to beta-amyloid. *J Exp Med* 197: 1657–1666.

Elmslie, K. S. 2004. Calcium channel blockers in the treatment of disease. *J Neurosci Res* 75: 733–741.

Engel, T., Hernandez, F., Avila, J., and Lucas, J. J. 2006. Full reversal of Alzheimer's disease-like phenotype in a mouse model with conditional overexpression of glycogen synthase kinase-3. *J Neurosci* 26: 5083–5090.

Fagan, A. M., Garber, M., Barbacid, M., Silos-Santiago, I., and Holtzman, D. M. 1997. A role for TrkA during maturation of striatal and basal forebrain cholinergic neurons in vivo. *J Neurosci* 17: 7644–7654.

Fahnestock, M., Michalski, B., Xu, B., and Coughlin, M. D. 2001. The precursor pro-nerve growth factor is the predominant form of nerve growth factor in brain and is increased in Alzheimer's disease. *Mol Cell Neurosci* 18: 210–220.

Fassbender, K., Masters, C., and Beyreuther, K. 2001. Alzheimer's disease: Molecular concepts and therapeutic targets. *Naturwissenschaften* 88: 261–267.

Fath, T., Eidenmuller, J., and Brandt, R. 2002. Tau-mediated cytotoxicity in a pseudohyperphosphorylation model of Alzheimer's disease. *J Neurosci* 22: 9733–9741.

Faux, N. G., Ritchie, C. W., Gunn, A., Rembach, A., Tsatsanis, A., Bedo, J., Harrison, J., Lannfelt, L., Blennow, K., Zetterberg, H., Ingelsson, M., Masters, C. L., Tanzi, R. E., Cummings, J. L., Herd, C. M., and Bush, A. I. 2010. PBT2 rapidly improves cognition in Alzheimer's Disease: additional phase II analyses. *J Alzheimers Dis* 20: 509–516.

Fisher, A. 2008. M1 muscarinic agonists target major hallmarks of Alzheimer's disease—the pivotal role of brain M1 receptors. *Neurodegener Dis* 5: 237–240.

Frost, B., Jacks, R. L., and Diamond, M. I. 2009. Propagation of tau misfolding from the outside to the inside of a cell. *J Biol Chem* 284: 12845–12852.

Gao, J., Wang, W. Y., Mao, Y. W., Graff, J., Guan, J. S., Pan, L., Mak, G., Kim, D., Su, S. C., and Tsai, L. H. 2010. A novel pathway regulates memory and plasticity via SIRT1 and miR-134. *Nature* 466: 1105–1109.

Gasparini, F., Bilbe, G., Gomez-Mancilla, B., and Spooren, W. 2008. mGluR5 antagonists: discovery, characterization and drug development. *Curr Opin Drug Discov Devel* 11: 655–665.

Ghosh, A. K., Gemma, S., and Tang, J. 2008. Beta-Secretase as a therapeutic target for Alzheimer's disease. *Neurotherapeutics* 5: 399–408.

Ginsberg, S. D., Che, S., Wuu, J., Counts, S. E., and Mufson, E. J. 2006. Down regulation of trk but not p75NTR gene expression in single cholinergic basal forebrain neurons mark the progression of Alzheimer's disease. *J Neurochem* 97: 475–487.

Glass, C. K., Saijo, K., Winner, B., Marchetto, M. C., and Gage, F. H. 2010. Mechanisms underlying inflammation in neurodegeneration. *Cell* 140: 918–934.

Glenner, G. G., and Wong, C. W. 1984. Alzheimer's disease: Initial report of the purification and characterization of a novel cerebrovascular amyloid protein. *Biochem Biophys Res Commun* 120: 885–890.

Goedert, M., and Jakes, R. 2005. Mutations causing neurodegenerative tauopathies. *Biochim Biophys Acta* 1739: 240–250.

Goedert, M., Spillantini, M. G., Jakes, R., Rutherford, D., and Crowther, R. A. 1989. Multiple isoforms of human microtubule-associated protein tau: Sequences and localization in neurofibrillary tangles of Alzheimer's disease. *Neuron* 3: 519–526.

Gong, C. X., Liu, F., Grundke-Iqbal, I., and Iqbal, K. 2005. Post-translational modifications of tau protein in Alzheimer's disease. *J Neural Transm* 112: 813–838.

Goodman, Y., and Mattson, M. P. 1994. Secreted forms of beta-amyloid precursor protein protect hippocampal neurons against amyloid beta-peptide-induced oxidative injury. *Exp Neurol* 128: 1–12.

Gotz, J., Chen, F., van Dorpe, J., and Nitsch, R. M. 2001. Formation of neurofibrillary tangles in P3011 tau transgenic mice induced by Abeta 42 fibrils. *Science* 293: 1491–1495.

Gozes, I., Stewart, A., Morimoto, B., Fox, A., Sutherland, K., and Schmeche, D. 2009. Addressing Alzheimer's disease tangles: From NAP to AL-108. *Curr Alzheimer Res* 6: 455–460.

Grigorev, V. V., Dranyi, O. A., and Bachurin, S. O. 2003. Comparative study of action mechanisms of dimebon and memantine on AMPA- and NMDA-subtypes glutamate receptors in rat cerebral neurons. *Bull Exp Biol Med* 136: 474–477.

Grober, E., Dickson, D., Sliwinski, M. J., Buschke, H., Katz, M., Crystal, H., and Lipton, R. B. 1999. Memory and mental status correlates of modified Braak staging. *Neurobiol Aging* 20: 573–579.

Haase, C., Stieler, J. T., Arendt, T., and Holzer, M. 2004. Pseudophosphorylation of tau protein alters its ability for self-aggregation. *J Neurochem* 88: 1509–1520.

Haass, C. 2010. Initiation and propagation of neurodegeneration. *Nat Med* 16: 1201–1204.

Haass, C., and Selkoe, D. J. 2007. Soluble protein oligomers in neurodegeneration: Lessons from the Alzheimer's amyloid beta-peptide. *Nat Rev Mol Cell Biol* 8: 101–112.

Hanger, D. P., Hughes, K., Woodgett, J. R., Brion, J. P., and Anderton, B. H. 1992. Glycogen synthase kinase-3 induces Alzheimer's disease-like phosphorylation of tau: Generation of paired helical filament epitopes and neuronal localisation of the kinase. *Neurosci Lett* 147: 58–62.

Hardy, J., and Selkoe, D. J. 2002. The amyloid hypothesis of Alzheimer's disease: Progress and problems on the road to therapeutics. *Science* 297: 353–356.

Hardy, J. A., and Higgins, G. A. 1992. Alzheimer's disease: The amyloid cascade hypothesis. *Science* 256: 184–185.

Harkany, T., Abraham, I., Konya, C., Nyakas, C., Zarandi, M., Penke, B., and Luiten, P. G. 2000. Mechanisms of beta-amyloid neurotoxicity: perspectives of pharmacotherapy. *Rev Neurosci* 11: 329–382.

Hart, G. W., Housley, M. P., and Slawson, C. 2007. Cycling of O-linked beta-N-acetylglucosamine on nucleocytoplasmic proteins. *Nature* 446: 1017–1022.

Hartley, D. M., Walsh, D. M., Ye, C. P., Diehl, T., Vasquez, S., Vassilev, P. M., Teplow, D. B., and Selkoe, D. J. 1999. Protofibrillar intermediates of amyloid beta-protein induce acute electrophysiological changes and progressive neurotoxicity in cortical neurons. *J Neurosci* 19: 8876–8884.

He, G., Luo, W., Li, P., Remmers, C., Netzer, W. J., Hendrick, J., Bettayeb, K., Flajolet, M., Gorelick, F., Wennogle, L. P., and Greengard, P. 2010. Gamma-secretase activating protein is a therapeutic target for Alzheimer's disease. *Nature* 467: 95–98.

He, H. J., Wang, X. S., Pan, R., Wang, D. L., Liu, M. N., and He, R. Q. 2009. The proline-rich domain of tau plays a role in interactions with actin. *BMC Cell Biol* 10: 81.

Hefti, F., and Mash, D. C. 1989. Localization of nerve growth factor receptors in the normal human brain and in Alzheimer's disease. *Neurobiol Aging* 10: 75–87.

Hemming, M. L., Elias, J. E., Gygi, S. P., and Selkoe, D. J. 2008. Proteomic profiling of gamma-secretase substrates and mapping of substrate requirements. *PLoS Biol* 6: e257, doi:10.1371/journal.pbio.0060257.

Hensley, K. 2010. Neuroinflammation in Alzheimer's disease: Mechanisms, pathologic consequences, and potential for therapeutic manipulation. *J Alzheimers Dis* 21: 1–14.

Hernandez, C. M., Kayed, R., Zheng, H., Sweatt, J. D., and Dineley, K. T. 2010. Loss of alpha7 nicotinic receptors enhances beta-amyloid oligomer accumulation, exacerbating early-stage cognitive decline and septohippocampal pathology in a mouse model of Alzheimer's disease. *J Neurosci* 30: 2442–2453.

Herreman, A., Serneels, L., Annaert, W., Collen, D., Schoonjans, L., and De Strooper, B. 2000. Total inactivation of gamma-secretase activity in presenilin-deficient embryonic stem cells. *Nat Cell Biol* 2: 461–462.

Hock, C., Maddalena, A., Raschig, A., Muller-Spahn, F., Eschweiler, G., Hager, K., Heuser, I., Hampel, H., Muller-Thomsen, T., Oertel, W., Wienrich, M., Signorell, A., Gonzalez-Agosti, C., and Nitsch, R. M. 2003. Treatment with the selective muscarinic m1 agonist talsaclidine decreases cerebrospinal fluid levels of A beta 42 in patients with Alzheimer's disease. *Amyloid* 10: 1–6.

Hong, L., Koelsch, G., Lin, X., Wu, S., Terzyan, S., Ghosh, A. K., Zhang, X. C., and Tang, J. 2000. Structure of the protease domain of memapsin 2 (beta-secretase) complexed with inhibitor. *Science* 290: 150–153.

Hong, L., Turner, R. T., 3rd, Koelsch, G., Shin, D., Ghosh, A. K., and Tang, J. 2002. Crystal structure of memapsin 2 (beta-secretase) in complex with an inhibitor OM00-3. *Biochemistry* 41: 10963–10967.

Hong, M., Chen, D. C., Klein, P. S., and Lee, V. M. 1997. Lithium reduces tau phosphorylation by inhibition of glycogen synthase kinase-3. *J Biol Chem* 272: 25326–25332.

Hoover, B. R., Reed, M. N., Su, J., Penrod, R. D., Kotilinek, L. A., Grant, M. K., Pitstick, R., Carlson, G. A., Lanier, L. M., Yuan, L. L., Ashe, K. H., and Liao, D. 2010. Tau mislocalization to dendritic spines mediates synaptic dysfunction independently of neurodegeneration. *Neuron* 68: 1067–1081.

Hsieh, H., Boehm, J., Sato, C., Iwatsubo, T., Tomita, T., Sisodia, S., and Malinow, R. 2006. AMPAR removal underlies Abeta-induced synaptic depression and dendritic spine loss. *Neuron* 52: 831–843.

Hu, X., Hicks, C. W., He, W., Wong, P., Macklin, W. B., Trapp, B. D., and Yan, R. 2006. BACE1 modulates myelination in the central and peripheral nervous system. *Nat Neurosci* 9: 1520–1525.

Hu, X., Zhou, X., He, W., Yang, J., Xiong, W., Wong, P., Wilson, C. G., and Yan, R. 2010. BACE1 deficiency causes altered neuronal activity and neurodegeneration. *J Neurosci* 30: 8819–8829.

Hu, X. Y., Zhang, H. Y., Qin, S., Xu, H., Swaab, D. F., and Zhou, J. N. 2002. Increased p75(NTR) expression in hippocampal neurons containing hyperphosphorylated tau in Alzheimer patients. *Exp Neurol* 178: 104–111.

Hu, Y., Wang, Z., Zhang, R., Wu, P., Xia, Z., Orsi, A., and Rees, D. 2008. Regulation of M1-receptor mRNA stability by smilagenin and its significance in improving memory of aged rats. *Neurobiol Aging* 31: 1010–1019.

Hu, Y., Xia, Z., Sun, Q., Orsi, A., and Rees, D. 2005. A new approach to the pharmacological regulation of memory: Sarsasapogenin improves memory by elevating the low muscarinic acetylcholine receptor density in brains of memory-deficit rat models. *Brain Res* 1060: 26–39.

Hyman, B. T., and Trojanowski, J. Q. 1997. Consensus recommendations for the postmortem diagnosis of Alzheimer disease from the National Institute on Aging and the Reagan Institute Working Group on diagnostic criteria for the neuropathological assessment of Alzheimer disease. *J Neuropathol Exp Neurol* 56: 1095–1097.

Ikeda, K., Urakami, K., Arai, H., Wada, K., Wakutani, Y., Ji, Y., Adachi, Y., Okada, A., Kowa, H., Sasaki, H., Ohno, K., Ohtsuka, Y., Ishikawa, Y., and Nakashima, K. 2000. The expression of presenilin 1 mRNA in skin fibroblasts and brains from sporadic Alzheimer's disease. *Dement Geriatr Cogn Disord* 11: 245–250.

Imbimbo, B. P. 2008. Therapeutic potential of gamma-secretase inhibitors and modulators. *Curr Top Med Chem* 8: 54–61.

Ittner, L. M., Ke, Y. D., Delerue, F., Bi, M., Gladbach, A., van Eersel, J., Wolfing, H., Chieng, B. C., Christie, M. J., Napier, I. A., Eckert, A., Staufenbiel, M., Hardeman, E., and Gotz, J. 2010. Dendritic function of tau mediates amyloid-beta toxicity in Alzheimer's disease mouse models. *Cell* 142: 387–397.

Jaen, J. C., Laborde, E., Bucsh, R. A., Caprathe, B. W., Sorenson, R. J., Fergus, J., Spiegel, K., Marks, J., Dickerson, M. R., and Davis, R. E. 1995. Kynurenic acid derivatives inhibit the binding of nerve growth factor (NGF) to the low-affinity p75 NGF receptor. *J Med Chem* 38: 4439–4445.

Jang, S. W., Liu, X., Chan, C. B., France, S. A., Sayeed, I., Tang, W., Lin, X., Xiao, G., Andero, R., Chang, Q., Ressler, K. J., and Ye, K. 2010a. Deoxygedunin, a natural product with potent neurotrophic activity in mice. *PLoS One* 5: e11528, doi:10.1371/journal.pone.0011528.

Jang, S. W., Liu, X., Chan, C. B., Weinshenker, D., Hall, R. A., Xiao, G., and Ye, K. 2009. Amitriptyline is a TrkA and TrkB receptor agonist that promotes TrkA/TrkB heterodimerization and has potent neurotrophic activity. *Chem Biol* 16: 644–656.

Jang, S. W., Liu, X., Yepes, M., Shepherd, K. R., Miller, G. W., Liu, Y., Wilson, W. D., Xiao, G., Blanchi, B., Sun, Y. E., and Ye, K. 2010b. A selective TrkB agonist with potent neurotrophic activities by 7,8-dihydroxyflavone. *Proc Natl Acad Sci USA* 107: 2687–2692.

Jang, S. W., Okada, M., Sayeed, I., Xiao, G., Stein, D., Jin, P., and Ye, K. 2007. Gambogic amide, a selective agonist for TrkA receptor that possesses robust neurotrophic activity, prevents neuronal cell death. *Proc Natl Acad Sci USA* 104: 16329–16334.

Jones, C. K., Brady, A. E., Davis, A. A., Xiang, Z., Bubser, M., Tantawy, M. N., Kane, A. S., Bridges, T. M., Kennedy, J. P., Bradley, S. R., Peterson, T. E., Ansari, M. S., Baldwin, R. M., Kessler, R. M., Deutch, A. Y., Lah, J. J., Levey, A. I., Lindsley, C. W., and Conn, P. J. 2008. Novel selective allosteric activator of the M1 muscarinic acetylcholine receptor regulates amyloid processing and produces antipsychotic-like activity in rats. *J Neurosci* 28: 10422–10433.

Jorissen, E., and De Strooper, B. 2010. Gamma-secretase and the intramembrane proteolysis of Notch. *Curr Top Dev Biol* 92: 201–230.

Kadir, A., Marutle, A., Gonzalez, D., Scholl, M., Almkvist, O., Mousavi, M., Mustafiz, T., Darreh-Shori, T., Nennesmo, I., and Nordberg, A. 2011. Positron emission tomography imaging and clinical progression in relation to molecular pathology in the first Pittsburgh Compound B positron emission tomography patient with Alzheimer's disease. *Brain* 134: 301–317.

Kagan, B. L., Hirakura, Y., Azimov, R., Azimova, R., and Lin, M. C. 2002. The channel hypothesis of Alzheimer's disease: Current status. *Peptides* 23: 1311–1315.

Kang, D. E., Soriano, S., Xia, X., Eberhart, C. G., De Strooper, B., Zheng, H., and Koo, E. H. 2002. Presenilin couples the paired phosphorylation of beta-catenin independent of axin: Implications for beta-catenin activation in tumorigenesis. *Cell* 110: 751–762.

Kayed, R., Head, E., Thompson, J. L., McIntire, T. M., Milton, S. C., Cotman, C. W., and Glabe, C. G. 2003. Common structure of soluble amyloid oligomers implies common mechanism of pathogenesis. *Science* 300: 486–489.

Kessels, H. W., Nguyen, L. N., Nabavi, S., and Malinow, R. 2010. The prion protein as a receptor for amyloid-beta. *Nature* 466: E3–4; discussion E4–5.

Kim, D., Nguyen, M. D., Dobbin, M. M., Fischer, A., Sananbenesi, F., Rodgers, J. T., Delalle, I., Baur, J. A., Sui, G., Armour, S. M., Puigserver, P., Sinclair, D. A., and Tsai, L. H. 2007. SIRT1 deacetylase protects against neurodegeneration in models for Alzheimer's disease and amyotrophic lateral sclerosis. *EMBO J* 26: 3169–3179.

Kimberly, W. T., LaVoie, M. J., Ostaszewski, B. L., Ye, W., Wolfe, M. S., and Selkoe, D. J. 2003. Gamma-secretase is a membrane protein complex comprised of presenilin, nicastrin, Aph-1, and Pen-2. *Proc Natl Acad Sci USA* 100: 6382–6387.

Kimura, H., Yukitake, H., Tajima, Y., Suzuki, H., Chikatsu, T., Morimoto, S., Funabashi, Y., Omae, H., Ito, T., Yoneda, Y., and Takizawa, M. 2010. ITZ-1, a client-selective Hsp90 inhibitor, efficiently induces heat shock factor 1 activation. *Chem Biol* 17: 18–27.

Kitazawa, M., Oddo, S., Yamasaki, T. R., Green, K. N., and LaFerla, F. M. 2005. Lipopolysaccharide-induced inflammation exacerbates tau pathology by a cyclin-dependent kinase 5-mediated pathway in a transgenic model of Alzheimer's disease. *J Neurosci* 25: 8843–8853.

Klein, W. L. 2002. Abeta toxicity in Alzheimer's disease: Globular oligomers (ADDLs) as new vaccine and drug targets. *Neurochem Int* 41: 345–352.

Knoth, R., Singec, I., Ditter, M., Pantazis, G., Capetian, P., Meyer, R. P., Horvat, V., Volk, B., and Kempermann, G. 2010. Murine features of neurogenesis in the human hippocampus across the lifespan from 0 to 100 years. *PLoS One* 5: e8809, doi:10.1371/journal.pone.0008809.

Knowles, J. K., Rajadas, J., Nguyen, T. V., Yang, T., LeMieux, M. C., Vander Griend, L., Ishikawa, C., Massa, S. M., Wyss-Coray, T., and Longo, F. M. 2009. The p75 neurotrophin receptor promotes amyloid-beta(1-42)-induced neuritic dystrophy in vitro and in vivo. *J Neurosci* 29: 10627–10637.

Kochegarov, A. A. 2003. Pharmacological modulators of voltage-gated calcium channels and their therapeutical application. *Cell Calcium* 33: 145–162.

Kordower, J. H., Gash, D. M., Bothwell, M., Hersh, L., and Mufson, E. J. 1989. Nerve growth factor receptor and choline acetyltransferase remain colocalized in the nucleus basalis (Ch4) of Alzheimer's patients. *Neurobiol Aging* 10: 67–74.

Kordower, J. H., Winn, S. R., Liu, Y. T., Mufson, E. J., Sladek, J. R., Jr., Hammang, J. P., Baetge, E. E., and Emerich, D. F. 1994. The aged monkey basal forebrain: rescue and sprouting of axotomized basal forebrain neurons after grafts of encapsulated cells secreting human nerve growth factor. *Proc Natl Acad Sci USA* 91: 10898–10902.

Kounnas, M. Z., Danks, A. M., Cheng, S., Tyree, C., Ackerman, E., Zhang, X., Ahn, K., Nguyen, P., Comer, D., Mao, L., Yu, C., Pleynet, D., Digregorio, P. J., Velicelebi, G., Stauderman, K. A., Comer, W. T., Mobley, W. C., Li, Y. M., Sisodia, S. S., Tanzi, R. E., and Wagner, S. L. 2010. Modulation of gamma-secretase reduces beta-amyloid deposition in a transgenic mouse model of Alzheimer's disease. *Neuron* 67: 769–780.

Kourie, J. I., Henry, C. L., and Farrelly, P. 2001. Diversity of amyloid beta protein fragment [1-40]-formed channels. *Cell Mol Neurobiol* 21: 255–284.

Kremer, J. J., Pallitto, M. M., Sklansky, D. J., and Murphy, R. M. 2000. Correlation of beta-amyloid aggregate size and hydrophobicity with decreased bilayer fluidity of model membranes. *Biochemistry* 39: 10309–10318.

Kukar, T. L., Ladd, T. B., Bann, M. A., Fraering, P. C., Narlawar, R., Maharvi, G. M., Healy, B., Chapman, R., Welzel, A. T., Price, R. W., Moore, B., Rangachari, V., Cusack, B., Eriksen, J., Jansen-West, K., Verbeeck, C., Yager, D., Eckman, C., Ye, W., Sagi, S., Cottrell, B. A., Torpey, J., Rosenberry, T. L., Fauq, A., Wolfe, M. S., Schmidt, B., Walsh, D. M., Koo, E. H., and Golde, T. E. 2008. Substrate-targeting gamma-secretase modulators. *Nature* 453: 925–929.

Kuner, P., Schubenel, R., and Hertel, C. 1998. Beta-amyloid binds to p57NTR and activates NFkappaB in human neuroblastoma cells. *J Neurosci Res* 54: 798–804.

Laird, F. M., Cai, H., Savonenko, A. V., Farah, M. H., He, K., Melnikova, T., Wen, H., Chiang, H. C., Xu, G., Koliatsos, V. E., Borchelt, D. R., Price, D. L., Lee, H. K., and Wong, P. C. 2005. BACE1, a major determinant of selective vulnerability of the brain to amyloid-beta amyloidogenesis, is essential for cognitive, emotional, and synaptic functions. *J Neurosci* 25: 11693–11709.

Lambert, M. P., Barlow, A. K., Chromy, B. A., Edwards, C., Freed, R., Liosatos, M., Morgan, T. E., Rozovsky, I., Trommer, B., Viola, K. L., Wals, P., Zhang, C., Finch, C. E., Krafft, G. A., and Klein, W. L. 1998. Diffusible, nonfibrillar ligands derived from Abeta1-42 are potent central nervous system neurotoxins. *Proc Natl Acad Sci USA* 95: 6448–6453.

Langmead, C. J., Austin, N. E., Branch, C. L., Brown, J. T., Buchanan, K. A., Davies, C. H., Forbes, I. T., Fry, V. A., Hagan, J .J., Herdon, H. J., Jones, G. A., Jeggo, R., Kew, J. N., Mazzali, A., Melarange, R., Patel, N., Pardoe, J., Randall, A. D., Roberts, C., Roopun, A., Starr, K. R., Teriakidis, A., Wood, M. D., Whittington, M., Wu, Z., and Watson, J. 2008. Characterization of a CNS penetrant, selective M1 muscarinic receptor agonist, 77-LH-28-1. *Br J Pharmacol* 154: 1104–1115.

Lanz, T. A., Hosley, J. D., Adams, W. J., and Merchant, K. M. 2004. Studies of Abeta pharmacodynamics in the brain, cerebrospinal fluid, and plasma in young (plaque-free) Tg2576 mice using the gamma-secretase inhibitor N2-[(2S)-2-(3,5-difluorophenyl)-2-hydroxyethanoyl]-N1-[(7S)-5-methyl-6-oxo-6,7-dihydro-5H-dibenzo[b,d]azepin-7-yl]-L-alaninamide (LY-411575). *J Pharmacol Exp Ther* 309: 49–55.

Lanz, T. A., Karmilowicz, M. J., Wood, K. M., Pozdnyakov, N., Du, P., Piotrowski, M. A., Brown, T. M., Nolan, C. E., Richter, K. E., Finley, J. E., Fei, Q., Ebbinghaus, C. F., Chen, Y. L., Spracklin, D. K., Tate, B., Geoghegan, K. F., Lau, L. F., Auperin, D. D., and Schachter, J. B. 2006. Concentration-dependent modulation of amyloid-beta in vivo and in vitro using the gamma-secretase inhibitor, LY-450139. *J Pharmacol Exp Ther* 319: 924–933.

Larbig, G., Pickhardt, M., Lloyd, D. G., Schmidt, B., and Mandelkow, E. 2007. Screening for inhibitors of tau protein aggregation into Alzheimer paired helical filaments: A ligand based approach results in successful scaffold hopping. *Curr Alzheimer Res* 4: 315–323.

Lasagna-Reeves, C. A., Castillo-Carranza, D. L., Guerrero-Muoz, M. J., Jackson, G. R., and Kayed, R. 2010. Preparation and characterization of neurotoxic tau oligomers. *Biochemistry* 49: 10039–10041.

Lauren, J., Gimbel, D. A., Nygaard, H. B., Gilbert, J. W., and Strittmatter, S. M. 2009. Cellular prion protein mediates impairment of synaptic plasticity by amyloid-beta oligomers. *Nature* 457: 1128–1132.

Lebon, G., Langmead, C. J., Tehan, B. G., and Hulme, E. C. 2009. Mutagenic mapping suggests a novel binding mode for selective agonists of M1 muscarinic acetylcholine receptors. *Mol Pharmacol* 75: 331–341.

Lee, B. H., Lee, M. J., Park, S., Oh, D. C., Elsasser, S., Chen, P. C., Gartner, C., Dimova, N., Hanna, J., Gygi, S. P., Wilson, S. M., King, R. W., and Finley, D. 2010. Enhancement of proteasome activity by a small-molecule inhibitor of USP14. *Nature* 467: 179–184.

Lee, D. H., and Wang, H. Y. 2003. Differential physiologic responses of alpha7 nicotinic acetylcholine receptors to beta-amyloid1-40 and beta-amyloid1-42. *J Neurobiol* 55: 25–30.

Lee, G., Newman, S. T., Gard, D. L., Band, H., and Panchamoorthy, G. 1998. Tau interacts with src-family non-receptor tyrosine kinases. *J Cell Sci* 111 (Pt 21): 3167–3177.

Lermontova, N. N., Redkozubov, A. E., Shevtsova, E. F., Serkova, T. P., Kireeva, E. G., and Bachurin, S. O. 2001. Dimebon and tacrine inhibit neurotoxic action of beta-amyloid in culture and block L-type Ca(2+) channels. *Bull Exp Biol Med* 132: 1079–1083.

LeSauteur, L., Maliartchouk, S., Le Jeune, H., Quirion, R., and Saragovi, H. U. 1996. Potent human p140-TrkA agonists derived from an anti-receptor monoclonal antibody. *J Neurosci* 16: 1308–1316.

Lesne, S., Koh, M. T., Kotilinek, L., Kayed, R., Glabe, C. G., Yang, A., Gallagher, M., and Ashe, K. H. 2006. A specific amyloid-beta protein assembly in the brain impairs memory. *Nature* 440: 352–357.

Li, K., Dai, D., Zhao, B., Yao, L., Yao, S., Wang, B., and Yang, Z. 2010. Association between the RAGE G82S polymorphism and Alzheimer's disease. *J Neural Transm* 117: 97–104.

Li, M., Guo, H., and Damuni, Z. 1995. Purification and characterization of two potent heat-stable protein inhibitors of protein phosphatase 2A from bovine kidney. *Biochemistry* 34: 1988–1996.

Li, M., Makkinje, A., and Damuni, Z. 1996. Molecular identification of I1PP2A, a novel potent heat-stable inhibitor protein of protein phosphatase 2A. *Biochemistry* 35: 6998–7002.

Li, R., Lindholm, K., Yang, L. B., Yue, X., Citron, M., Yan, R., Beach, T., Sue, L., Sabbagh, M., Cai, H., Wong, P., Price, D., and Shen, Y. 2004. Amyloid beta peptide load is correlated with increased beta-secretase activity in sporadic Alzheimer's disease patients. *Proc Natl Acad Sci USA* 101: 3632–3637.

Lin, X., Koelsch, G., Wu, S., Downs, D., Dashti, A., and Tang, J. 2000. Human aspartic protease memapsin 2 cleaves the beta-secretase site of beta-amyloid precursor protein. *Proc Natl Acad Sci USA* 97: 1456–1460.

Li, X. D., and Buccafusco, J. J. 2003. Effect of beta-amyloid peptide 1-42 on the cytoprotective action mediated by alpha7 nicotinic acetylcholine receptors in growth factor-deprived differentiated PC-12 cells. *J Pharmacol Exp Ther* 307: 670–675.

Lindsley, C. W., and Emmitte, K. A. 2009. Recent progress in the discovery and development of negative allosteric modulators of mGluR5. *Curr Opin Drug Discov Devel* 12: 446–457.

Lindwall, G., and Cole, R. D. 1984. Phosphorylation affects the ability of tau protein to promote microtubule assembly. *J Biol Chem* 259: 5301–5305.

Liu, F., Iqbal, K., Grundke-Iqbal, I., Hart, G. W., and Gong, C. X. 2004. O-GlcNAcylation regulates phosphorylation of tau: A mechanism involved in Alzheimer's disease. *Proc Natl Acad Sci USA* 101: 10804–10809.

Liu, Q., Kawai, H., and Berg, D. K. 2001. Beta-amyloid peptide blocks the response of alpha 7-containing nicotinic receptors on hippocampal neurons. *Proc Natl Acad Sci USA* 98: 4734–4739.

Liu, X., Chan, C. B., Jang, S. W., Pradoldej, S., Huang, J., He, K., Phun, L. H., France, S., Xiao, G., Jia, Y., Luo, H. R., and Ye, K. 2010. A synthetic 7,8-dihydroxyflavone derivative promotes neurogenesis and exhibits potent antidepressant effect. *J Med Chem* [Epub ahead of print].

Liu, Y., Dargusch, R., and Schubert, D. 1997. Beta amyloid toxicity does not require RAGE protein. *Biochem Biophys Res Commun* 237: 37–40.

Lopez-Arrieta, J. M., and Birks, J. 2002. Nimodipine for primary degenerative, mixed and vascular dementia. *Cochrane Database Syst Rev*, article no. CD000147, doi: 10.1002/14651858.CD000147.

Lowry, K. S., Murray, S. S., McLean, C. A., Talman, P., Mathers, S., Lopes, E. C., and Cheema, S. S. 2001. A potential role for the p75 low-affinity neurotrophin receptor in spinal motor neuron degeneration in murine and human amyotrophic lateral sclerosis. *Amyotroph Lateral Scler Other Motor Neuron Disord* 2: 127–134.

Lue, L. F., Walker, D. G., Brachova, L., Beach, T. G., Rogers, J., Schmidt, A. M., Stern, D. M., and Yan, S. D. 2001. Involvement of microglial receptor for advanced glycation end products (RAGE) in Alzheimer's disease: Identification of a cellular activation mechanism. *Exp Neurol* 171: 29–45.

Luo, W., Dou, F., Rodina, A., Chip, S., Kim, J., Zhao, Q., Moulick, K., Aguirre, J., Wu, N., Greengard, P., and Chiosis, G. 2007. Roles of heat-shock protein 90 in maintaining and facilitating the neurodegenerative phenotype in tauopathies. *Proc Natl Acad Sci USA* 104: 9511–9516.

Luo, Y., Bolon, B., Damore, M. A., Fitzpatrick, D., Liu, H., Zhang, J., Yan, Q., Vassar, R., and Citron, M. 2003. BACE1 (beta-secretase) knockout mice do not acquire compensatory gene expression changes or develop neural lesions over time. *Neurobiol Dis* 14: 81–88.

Luo, Y., Bolon, B., Kahn, S., Bennett, B. D., Babu-Khan, S., Denis, P., Fan, W., Kha, H., Zhang, J., Gong, Y., Martin, L., Louis, J.C., Yan, Q., Richards, W. G., Citron, M., and Vassar, R. 2001. Mice deficient in BACE1, the Alzheimer's beta-secretase, have normal phenotype and abolished beta-amyloid generation. *Nat Neurosci* 4: 231–232.

Ma, L., Seager, M. A., Wittmann, M., Jacobson, M., Bickel, D., Burno, M., Jones, K., Graufelds, V. K., Xu, G., Pearson, M., McCampbell, A., Gaspar, R., Shughrue, P., Danziger, A., Regan, C., Flick, R., Pascarella, D., Garson, S., Doran, S., Kreatsoulas, C., Veng, L.,

Lindsley, C. W., Shipe, W., Kuduk, S., Sur, C., Kinney, G., Seabrook, G. R., and Ray, W. J. 2009. Selective activation of the M1 muscarinic acetylcholine receptor achieved by allosteric potentiation. *Proc Natl Acad Sci USA* 106: 15950–15955.

Macdonald, A., Briggs, K., Poppe, M., Higgins, A., Velayudhan, L., and Lovestone, S. 2008. A feasibility and tolerability study of lithium in Alzheimer's disease. *Int J Geriatr Psychiatry* 23: 704–711.

Maeda, S., Sahara, N., Saito, Y., Murayama, S., Ikai, A., and Takashima, A. 2006. Increased levels of granular tau oligomers: An early sign of brain aging and Alzheimer's disease. *Neurosci Res* 54: 197–201.

Maillard, I., Adler, S. H., and Pear, W. S. 2003. Notch and the immune system. *Immunity* 19: 781–791.

Maliartchouk, S., Feng, Y., Ivanisevic, L., Debeir, T., Cuello, A. C., Burgess, K., and Saragovi, H. U. 2000. A designed peptidomimetic agonistic ligand of TrkA nerve growth factor receptors. *Mol Pharmacol* 57: 385–391.

Malouitre, S., Dube, H., Selwood, D., and Crompton, M. 2009. Mitochondrial targeting of cyclosporin A enables selective inhibition of cyclophilin-D and enhanced cytoprotection after glucose and oxygen deprivation. *Biochem J* 425: 137–148.

Mandelkow, E. M., Drewes, G., Biernat, J., Gustke, N., Van Lint, J., Vandenheede, J. R., and Mandelkow, E. 1992. Glycogen synthase kinase-3 and the Alzheimer-like state of microtubule-associated protein tau. *FEBS Lett* 314: 315–321.

Marlo, J. E., Niswender, C. M., Days, E. L., Bridges, T. M., Xiang, Y., Rodriguez, A. L., Shirey, J. K., Brady, A. E., Nalywajko, T., Luo, Q., Austin, C. A., Williams, M. B., Kim, K., Williams, R., Orton, D., Brown, H. A., Lindsley, C. W., Weaver, C. D., and Conn, P. J. 2009. Discovery and characterization of novel allosteric potentiators of M1 muscarinic receptors reveals multiple modes of activity. *Mol Pharmacol* 75: 577–588.

Martinez, A., Alonso, M., Castro, A., Dorronsoro, I., Gelpi, J. L., Luque, F. J., Perez, C., and Moreno, F. J. 2005. SAR and 3D-QSAR studies on thiadiazolidinone derivatives: Exploration of structural requirements for glycogen synthase kinase 3 inhibitors. *J Med Chem* 48: 7103–7112.

Mason, R. P., Jacob, R. F., Walter, M. F., Mason, P. E., Avdulov, N. A., Chochina, S. V., Igbavboa, U., and Wood, W. G. 1999. Distribution and fluidizing action of soluble and aggregated amyloid beta-peptide in rat synaptic plasma membranes. *J Biol Chem* 274: 18801–18807.

Massa, S. M., Xie, Y., Yang, T., Harrington, A. W., Kim, M. L., Yoon, S. O., Kraemer, R., Moore, L. A., Hempstead, B. L., and Longo, F. M. 2006. Small, nonpeptide p75NTR ligands induce survival signaling and inhibit proNGF-induced death. *J Neurosci* 26: 5288–5300.

Massa, S. M., Yang, T., Xie, Y., Shi, J., Bilgen, M., Joyce, J. N., Nehama, D., Rajadas, J., and Longo, F. M. 2010. Small molecule BDNF mimetics activate TrkB signaling and prevent neuronal degeneration in rodents. *J Clin Invest* 120: 1774–1785.

Medina, M., and Castro, A. 2008. Glycogen synthase kinase-3 (GSK-3) inhibitors reach the clinic. 2008. *Curr Opin Drug Discov Devel* 11: 533–543.

Michikawa, M., Gong, J. S., Fan, Q. W., Sawamura, N., and Yanagisawa, K. 2001. A novel action of alzheimer's amyloid beta-protein (Abeta): Oligomeric Abeta promotes lipid release. *J Neurosci* 21: 7226–7235.

Milano, J., McKay, J., Dagenais, C., Foster-Brown, L., Pognan, F., Gadient, R., Jacobs, R. T., Zacco, A., Greenberg, B., and Ciaccio, P. J. 2004. Modulation of notch processing by gamma-secretase inhibitors causes intestinal goblet cell metaplasia and induction of genes known to specify gut secretory lineage differentiation. *Toxicol Sci* 82: 341–358.

Millay, D. P., Sargent, M. A., Osinska, H., Baines, C. P., Barton, E. R., Vuagniaux, G., Sweeney, H. L., Robbins, J., and Molkentin, J. D. 2008. Genetic and pharmacologic inhibition of mitochondrial-dependent necrosis attenuates muscular dystrophy. *Nat Med* 14: 442–447.

Mimuro, M., Yoshida, M., Miyao, S., Harada, T., Ishiguro, K., and Hashizume, Y. 2010. Neuronal and glial tau pathology in early frontotemporal lobar degeneration-tau, Pick's disease subtype. *J Neurol Sci* 290: 177–182.

Min, S. W., Cho, S. H., Zhou, Y., Schroeder, S., Haroutunian, V., Seeley, W. W., Huang, E. J., Shen, Y., Masliah, E., Mukherjee, C., Meyers, D., Cole, P. A., Ott, M., and Gan, L. 2010. Acetylation of tau inhibits its degradation and contributes to tauopathy. *Neuron* 67: 953–966.

Mocanu, M. M., Nissen, A., Eckermann, K., Khlistunova, I., Biernat, J., Drexler, D., Petrova, O., Schonig, K., Bujard, H., Mandelkow, E., Zhou, L., Rune, G., and Mandelkow, E. M. 2008. The potential for beta-structure in the repeat domain of tau protein determines aggregation, synaptic decay, neuronal loss, and coassembly with endogenous tau in inducible mouse models of tauopathy. *J Neurosci* 28: 737–748.

Mohajeri, M. H., Saini, K. D., and Nitsch, R. M. 2004. Transgenic BACE expression in mouse neurons accelerates amyloid plaque pathology. *J Neural Transm* 111: 413–425.

Morishima-Kawashima, M., Hasegawa, M., Takio, K., Suzuki, M., Yoshida, H., Watanabe, A., Titani, K., and Ihara, Y. 1995. Hyperphosphorylation of tau in PHF. *Neurobiol Aging* 16: 365–371; discussion 371–380.

Muehlhauser, F., Liebl, U., Kuehl, S., Walter, S., Bertsch, T., and Fassbender, K. 2001. Aggregation-dependent interaction of the Alzheimer's beta-amyloid and microglia. *Clin Chem Lab Med* 39: 313–316.

Mufson, E. J., Bothwell, M., Hersh, L. B., and Kordower, J. H. 1989a. Nerve growth factor receptor immunoreactive profiles in the normal, aged human basal forebrain: Colocalization with cholinergic neurons. *J Comp Neurol* 285: 196–217.

Mufson, E. J., Bothwell, M., and Kordower, J. H. 1989b. Loss of nerve growth factor receptor-containing neurons in Alzheimer's disease: A quantitative analysis across subregions of the basal forebrain. *Exp Neurol* 105: 221–232.

Nagahara, A. H., Merrill, D. A., Coppola, G., Tsukada, S., Schroeder, B. E., Shaked, G. M., Wang, L., Blesch, A., Kim, A., Conner, J. M., Rockenstein, E., Chao, M. V., Koo, E. H., Geschwind, D., Masliah, E., Chiba, A. A., and Tuszynski, M. H. 2009. Neuroprotective effects of brain-derived neurotrophic factor in rodent and primate models of Alzheimer's disease. *Nat Med* 15: 331–337.

Nagele, R. G., D'Andrea, M. R., Anderson, W. J., and Wang, H. Y. 2002. Intracellular accumulation of beta-amyloid(1-42) in neurons is facilitated by the alpha 7 nicotinic acetylcholine receptor in Alzheimer's disease. *Neuroscience* 110: 199–211.

Naumann, T., Casademunt, E., Hollerbach, E., Hofmann, J., Dechant, G., Frotscher, M., and Barde, Y. A. 2002. Complete deletion of the neurotrophin receptor p75NTR leads to long-lasting increases in the number of basal forebrain cholinergic neurons. *J Neurosci* 22: 2409–2418.

Neve, R. L., Harris, P., Kosik, K. S., Kurnit, D. M., and Donlon, T. A. 1986. Identification of cDNA clones for the human microtubule-associated protein tau and chromosomal localization of the genes for tau and microtubule-associated protein 2. *Brain Res* 387: 271–280.

Niederhauser, O., Mangold, M., Schubenel, R., Kusznir, E. A., Schmidt, D., and Hertel, C. 2000. NGF ligand alters NGF signaling via p75(NTR) and trkA. *J Neurosci Res* 61: 263–272.

Nishitomi, K., Sakaguchi, G., Horikoshi, Y., Gray, A. J., Maeda, M., Hirata-Fukae, C., Becker, A. G., Hosono, M., Sakaguchi, I., Minami, S. S., Nakajima, Y., Li, H. F., Takeyama, C., Kihara, T., Ota, A., Wong, P. C., Aisen, P. S., Kato, A., Kinoshita, N., and Matsuoka, Y. 2006. BACE1 inhibition reduces endogenous Abeta and alters APP processing in wild-type mice. *J Neurochem* 99: 1555–1563.

Noble, W., Olm, V., Takata, K., Casey, E., Mary, O., Meyerson, J., Gaynor, K., LaFrancois, J., Wang, L., Kondo, T., Davies, P., Burns, M., Veeranna, Nixon, R., Dickson, D., Matsuoka, Y., Ahlijanian, M., Lau, L. F., and Duff, K. 2003. Cdk5 is a key factor in tau aggregation and tangle formation in vivo. *Neuron* 38: 555–565.

Ohsawa, I., Takamura, C., Morimoto, T., Ishiguro, M., and Kohsaka, S. 1999. Amino-terminal region of secreted form of amyloid precursor protein stimulates proliferation of neural stem cells. *Eur J Neurosci* 11: 1907–1913.

Oz, M., Lorke, D. E., Hasan, M., and Petroianu, G. A. 2011. Cellular and molecular actions of methylene blue in the nervous system. *Med Res Rev* 31: 93–117.

Ozmen, L., Woolley, M., Albientz, A., Miss, M. T., Nelboeck, P., Malherbe, P., Czech, C., Gruninger-Leitch, F., Brockhaus, M., Ballard, T., and Jacobsen, H. 2005. BACE/APPV717F double-transgenic mice develop cerebral amyloidosis and inflammation. *Neurodegener Dis* 2: 284–298.

Pacholec, M., Bleasdale, J. E., Chrunyk, B., Cunningham, D., Flynn, D., Garofalo, R. S., Griffith, D., Griffor, M., Loulakis, P., Pabst, B., Qiu, X., Stockman, B., Thanabal, V., Varghese, A., Ward, J., Withka, J., and Ahn, K. 2010. SRT1720, SRT2183, SRT1460, and resveratrol are not direct activators of SIRT1. *J Biol Chem* 285: 8340–8351.

Panda, D., Samuel, J.C., Massie, M., Feinstein, S. C., and Wilson, L. 2003. Differential regulation of microtubule dynamics by three- and four-repeat tau: implications for the onset of neurodegenerative disease. *Proc Natl Acad Sci USA* 100: 9548–9553.

Patrick, G. N., Zukerberg, L., Nikolic, M., de la Monte, S., Dikkes, P., and Tsai, L. H. 1999. Conversion of p35 to p25 deregulates Cdk5 activity and promotes neurodegeneration. *Nature* 402: 615–622.

Pedraza, C. E., Podlesniy, P., Vidal, N., Arevalo, J. C., Lee, R., Hempstead, B., Ferrer, I., Iglesias, M., and Espinet, C. 2005. Pro-NGF isolated from the human brain affected by Alzheimer's disease induces neuronal apoptosis mediated by p75NTR. *Am J Pathol* 166: 533–543.

Pei, J. J., Grundke-Iqbal, I., Iqbal, K., Bogdanovic, N., Winblad, B., and Cowburn, R. F. 1998. Accumulation of cyclin-dependent kinase 5 (cdk5) in neurons with early stages of Alzheimer's disease neurofibrillary degeneration. *Brain Res* 797: 267–277.

Pei, J. J., Tanaka, T., Tung, Y. C., Braak, E., Iqbal, K., and Grundke-Iqbal, I. 1997. Distribution, levels, and activity of glycogen synthase kinase-3 in the Alzheimer disease brain. *J Neuropathol Exp Neurol* 56: 70–78.

Petty, B. G., Cornblath, D. R., Adornato, B. T., Chaudhry, V., Flexner, C., Wachsman, M., Sinicropi, D., Burton, L. E., and Peroutka, S. J. 1994. The effect of systemically administered recombinant human nerve growth factor in healthy human subjects. *Ann Neurol* 36: 244–246.

Phiel, C. J., Wilson, C. A., Lee, V. M., and Klein, P. S. 2003. GSK-3alpha regulates production of Alzheimer's disease amyloid-beta peptides. *Nature* 423: 435–439.

Piedrahita, D., Hernandez, I., Lopez-Tobon, A., Fedorov, D., Obara, B., Manjunath, B. S., Boudreau, R. L., Davidson, B., Laferla, F., Gallego-Gomez, J. C., Kosik, K. S., and Cardona-Gomez, G. P. 2010. Silencing of CDK5 reduces neurofibrillary tangles in transgenic alzheimer's mice. *J Neurosci* 30: 13966–13976.

Pieper, A. A., Xie, S., Capota, E., Estill, S. J., Zhong, J., Long, J. M., Becker, G. L., Huntington, P., Goldman, S. E., Shen, C. H., Capota, M., Britt, J. K., Kotti, T., Ure, K., Brat, D. J., Williams, N. S., MacMillan, K. S., Naidoo, J., Melito, L., Hsieh, J., De Brabander, J., Ready, J. M., and McKnight, S. L. 2010. Discovery of a proneurogenic, neuroprotective chemical. *Cell* 142: 39–51.

Plattner, F., Angelo, M., and Giese, K. P. 2006. The roles of cyclin-dependent kinase 5 and glycogen synthase kinase 3 in tau hyperphosphorylation. *J Biol Chem* 281: 25457–25465.

Podlesniy, P., Kichev, A., Pedraza, C., Saurat, J., Encinas, M., Perez, B., Ferrer, I., and Espinet, C. 2006. Pro-NGF from Alzheimer's disease and normal human brain displays distinctive abilities to induce processing and nuclear translocation of intracellular domain of p75NTR and apoptosis. *Am J Pathol* 169: 119–131.

Podlisny, M. B., Walsh, D. M., Amarante, P., Ostaszewski, B. L., Stimson, E. R., Maggio, J. E., Teplow, D. B., and Selkoe, D. J. 1998. Oligomerization of endogenous and synthetic amyloid beta-protein at nanomolar levels in cell culture and stabilization of monomer by Congo red. *Biochemistry* 37: 3602–3611.

Preuss, U., Biernat, J., Mandelkow, E. M., and Mandelkow, E. 1997. The "jaws" model of tau-microtubule interaction examined in CHO cells. *J Cell Sci* 110 (Pt 6): 789–800.

Rapoport, M., Dawson, H. N., Binder, L. I., Vitek, M. P., and Ferreira, A. 2002. Tau is essential to beta-amyloid-induced neurotoxicity. *Proc Natl Acad Sci USA* 99: 6364–6369.

Ravikumar, B., Berger, Z., Vacher, C., O'Kane, C. J., and Rubinsztein, D. C. 2006. Rapamycin pre-treatment protects against apoptosis. *Hum Mol Genet* 15: 1209–1216.

Ravikumar, B., Vacher, C., Berger, Z., Davies, J. E., Luo, S., Oroz, L. G., Scaravilli, F., Easton, D. F., Duden, R., O'Kane, C. J., and Rubinsztein, D. C. 2004. Inhibition of mTOR induces autophagy and reduces toxicity of polyglutamine expansions in fly and mouse models of Huntington disease. *Nat Genet* 36: 585–595.

Rayasam, G. V., Tulasi, V. K., Sodhi, R., Davis, J. A., and Ray, A. 2009. Glycogen synthase kinase 3: More than a namesake. *Br J Pharmacol* 156: 885–898.

Renner, M., Lacor, P. N., Velasco, P. T., Xu, J., Contractor, A., Klein, W. L., and Triller, A. 2010. Deleterious effects of amyloid beta oligomers acting as an extracellular scaffold for mGluR5. *Neuron* 66: 739–754.

Roberds, S. L., Anderson, J., Basi, G., Bienkowski, M. J., Branstetter, D. G., Chen, K. S., Freedman, S. B., Frigon, N. L., Games, D., Hu, K., Johnson-Wood, K., Kappenman, K. E., Kawabe, T. T., Kola, I., Kuehn, R., Lee, M., Liu, W., Motter, R., Nichols, N. F., Power, M., Robertson, D. W., Schenk, D., Schoor, M., Shopp, G. M., Shuck, M. E., Sinha, S., Svensson, K. A., Tatsuno, G., Tintrup, H., Wijsman, J., Wright, S., and McConlogue, L. 2001. BACE knockout mice are healthy despite lacking the primary beta-secretase activity in brain: Implications for Alzheimer's disease therapeutics. *Hum Mol Genet* 10: 1317–1324.

Roberson, E. D., Scearce-Levie, K., Palop, J. J., Yan, F., Cheng, I. H., Wu, T., Gerstein, H., Yu, G. Q., and Mucke, L. 2007. Reducing endogenous tau ameliorates amyloid beta-induced deficits in an Alzheimer's disease mouse model. *Science* 316: 750–754.

Rochette, M. J., and Murphy, M. P. 2002. Gamma-secretase: Substrates and inhibitors. *Mol Neurobiol* 26: 81–95.

Ryder, J., Su, Y., Liu, F., Li, B., Zhou, Y., and Ni, B. 2003. Divergent roles of GSK3 and CDK5 in APP processing. *Biochem Biophys Res Commun* 312: 922–929.

Sarkar, S., Floto, R. A., Berger, Z., Imarisio, S., Cordenier, A., Pasco, M., Cook, L. J., and Rubinsztein, D. C. 2005. Lithium induces autophagy by inhibiting inositol monophosphatase. *J Cell Biol* 170: 1101–1111.

Sarkar, S., and Rubinsztein, D. C. 2006. Inositol and IP3 levels regulate autophagy: Biology and therapeutic speculations. *Autophagy* 2: 132–134.

Sarkar, S., and Rubinsztein, D. C. 2008. Small molecule enhancers of autophagy for neurodegenerative diseases. *Mol Biosyst* 4: 895–901.

Sasaki, N., Toki, S., Chowei, H., Saito, T., Nakano, N., Hayashi, Y., Takeuchi, M., and Makita, Z. 2001. Immunohistochemical distribution of the receptor for advanced glycation end products in neurons and astrocytes in Alzheimer's disease. *Brain Res* 888: 256–262.

Saura, C. A., Choi, S. Y., Beglopoulos, V., Malkani, S., Zhang, D., Shankaranarayana Rao, B. S., Chattarji, S., Kelleher, R. J., 3rd, Kandel, E. R., Duff, K., Kirkwood, A., and Shen, J. 2004. Loss of presenilin function causes impairments of memory and synaptic plasticity followed by age-dependent neurodegeneration. *Neuron* 42: 23–36.

Schild, A., Ittner, L. M., and Gotz, J. 2006. Altered phosphorylation of cytoskeletal proteins in mutant protein phosphatase 2A transgenic mice. *Biochem Biophys Res Commun* 343: 1171–1178.

Seeburger, J. L., Tarras, S., Natter, H., and Springer, J. E. 1993. Spinal cord motoneurons express p75NGFR and p145trkB mRNA in amyotrophic lateral sclerosis. *Brain Res* 621: 111–115.

Selkoe, D. J. 2001. Alzheimer's disease: Genes, proteins, and therapy. *Physiol Rev* 81: 741–766.

Selkoe, D. J. 2002. Alzheimer's disease is a synaptic failure. *Science* 298: 789–791.

Selkoe, D. J. 2008. Soluble oligomers of the amyloid beta-protein impair synaptic plasticity and behavior. *Behav Brain Res* 192: 106–113.

Sinha, S., Anderson, J. P., Barbour, R., Basi, G. S., Caccavello, R., Davis, D., Doan, M., Dovey, H. F., Frigon, N., Hong, J., Jacobson-Croak, K., Jewett, N., Keim, P., Knops, J., Lieberburg, I., Power, M., Tan, H., Tatsuno, G., Tung, J., Schenk, D., Seubert, P., Suomensaari, S. M., Wang, S., Walker, D., Zhao, J., McConlogue, L., and John, V. 1999. Purification and cloning of amyloid precursor protein beta-secretase from human brain. *Nature* 402: 537–540.

Siwak-Tapp, C. T., Head, E., Muggenburg, B. A., Milgram, N. W., and Cotman, C. W. 2007. Neurogenesis decreases with age in the canine hippocampus and correlates with cognitive function. *Neurobiol Learn Mem* 88: 249–259.

Slutsky, I., Abumaria, N., Wu, L. J., Huang, C., Zhang, L., Li, B., Zhao, X., Govindarajan, A., Zhao, M. G., Zhuo, M., Tonegawa, S., and Liu, G. 2010. Enhancement of learning and memory by elevating brain magnesium. *Neuron* 65: 165–177.

Smith, M. J., Sharples, R. A., Evin, G., McLean, C. A., Dean, B., Pavey, G., Fantino, E., Cotton, R. G., Imaizumi, K., Masters, C. L., Cappai, R., and Culvenor, J. G. 2004. Expression of truncated presenilin 2 splice variant in Alzheimer's disease, bipolar disorder, and schizophrenia brain cortex. *Brain Res Mol Brain Res* 127: 128–135.

Sontag, E., Luangpirom, A., Hladik, C., Mudrak, I., Ogris, E., Speciale, S., and White, C. L., III. 2004. Altered expression levels of the protein phosphatase 2A ABalphaC enzyme are associated with Alzheimer disease pathology. *J Neuropathol Exp Neurol* 63: 287–301.

Sontag, E., Nunbhakdi-Craig, V., Lee, G., Bloom, G. S., and Mumby, M. C. 1996. Regulation of the phosphorylation state and microtubule-binding activity of tau by protein phosphatase 2A. *Neuron* 17: 1201–1207.

Sotthibundhu, A., Sykes, A. M., Fox, B., Underwood, C. K., Thangnipon, W., and Coulson, E. J. 2008. Beta-amyloid(1-42) induces neuronal death through the p75 neurotrophin receptor. *J Neurosci* 28: 3941–3946.

Spooren, W. P., Gasparini, F., Bergmann, R., and Kuhn, R. 2000. Effects of the prototypical mGlu(5) receptor antagonist 2-methyl-6-(phenylethynyl)-pyridine on rotarod, locomotor activity and rotational responses in unilateral 6-OHDA-lesioned rats. *Eur J Pharmacol* 406: 403–410.

Stanger, B. Z., Datar, R., Murtaugh, L. C., and Melton, D. A. 2005. Direct regulation of intestinal fate by Notch. *Proc Natl Acad Sci USA* 102: 12443–12448.

Stoothoff, W., Jones, P. B., Spires-Jones, T. L., Joyner, D., Chhabra, E., Bercury, K., Fan, Z., Xie, H., Bacskai, B., Edd, J., Irimia, D., and Hyman, B. T. 2009. Differential effect of three-repeat and four-repeat tau on mitochondrial axonal transport. *J Neurochem* 111: 417–427.

Supnet, C., and Bezprozvanny, I. 2010a. The dysregulation of intracellular calcium in Alzheimer disease. *Cell Calcium* 47: 183–189.

Supnet, C., and Bezprozvanny, I. 2010b. Neuronal calcium signaling, mitochondrial dysfunction, and Alzheimer's disease. *J Alzheimers Dis* 20 Suppl 2: S487–498.

Supnet, C., Noonan, C., Richard, K., Bradley, J., and Mayne, M. 2010. Up-regulation of the type 3 ryanodine receptor is neuroprotective in the TgCRND8 mouse model of Alzheimer's disease. *J Neurochem* 112: 356–365.

Takasugi, N., Tomita, T., Hayashi, I., Tsuruoka, M., Niimura, M., Takahashi, Y., Thinakaran, G., and Iwatsubo, T. 2003. The role of presenilin cofactors in the gamma-secretase complex. *Nature* 422: 438–441.

Tanimukai, H., Grundke-Iqbal, I., and Iqbal, K. 2005. Up-regulation of inhibitors of protein phosphatase-2A in Alzheimer's disease. *Am J Pathol* 166: 1761–1771.

Tapiola, T., Overmyer, M., Lehtovirta, M., Helisalmi, S., Ramberg, J., Alafuzoff, I., Riekkinen, P., Sr., and Soininen, H. 1997. The level of cerebrospinal fluid tau correlates with neurofibrillary tangles in Alzheimer's disease. *Neuroreport* 8: 3961–3963.

Thathiah, A., and De Strooper, B. 2009. G protein-coupled receptors, cholinergic dysfunction, and Abeta toxicity in Alzheimer's disease. *Sci Signal* 2: re8.

Thathiah, A., Spittaels, K., Hoffmann, M., Staes, M., Cohen, A., Horre, K., Vanbrabant, M., Coun, F., Baekelandt, V., Delacourte, A., Fischer, D. F., Pollet, D., De Strooper, B., and Merchiers, P. 2009. The orphan G protein-coupled receptor 3 modulates amyloid-beta peptide generation in neurons. *Science* 323: 946–951.

Thies, E., and Mandelkow, E. M. 2007. Missorting of tau in neurons causes degeneration of synapses that can be rescued by the kinase MARK2/Par-1. *J Neurosci* 27: 2896–2907.

Thomas, R. L., Mistry, R., Langmead, C. J., Wood, M. D., and Challiss, R. A. 2008. G protein coupling and signaling pathway activation by m1 muscarinic acetylcholine receptor orthosteric and allosteric agonists. *J Pharmacol Exp Ther* 327: 365–374.

Tomita, T. 2009. Secretase inhibitors and modulators for Alzheimer's disease treatment. *Expert Rev Neurother* 9: 661–679.

Tran, M. H., Yamada, K., and Nabeshima, T. 2002. Amyloid beta-peptide induces cholinergic dysfunction and cognitive deficits: a minireview. *Peptides* 23: 1271–1283.

Tsukamoto, E., Hashimoto, Y., Kanekura, K., Niikura, T., Aiso, S., and Nishimoto, I. 2003. Characterization of the toxic mechanism triggered by Alzheimer's amyloid-beta peptides via p75 neurotrophin receptor in neuronal hybrid cells. *J Neurosci Res* 73: 627–636.

Turner, B. J., Murray, S. S., Piccenna, L. G., Lopes, E. C., Kilpatrick, T. J., and Cheema, S. S. 2004. Effect of p75 neurotrophin receptor antagonist on disease progression in transgenic amyotrophic lateral sclerosis mice. *J Neurosci Res* 78: 193–199.

Tuszynski, M. H., Thal, L., Pay, M., Salmon, D. P., Hoi, S. U., Bakay, R., Patel, P., Blesch, A., Vahlsing, H. L., Ho, G., Tong, G., Potkin, S. G., Fallon, J., Hansen, L., Mufson, E. J., Kordower, J. H., Gall, C., and Conner, J. 2005. A phase 1 clinical trial of nerve growth factor gene therapy for Alzheimer disease. *Nat Med* 11: 551–555.

Ueno, M., Nakagawa, T., Wu, B., Onodera, M., Huang, C. L., Kusaka, T., Araki, N., and Sakamoto, H. 2010. Transporters in the brain endothelial barrier. *Curr Med Chem* 17: 1125–1138.

Varney, M. A., Cosford, N. D., Jachec, C., Rao, S. P., Sacaan, A., Lin, F. F., Bleicher, L., Santori, E. M., Flor, P. J., Allgeier, H., Gasparini, F., Kuhn, R., Hess, S. D., Velicelebi, G., and Johnson, E. C. 1999. SIB-1757 and SIB-1893: Selective, noncompetitive antagonists of metabotropic glutamate receptor type 5. *J Pharmacol Exp Ther* 290: 170–181.

Vassar, R., Bennett, B. D., Babu-Khan, S., Kahn, S., Mendiaz, E. A., Denis, P., Teplow, D. B., Ross, S., Amarante, P., Loeloff, R., Luo, Y., Fisher, S., Fuller, J., Edenson, S., Lile, J., Jarosinski, M. A., Biere, A. L., Curran, E., Burgess, T., Louis, J. C., Collins, F., Treanor, J., Rogers, G., and Citron, M. 1999. Beta-secretase cleavage of Alzheimer's amyloid precursor protein by the transmembrane aspartic protease BACE. *Science* 286: 735–741.

Verdier, Y., Zarandi, M., and Penke, B. 2004. Amyloid beta-peptide interactions with neuronal and glial cell plasma membrane: Binding sites and implications for Alzheimer's disease. *J Pept Sci* 10: 229–248.

Virshup, D. M., and Shenolikar, S. 2009. From promiscuity to precision: Protein phosphatases get a makeover. *Mol Cell* 33: 537–545.

von Bergen, M., Friedhoff, P., Biernat, J., Heberle, J., Mandelkow, E. M., and Mandelkow, E. 2000. Assembly of tau protein into Alzheimer paired helical filaments depends on a local sequence motif ((306)VQIVYK(311)) forming beta structure. *Proc Natl Acad Sci USA* 97: 5129–5134.

Walsh, D. M., Klyubin, I., Fadeeva, J. V., Cullen, W. K., Anwyl, R., Wolfe, M. S., Rowan, M. J., and Selkoe, D. J. 2002. Naturally secreted oligomers of amyloid beta protein potently inhibit hippocampal long-term potentiation in vivo. *Nature* 416: 535–539.

Wang, H., Song, L., Laird, F., Wong, P. C., and Lee, H. K. 2008. BACE1 knock-outs display deficits in activity-dependent potentiation of synaptic transmission at mossy fiber to CA3 synapses in the hippocampus. *J Neurosci* 28: 8677–8681.

Wang, H. Y., Lee, D. H., D'Andrea, M. R., Peterson, P. A., Shank, R. P., and Reitz, A. B. 2000a. Beta-amyloid(1-42) binds to alpha7 nicotinic acetylcholine receptor with high affinity: Implications for Alzheimer's disease pathology. *J Biol Chem* 275: 5626–5632.

Wang, H. Y., Lee, D. H., Davis, C. B., and Shank, R. P. 2000b. Amyloid peptide Abeta(1-42) binds selectively and with picomolar affinity to alpha7 nicotinic acetylcholine receptors. *J Neurochem* 75: 1155–1161.

Wang, H. Y., Li, W., Benedetti, N. J., and Lee, D. H. 2003. Alpha 7 nicotinic acetylcholine receptors mediate beta-amyloid peptide-induced tau protein phosphorylation. *J Biol Chem* 278: 31547–31553.

Wang, J. M., Singh, C., Liu, L., Irwin, R. W., Chen, S., Chung, E. J., Thompson, R. F., and Brinton, R. D. 2010. Allopregnanolone reverses neurogenic and cognitive deficits in mouse model of Alzheimer's disease. *Proc Natl Acad Sci USA* 107: 6498–6503.

Wang, X., Blanchard, J., Kohlbrenner, E., Clement, N., Linden, R. M., Radu, A., Grundke-Iqbal, I., and Iqbal, K. 2010. The carboxy-terminal fragment of inhibitor-2 of protein phosphatase-2A induces Alzheimer disease pathology and cognitive impairment. *Faseb J* 24: 4420–4432.

Weggen, S., Eriksen, J. L., Das, P., Sagi, S. A., Wang, R., Pietrzik, C. U., Findlay, K. A., Smith, T. E., Murphy, M. P., Bulter, T., Kang, D. E., Marquez-Sterling, N., Golde, T. E., and Koo, E. H. 2001. A subset of NSAIDs lower amyloidogenic Abeta42 independently of cyclooxygenase activity. *Nature* 414: 212–216.

Weingarten, M. D., Lockwood, A. H., Hwo, S. Y., and Kirschner, M. W. 1975. A protein factor essential for microtubule assembly. *Proc Natl Acad Sci USA* 72: 1858–1862.

Willem, M., Dewachter, I., Smyth, N., Van Dooren, T., Borghgraef, P., Haass, C., and Van Leuven, F. 2004. Beta-site amyloid precursor protein cleaving enzyme 1 increases amyloid deposition in brain parenchyma but reduces cerebrovascular amyloid angiopathy in aging BACE x APP[V717I] double-transgenic mice. *Am J Pathol* 165: 1621–1631.

Wischik, C. M., Edwards, P. C., Lai, R. Y., Roth, M., and Harrington, C. R. 1996. Selective inhibition of Alzheimer disease-like tau aggregation by phenothiazines. *Proc Natl Acad Sci USA* 93: 11213–11218.

Wolfe, M. S. 2008. Gamma-secretase: Structure, function, and modulation for Alzheimer's disease. *Curr Top Med Chem* 8: 2–8.

Xia, X., Qian, S., Soriano, S., Wu, Y., Fletcher, A. M., Wang, X. J., Koo, E. H., Wu, X., and Zheng, H. 2001. Loss of presenilin 1 is associated with enhanced beta-catenin signaling and skin tumorigenesis. *Proc Natl Acad Sci USA* 98: 10863–10868.

Yaar, M., Zhai, S., Fine, R. E., Eisenhauer, P. B., Arble, B. L., Stewart, K. B., and Gilchrest, B. A. 2002. Amyloid beta binds trimers as well as monomers of the 75-kDa neurotrophin receptor and activates receptor signaling. *J Biol Chem* 277: 7720–7725.

Yaar, M., Zhai, S., Panova, I., Fine, R. E., Eisenhauer, P. B., Blusztajn, J. K., Lopez-Coviella, I., and Gilchrest, B. A. 2007. A cyclic peptide that binds p75(NTR) protects neurones from beta amyloid (1-40)-induced cell death. *Neuropathol Appl Neurobiol* 33: 533–543.

Yaar, M., Zhai, S., Pilch, P. F., Doyle, S. M., Eisenhauer, P. B., Fine, R. E., and Gilchrest, B. A. 1997. Binding of beta-amyloid to the p75 neurotrophin receptor induces apoptosis: A possible mechanism for Alzheimer's disease. *J Clin Invest* 100: 2333–2340.

Yan, R., Bienkowski, M. J., Shuck, M. E., Miao, H., Tory, M. C., Pauley, A. M., Brashier, J. R., Stratman, N. C., Mathews, W. R., Buhl, A. E., Carter, D. B., Tomasselli, A. G., Parodi, L. A., Heinrikson, R. L., and Gurney, M. E. 1999. Membrane-anchored aspartyl protease with Alzheimer's disease beta-secretase activity. *Nature* 402: 533–537.

Yan, S. D., Chen, X., Fu, J., Chen, M., Zhu, H., Roher, A., Slattery, T., Zhao, L., Nagashima, M., Morser, J., Migheli, A., Nawroth, P., Stern, D., and Schmidt, A. M. 1996. RAGE and amyloid-beta peptide neurotoxicity in Alzheimer's disease. *Nature* 382: 685–691.

Yang, T., Knowles, J. K., Lu, Q., Zhang, H., Arancio, O., Moore, L. A., Chang, T., Wang, Q., Andreasson, K., Rajadas, J., Fuller, G. G., Xie, Y., Massa, S. M., and Longo, F. M. 2008. Small molecule, non-peptide p75 ligands inhibit Abeta-induced neurodegeneration and synaptic impairment. *PLoS One* 3: e3604, doi:10.1371/journal.pone.0003604.

Yuzwa, S. A., Macauley, M. S., Heinonen, J. E., Shan, X., Dennis, R. J., He, Y., Whitworth, G. E., Stubbs, K. A., McEachern, E. J., Davies, G. J., and Vocadlo, D. J. 2008. A potent mechanism-inspired O-GlcNAcase inhibitor that blocks phosphorylation of tau in vivo. *Nat Chem Biol* 4: 483–490.

Zhang, Y., Hong, Y., Bounhar, Y., Blacker, M., Roucou, X., Tounekti, O., Vereker, E., Bowers, W. J., Federoff, H. J., Goodyer, C. G., and LeBlanc, A. 2003. p75 neurotrophin receptor protects primary cultures of human neurons against extracellular amyloid beta peptide cytotoxicity. *J Neurosci* 23: 7385–7394.

Zhao, J., Fu, Y., Yasvoina, M., Shao, P., Hitt, B., O'Connor, T., Logan, S., Maus, E., Citron, M., Berry, R., Binder, L., and Vassar, R. 2007. Beta-site amyloid precursor protein cleaving enzyme 1 levels become elevated in neurons around amyloid plaques: Implications for Alzheimer's disease pathogenesis. *J Neurosci* 27: 3639–3649.

Zhou, S., Zhou, H., Walian, P. J., and Jap, B. K. 2005. CD147 is a regulatory subunit of the gamma-secretase complex in Alzheimer's disease amyloid beta-peptide production. *Proc Natl Acad Sci USA* 102: 7499–7504.

Zhu, H., Young, M. B., Nantermet, P. G., Graham, S. L., Colussi, D., Lai, M. T., Pietrak, B., Price, E. A., Sankaranarayanan, S., Shi, X. P., Tugusheva, K., Holahan, M. A., Michener, M. S., Cook, J. J., Simon, A., Hazuda, D. J., Vacca, J. P., and Rajapakse, H. A. 2010. Rapid P1 SAR of brain penetrant tertiary carbinamine derived BACE inhibitors. *Bioorg Med Chem Lett* 20: 1779–1782.

6 Alzheimer's Disease: Clinical Aspects

R. Scott Turner

CONTENTS

6.1 CASE REPORT

A 75-year-old well-appearing widowed woman presents to a Memory Disorders Clinic. She is well-kempt and accompanied by her daughter and son-in-law, who report a 1–2 year history of gradual memory decline with insidious onset. The daughter has more recent concerns regarding her mother's handling of her own financial and medical affairs and these led to a concern regarding her mother's ability to continue driving and living independently. The daughter reports that her mother is repeating questions and forgetting conversations and appointments. These concerns prompted the clinic evaluation today. The patient denies any medical problems, and reports no difficulties in handling her own affairs; she wishes to continue driving and living in her home of many years, and agreed reluctantly to neurologic evaluation. This is the first time in her life she has consulted with a neurologist. She reports that she does forget at times, but this is "normal for her age," and "all my friends have the same problem—senior moments."

The social history is significant for a formal education of 14 years and employment as an administrator until voluntary retirement 12 years ago. There is a history of hypertension and hypercholesterolemia, requiring two prescription medications daily. More recently, depression was suspected, but unchanged by a 2-month treatment trial with a prescription antidepressant. There is no history of prior depression, anxiety, seizures, syncope, traumatic brain injury with loss of consciousness, stroke or transient ischemic attack, falls, incontinence, thyroid disorder, vitamin B12 deficiency, alcoholism, syphilis, HIV, or a family history of dementia, Parkinson's disease or Alzheimer's disease (AD), or other psychiatric or neurologic illness. She reports some recent weight loss ("a few pounds") but not enough to raise concern, and she remains slightly above ideal body weight. There is a recent history of decreased social activities and engagements, especially those requiring driving, and some loss of interest in maintaining her usual hobbies and interests. Sleep is more fragmented in recent years but there are no sleep complaints. She denies recent hospitalization or emergency room visits. There is no history of paranoid delusions (stealing or hiding things, or money, for example). She denies visual hallucinations, and the family denies significant fluctuations in her cognitive and functional abilities—symptoms that would be more consistent with Lewy body dementia than AD. There is no history of inappropriate behaviors or disinhibition, or a significant language disorder to suggest a frontotemporal dementia.

On physical examination, the vital signs and general medical examination were normal. Neurologic examination revealed intact strength, muscle tone, sensation, coordination, gait, and reflexes. A mild intention tremor was noted with outstretched hands. There was no evidence of myoclonus or spastic paraparesis. Language was fluent but marked by occasional word-finding pauses and circumlocutions (especially with low-frequency words). Language, both spontaneous and in response to direct questioning of current events, was somewhat deficient in facts, despite her "keeping up with the news." Memory was impaired, including memory of recent medical history (including reasons for her taking daily medications). The Mini-Mental State Examination score was 23 out of 30, with points subtracted for errors in orientation, memory, and calculations (serial 7 subtractions). She could not copy a Necker cube, and could not correctly draw a clock showing "11:10." She had some difficulty naming parts of a watch, and she struggled with an executive task, namely, oral trails ("continue this pattern, all the way to the end: A1, B2, C3 ...").

Mild deficits in executive function, visuospatial skills, and a mild dysnomia, accompanied by readily apparent memory deficits, were consistent with a mild dementia. There were no signs of asymmetry to suggest a stroke, and no evidence of Parkinsonism (bradykinesia, rigidity, resting tremor, etc.) to suggest Lewy body dementia. The examiner suspected mild dementia due to AD, and ordered blood tests (to include a vitamin B12 level and thyroid function test [thyroid-stimulating hormone or TSH]), a neuroimaging study (brain magnetic resonance imaging [MRI]), and neuropsychometric testing. ApoE genotyping, cerebrospinal fluid collection for proteomic analysis (particularly Aβ and tau levels), and ^{18}F-2-fluoro-2-deoxy-d-glucose positron emission tomography (FDG-PET) imaging were not ordered. Despite the fact that FDG-PET is approved in the United States as a diagnostic study for individuals with AD versus a frontotemporal dementia, third-party payers are resisting coverage due to lack of evidence that obtaining this test significantly alters clinical management or patient outcomes.

At the return visit one month later, there were no significant interval changes in either history or physical examination. All blood tests obtained were normal or negative. The MRI revealed atrophy and white matter changes (interpreted by the neuroradiologist as ischemic in etiology)—all changes were considered normal for her age. Neuropsychometric testing was abnormal and confirmed deficits in several cognitive domains—memory, language, visuospatial skills, and executive function—consistent with a mild dementia; there was no evidence of depression using standard scales. After review of the history, examination, and diagnostic testing, a mild dementia due to AD was diagnosed, and a cholinesterase inhibitor was prescribed. The possibility of coexistent mild depression (versus the apathy of AD) was considered, but postponed to address in a follow-up visit. The effects and side effects of cholinesterase inhibitors were reviewed with the patient and family. The patient was advised to continue monitoring and treatment of hypertension and hypercholesterolemia with her primary care provider, and a suggestion was made to begin investigating options for living alternatives. Discontinuation of driving was recommended, as well as more supervision regarding her day-to-day medical and financial affairs. Initiation of discussion of advance directives was also suggested. The patient was resistant to the diagnosis of AD, and reluctant to take any advice. Although the daughter suggested denial, the examiner instead suspected anosagnosia (a lack of awareness of one's own signs and symptoms) as an alternative explanation for the patient's indifference to the diagnosis.

At the next follow-up visit in four months, there was no significant interval change in history or physical examination, and she was tolerating the cholinesterase medication well (denying nausea, vomiting, diarrhea, muscle cramps, nightmares, vivid dreams, and syncope). Since she was qualified and interested, enrollment in a clinical trial for individuals with mild to moderate dementia due to AD was discussed. She and her family declined participation at this time, but would discuss this option with friends, family, and her primary care provider. Over the next several years, her dementia progressed into moderate and then severe stages, and her Mini-Mental State Exam (MMSE) score declined at the anticipated rate of about 2.5 points per year. Behavioral symptoms became more prominent, and included worsening apathy, and later agitation, anxiety, pacing, wandering, and delusions, particularly at nighttime (sundowning). She required more supervision, encouragement, and assistance at first with complex activities of daily living (ADLs) such as handling finances and daily medications, and driving and shopping independently, and then later with basic ADLs (dressing, grooming, bathing, walking, transfers, toileting, and finally, eating). Antidepressant medications had no noticeable effect on apathy, depressive symptoms, or anxiety. She was transferred to a nursing home when she became persistently incontinent of bladder and then bowel, and behavioral difficulties became unmanageable to the family caregivers. A daily evening atypical antipsychotic improved sundowning symptoms—particularly agitation, anxiety, and delusions. Weight loss continued, and she fell and suffered a hip fracture in the nursing home. Hospice care was initiated as she became progressively vegetative, mute, and bedbound. At this point, medications were withdrawn and aggressive life-sustaining measures were declined, per advanced directives of the patient and her family. She died peacefully with inanition, dehydration, pneumonia, a sacral decubitus ulcer, and sepsis, about

8 years from the onset of dementia. A brain-only autopsy was prearranged at the request of the family.

On gross examination, the brain was diffusely atrophic, and had lost approximately 1/3 of its estimated premorbid weight. There were no gross infarcts or hemorrhages. Silver-stained brain sections from several cortical regions revealed abundant neuritic plaques and neurofibrillary tangles—thus meeting Reagan criteria for high-probability AD. The Consortium to Establish a Registry for Alzheimer's Disease (CERAD) criteria and the Braak and Braak staging were both consistent with a high probability of AD. Examination of the white matter revealed rarefaction, but no evidence of lacunar infarcts or other focal ischemic events. Brain sections examined for α-synuclein (Lewy bodies and Lewy neurites) and TAR DNA binding protein 43 (TPD-43) immunostains were negative, thus ruling out Lewy body dementia or a frontotemporal dementia linked to TDP-43 as the dementia etiology. These findings were reviewed with the daughter, who became concerned about her own risk of developing AD, and asked about any steps she may take now or later to lower this risk.

6.2 QUESTIONS

This relatively straightforward and fictional individual with progressive dementia due to AD raises many questions and issues, some of which remain controversial or unanswered. What are the key presenting signs and symptoms of AD? How are they different from normal aging, from depression, or from mild cognitive impairment (MCI)? What is normal aging? Is it normal to develop AD with aging? How much memory loss and cognitive decline is considered normal with aging? Would we all develop dementia or AD should we live long enough? Why is aging the major risk factor for AD? What are the major genetic and environmental risk factors? What is the link with traumatic brain injury? Why is the ApoE4 gene a risk factor? What other genes modify risk? What are the effects of race and ethnicity on risk? Is the rare familial form of AD similar to or different from the far more common sporadic AD? What causes AD? How is AD different from the other major neurodegenerative dementias, particularly Lewy body dementia and the frontotemporal dementias? What is vascular dementia and how does this differ from AD? What are the current diagnostic criteria for AD, for MCI, and for asymptomatic (prodromal, preclinical) AD? How and why are these criteria evolving? What biomarkers of AD may be useful in screening, in diagnosis, in prognosis, and in evaluation of drug efficacy in clinical trials of new therapeutics? What treatments are available now and how do they work? What are the current approaches to drug discovery in AD? Are there any disease-modifying treatments currently, or are they only symptomatic? How does one prove a new treatment to be disease modifying? How good are the transgenic and other animal models of AD? What are the best ways to prove drug efficacy in individuals with dementia due to AD? What are the major behavioral and psychiatric signs and symptoms of AD, and what are the best ways to treat these? What nonpharmacologic treatments have proven beneficial for the behavioral manifestations of AD? What are the current pathologic criteria for AD? How and why are they evolving? How many plaques and tangles are normal for age? Are these biochemical pathologies linked in some way? What are plaques and tangles composed of and how do they develop? What are the other major pathologic features of AD? Does vascular amyloid play a role in AD pathogenesis, in microhemorrhages, in white matter changes? Why are some brain regions severely affected by AD, while other regions remain unaffected?

6.3 INTRODUCTION

Age-related and progressive cognitive decline have been known since antiquity. Shakespeare famously wrote of seven ages of man, with the last scene "second childishness and mere oblivion, sans teeth, sans eyes, sans taste, sans everything." Dr. Alois Alzheimer was the first to associate the 5-year clinical progressive dementia in a 51-year-old woman with brain autopsy findings of neuronal loss, neurofibrillary tangles, and miliary amyloid plaques upon light microscopic examination of Bielshowsky silver-stained brain sections (Figure 6.1). Thus, Dr. Alzheimer suggested a link, perhaps causal, between the progressive clinical dementia of this individual and the abnormal aggregates found on brain sections (Alzheimer, 1907). What later became known as Alzheimer's disease (AD) now afflicts 2% to 3% of individuals by age 65, with an approximate doubling of incidence for every 5 years of age afterward. The prevalence of AD in one study approaches 50% of those over age 85 (Evans et al., 1989). Currently, there are an estimated 5 million individuals in the United States with AD, and these numbers are projected to increase as the baby boomer population ages. For reasons that remain unclear, African Americans and Hispanics have a 2 times and 1.5 times higher risk of developing AD than Caucasians. Because of expanding populations and increasing life expectancy, the number of affected individuals will rise to more than 14 million in the United States and approximately 100 million worldwide by 2050. A large fraction of this increase will occur in countries such as India and China, where life expectancies are quickly advancing into the striking range of AD (usually > 65). Although AD is the most common cause of dementia in the elderly in the United States, it is not inevitable with aging, and escapees warrant further epidemiological and genetic study. In fact,

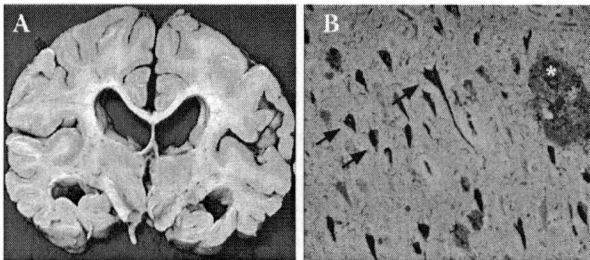

FIGURE 6.1 (See color insert.) Gross and histopathological hallmarks of Alzheimer's disease (AD). (A) A coronal slice demonstrates enlarged ventricles, a thinned cortical ribbon, and atrophy of hippocampi. (B) A silver-stained section of the hippocampal pyramidal layer CA1 reveals numerous neurofibrillary tangles (arrows) and a prominent neuritic plaque (*). (Photos courtesy of Dr. Brent Harris, Director of Neuropathology, Georgetown University Medical Center.)

many of the very old (90+) have significant AD-like pathologies in their brains yet are without clinical dementia (Savva et al., 2009). This dissociation points to flaws in our understanding of disease pathogenesis and flaws in current diagnostic criteria.

6.4 CLINICAL CRITERIA

The *Diagnostic and Statistical Manual*, 4th edition (1994) or the National Institute of Neurologic, Communicative Disorders and Stroke-AD and Related Disorders Association (NINCDS-ADRDA) (McKhann et al., 1984) criteria are currently used for the clinical diagnosis of AD. These criteria are similar and require a gradually progressive dementia of older adults severe enough to impair social or occupational functioning with other etiologies, including depression and delirium, excluded (Knopman et al., 2001). By definition, dementia requires a decline in memory and at least one other cognitive domain, typically visuospatial skills, language and calculation, praxis (learned motor skills), gnosis (higher-order sensory perceptions), or frontal executive functions (reasoning, insight, foresight, judgment, etc.). A diagnosis of definite AD requires light microscopic examination of brain sections obtained by either brain biopsy or autopsy—both of which are rarely performed. Thus, possible or probable AD is routinely diagnosed clinically. Possible AD is diagnosed when uncertainty arises from a putative secondary etiology, or the dementia has an atypical onset, course, or presentation. Diagnostic accuracies, compared with the gold-standard of autopsy, for possible and probable AD by NINCDS-ADRDA criteria are approximately 50% to 60% and 80% to 90%, respectively, at specialized centers. Confounding diagnoses of individuals who present to cognitive disorders clinics at specialized medical centers are often Lewy body dementia, the frontotemporal dementias, vascular dementia, and mixed dementias (especially AD plus vascular). Mild depression is often a comorbid diagnosis at the onset of AD. Dubois et al. (2007) propose an update to the well-established NINCDS-ADRDA criteria; the new criteria redefine AD to incorporate individuals with amnestic mild cognitive impairment (MCI) and supported by a positive molecular biomarker such as abnormal cerebrospinal fluid (CSF) proteomics or a positive amyloid PET neuroimaging study. Efforts are now underway to redefine AD, MCI due to AD, and preclinical (at risk, asymptomatic, or prodromal) AD. Thus, these criteria establish a new category—cognitively intact older individuals with a positive AD biomarker (Dubois et al., 2010). The natural history and clinical course of this population are as yet unclear.

6.5 PATHOLOGIC CRITERIA

The Khachaturian criteria for AD require that the density of neuritic plaques and neurofibrillary tangles in brain sections exceed a given threshold that increases with age (Khachaturian, 1985). In contrast, the Consortium to Establish a Registry for Alzheimer's Disease (CERAD) criteria focus exclusively on the density of neuritic plaques (the sine qua nonpathological marker of AD) in brain sections compared with the plaque density of given high-power microscopic fields. Because neurofibrillary tangles are not specific to AD, they were not considered essential to the diagnosis

(Mirra et al., 1991). The current Reagan criteria for AD, however, require both amyloid plaques and neurofibrillary tangles in multiple brain regions and declare all such pathology abnormal (the National Institute on Aging and Reagan Institute Working Group on Diagnostic Criteria for the Neuropathologic Assessment of Alzheimer's disease, 1997). These criteria incorporate the semiquantitative CERAD plaque density scale (Mirra et al., 1991) as well as Braak and Braak (1991) staging of the density and distribution of pathological abnormalities in AD brain. Despite numerous other neuropathological changes in brain, including neuronal and synaptic loss, gliosis (both microglial and astrocytic), inflammation, cholinergic and other neurotransmitter deficits, microvascular amyloid angiopathy (Figure 6.2), oxidative damage, and mitochondrial dysfunction, the mainstay of pathological diagnosis remains silver staining of brain sections and light microscopic examination of the density and distribution of neuritic plaques and neurofibrillary tangles in brain—in other words, methods similar to those utilized by Dr. Alzheimer in 1906 (published 1907). The neuropathology of AD is anatomically stereotypic and first affects the entorhinal cortex and hippocampus followed by other limbic structures and neocortex (Braak and Braak, 1991; Kretzschmar, 2009). This is consistent with the initial amnestic clinical presentation of subjects with AD followed by an average of 8 to 10 years of progressive decline in multiple cognitive domains ultimately resulting in mutism, inanition, a vegetative state, and death. As with other neurodegenerative diseases, the etiology of the selective vulnerability of distinct brain regions to AD pathologies remains obscure. Less common focal variants of AD, such as posterior cortical atrophy present atypically with prominent visual and visuospatial deficits (visual agnosias) leading to cortical blindness, with the focus of disease presentation localized to the occipito-parietal lobes.

6.6   RISK FACTORS

The major risk factor for AD is aging. Even those with Down's syndrome and individuals with genetic polymorphisms or mutations that increase risk of AD require a degree of aging before symptoms and signs commence. It is unclear, however, what specific factors associated with aging increase AD risk. One hypothesis for sporadic AD is that central nervous system (CNS) clearance mechanisms of Aβ/amyloid

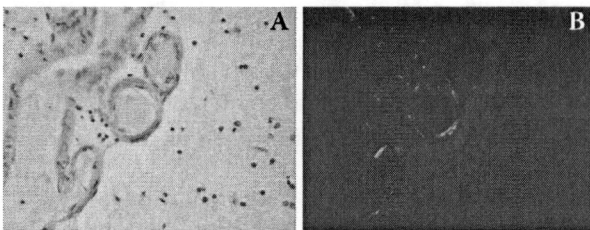

FIGURE 6.2 (See color insert.)   A Congo red–stained section highlights amyloid deposition within the wall of a small arteriole (orange/red) on brightfield microscopy (A) and demonstrates apple green birefringence by polarized light microscopy. (Photos courtesy of Dr. Brent Harris, Director of Neuropathology, Georgetown University Medical Center.)

decline with aging, with loss of the normal homeostasis of Aβ levels (in which generation equals clearance) (Mawuenyega et al., 2010). Having a first-degree relative with AD increases the risk approximately two- to fourfold, and this grows higher with increasing numbers of affected first-degree relatives. These data clearly implicate genetic factors. Certain environmental factors also affect AD risk. For example, a low level of educational or occupational attainment or a history of traumatic brain injury severe enough to induce loss of consciousness increase risk. Compared to males, females have a slightly higher risk of AD, and this is hypothesized to be related to a lack of postmenopausal estrogen (Tang et al., 1996). Risk factors for stroke, such as hypertension, diabetes, smoking, hypercholesterolemia, and hyperhomocysteinemia, also increase risk of AD. Whether these putative risk factors act directly on AD pathogenic mechanisms or indirectly by vascular compromise (cerebral infarcts), or both, remains unclear (Mayeux, 2003). Factors that may increase risk of both AD and cognitive decline with aging are as follows: having the ApoE4 genotype, having a diagnosis of diabetes or depression and currently smoking; factors that may decrease risk include physical activity, a Mediterranean diet, and cognitive training or maintaining cognitively engaging activities (Plassman et al., 2010).

Down's syndrome (trisomy 21), including translocation Down's (21q), is clearly a risk factor for AD (Evenhuis, 1990). The high prevalence of progressive dementia in individuals with Down's syndrome led to autopsy findings of typical AD pathologies, including neurofibrillary tangles and neuritic plaques, in aging brain. However, the onset of dementia typically occurs in the third to fifth decade of life, and neuropathology begins even sooner. The disease mechanism is likely a gene dosage effect since amyloid precursor protein (APP) is encoded at chromosome 21q. Cells from Down's syndrome subjects express approximately 1.5 times the normal level of APP, and thus secrete higher levels of Aβ derived from APP by the proteases β-secretase and γ-secretase. Aβ peptides, including Aβ40 and Aβ42, spontaneously alter their conformation to become insoluble neurotoxic aggregates and are the major component of the amyloid plaques in AD brain (Selkoe, 2008a). Analogous to the gene dosage effect of Down's syndrome, mutations and polymorphisms within promoter regions of APP may modulate its level of expression in vivo and thus risk of AD (Theuns et al., 2006). Duplication of the APP locus (also without mutations) causes autosomal dominant early onset AD with amyloid angiopathy (Rovelet-Lecrux et al., 2006).

6.7 FAMILIAL AD

Similar to other human diseases, the identification and analysis of probands and pedigrees with rare genetic forms of a common sporadic disease proved to be informative with regard to pathogenesis, development of transgenic animal models, and testing of new therapeutic strategies. Thus, much has been learned about the putative cause of AD by the study of rare individuals with early onset familial AD (Selkoe, 2008a). There are now more than 160 familial AD mutations reported in three genes. Other than pedigree analyses showing early onset (presenile) highly penetrant autosomal-dominant patterns of inheritance, these genetic forms of AD are similar, both clinically and pathologically, to the overwhelming majority (99%)

of individuals with sporadic (senile) AD. Thus, proposed pathogenic mechanisms of familial AD are extrapolated to sporadic AD, and vice versa. However, the more aggressive, earliest-onset, and rapidly progressive forms of familial AD are also associated with myoclonus, seizures, and spastic paraparesis—atypical signs and symptoms in individuals in the early stages of sporadic AD. On pathologic studies, these more aggressive familial AD genotypes may also be associated with atypical "cotton wool" amyloid plaques apparent on brain sections.

The first mutations identified in familial AD were missense mutations in APP. Not coincidentally, these mutations cluster near the β- and γ-cleavage sites that release Aβ from APP. The location of these APP mutations suggested a disease mechanism favoring amyloidogenic (producing Aβ) over nonamyloidogenic APP catabolism (a toxic gain of function). For example, a double missense mutation (K670N/M671L in the APP_{770} isoform) near the β-cleavage site promotes A β 40 and A β 42 generation by significantly improving beta-amyloid cleaving enzyme (BACE1) kinetics. In contrast, any one of several single missense mutations near the γ-cleavage site (including APP T714I or A; V715M or A; I716V or T; V717I, G, F, or L; and L723P) specifically promotes Aβ42 generation. Aβ42 is far more spontaneously amyloidogenic than Aβ40, again suggesting a disease mechanism for these APP mutations. The identification of these genetic mutations led to the notion that the progressive accumulation and deposition of Aβ/amyloid in brain causes AD—the amyloid hypothesis—and allowed the generation of human APP transgenic mice that develop age-dependent behavioral decline in learning and memory tasks as well as progressive CNS Aβ/amyloid accumulation and deposition in a pattern strikingly similar to that found with human AD (Games et al., 1995, Hsiao et al., 1996). However, these mice do not develop neurofibrillary tangles, significant loss of synaptic or cholinergic markers, or neuronal loss, making them at best partial AD-like models. Some investigators suggest that the modest memory deficits and minimal neuronal loss found in aged transgenic AD mice model human MCI but not true AD.

Pathogenic APP mutations within the Aβ sequence usually result in a different phenotype and present clinically with a combination of lobar hemorrhagic strokes or microvascular ischemic strokes and/or progressive dementia. The pattern of inheritance is also autosomal dominant with a high degree of penetrance. Pathologically, these disorders are characterized by a much greater Aβ/amyloid burden within blood vessel walls in addition to parenchymal amyloid deposits as typically found with AD. Pathogenic missense mutations are known within the Aβ sequence at positions 692, 693, and 694 near the α-cleavage site. Because these mutations are intrinsic to Aβ, they alter its propensity to form insoluble amyloid fibrils and shorter protofibrils. The APP A692G (Flemish) mutation promotes Aβ production but retards its fibrillogenesis; this mutation leads to a combination of microvascular amyloidopathy and AD-like pathology and presents with dementia and cerebral hemorrhages. The APP E693Q (Dutch), APP D694N (Iowa), and APP E693K (Italian) mutations promote amyloid fibril formation from Aβ and also present clinically with dementia and lobar cerebral hemorrhages. The APP E693G (Arctic) mutation retards Aβ40 and Aβ42 production but enhances protofibril formation and presents clinically as AD, suggesting that protofibril formation from soluble Aβ may be a unifying event in AD pathogenesis (Haass and Steiner, 2001).

Like all amyloidopathies, the β-pleated sheet conformation of Aβ in amyloid plaques and blood vessel walls results in their fluorescence with thioflavin-S staining, and apple-green birefringence with Congo red–stained brain sections visualized by polarized light microscopy. Hereditary cerebral congophilic angiopathies with dementia are not limited to mutations in APP, but include other potentially amyloidogenic proteins such as cystatin C (Icelandic) and transthyretin. Similar to AD, other cerebral amyloidopathies (with parenchymal amyloid deposition) cause progressive dementia, such as British familial dementia or Danish familial dementia caused by a point mutation, or a ten-base pair duplication, respectively, of the *BRI* gene on chromosome 13.

Most early-onset familial AD pedigrees do not carry a mutation in APP, implicating other affected genes. By study of these families, mutations were identified in *presenilin-1* (*PS-1*, for presenile dementia, or onset < 60 to 65 years of age) on chromosome 14 and the homologous *presenilin-2* (*PS-2*) on chromosome 1 (see Bertram et al., 2011, and Cruts and Rademakers, 2011 for a complete list of familial AD mutations). Of the rare early-onset familial forms of AD, the most commonly found mutation (~85% of familial AD) is in *PS-1*. The discovery of these mutations provided a test for the amyloid hypothesis: do they alter APP metabolism and Aβ generation? Again, studies of cells in culture, samples from affected patients (skin fibroblasts, serum, etc.), and new transgenic mice reveal that *PS* mutations promote Aβ42 generation from APP (a toxic gain of function) (Scheuner et al., 1996). Transgenic mice expressing both human mutant APP and human mutant PS-1 exhibit accelerated amyloid deposition in brain compared with single transgenic mice expressing only mutant human APP. Thus, common to almost all familial AD mutations is an increased generation of Aβ42 from APP. PS mutations likely also have other detrimental effects promoting AD neuropathologies, for example, by increasing susceptibility of neurons to apoptosis (a loss of γ-secretase function). Presenilin is the catalytic component of the γ-secretase complex (also composed of PEN-2, APH-1, and nicastrin) responsible for hydrolysis of APP and other proteins (including Notch) in the center of the lipid bilayer of cell membranes (known as regulated intramembranous proteolysis, or RIP).

6.8 SPORADIC AD

Apolipoprotein E (*ApoE*) polymorphisms on chromosome 19 are associated with risk of sporadic late-onset AD (Strittmatter et al., 1993). ApoE is synthesized in the liver and plays a role in lipid and cholesterol transport in lipoprotein particles in blood. In the brain, ApoE is secreted by glial cells, with receptors on neurons. Thus, ApoE is similarly involved in CNS lipid and cholesterol metabolism. The three major *ApoE* polymorphisms in man—2, 3, and 4—result in six possible genotypes. The gene frequency in the U.S. population is 3 > 4 > 2. Although only about 25% of the US population is *ApoE4*-positive, of those affected with AD, the *ApoE4* frequency is approximately 50%. Having one or two *ApoE4* alleles increases the risk of late-onset AD and lowers the average age of onset with a gene dosage effect. Thus, the hierarchy of AD risk is *ApoE4/4 > ApoE4/x > ApoEx/x*. The *ApoE2* allele is considered protective, with *ApoE3* intermediate in risk. Genetic risks may be additive; for example, the *ApoE4* allele lowers the age of AD onset in subjects with Down's syndrome or with *APP* or *PS-1* mutations.

The mechanisms whereby ApoE polymorphisms affect AD risk remain unclear. ApoE4 may promote the formation of insoluble fibrillar amyloid from soluble Aβ, thus acting as a pathological chaperone. In the brain, ApoE plays a complex dual role—in promoting Aβ transport and clearance, and in promoting Aβ deposition as amyloid (a pathologic chaperone). Double transgenic mice expressing human mutant APP causing AD and human ApoE4 develop a greater amyloid burden in brain compared with mice coexpressing human ApoE3. ApoE-deficient mice expressing human mutant APP develop fewer amyloid plaques, again consistent with a pathological chaperone role for ApoE in Aβ/amyloidogenesis. Additional mechanisms whereby ApoE4 increases risk of AD, including effects on APP metabolism, are likely. Interestingly, the *ApoE4* allele may be detrimental to individuals with other brain injuries such as ischemic stroke, traumatic brain injury, multiple sclerosis, and non-AD dementias (such as HIV encephalopathy). In fact, *ApoE2* is a human longevity gene, with few or no *ApoE4*-positive centenarians found in population studies. Other than *ApoE*, several genes confer a comparatively minor influence on AD risk, including clusterin, PICALM, and CR1. More than 100 other genetic associations in sporadic AD remain controversial and conflicting (see Bertram et al., 2011 for a complete and up-to-date listing of genes associated with AD, listed approximately in order of the quantity and quality of supportive evidence in the literature).

6.9   THE AMYLOID HYPOTHESIS

In support of the amyloid hypothesis of AD is evidence that Down's syndrome, *APP*, *PS-1*, and *PS-2* mutations, and the *ApoE4* polymorphism either promote Aβ generation, especially Aβ42, or its deposition in brain (Figure 6.3). Immunohistochemical stains reveal that the earliest Aβ deposits in aging brain are primarily Aβ42. These preamyloid deposits (diffuse plaques) are thought to evolve into mature neuritic plaques and thus are likened to the benign fatty streaks that subsequently evolve into pathogenic atherosclerotic plaques within blood vessels. Diffuse Aβ/amyloid plaques, unlike neuritic plaques, were considered benign since they are not surrounded by dystrophic neurites (swollen and deformed neuronal processes filled with phospho-tau aggregates), reactive gliosis (microglial and astrocytic), and inflammation and are not associated with clinical dementia. However, soluble Aβ aggregates (oligomers) may be the most neurotoxic species of amyloid (Selkoe, 2008b). These soluble oligomeric species of Aβ are not apparent with the routine neuropathologic methods used to diagnose AD. Neither are they apparent on amyloid ligand–based PET imaging techniques that detect CNS plaque load. This revision of the amyloid hypothesis may help to explain clinical dissociations found with neuropathologic correlation studies and serial amyloid PET imaging.

Evidence against the amyloid hypothesis of AD is the poor correlation of neuritic plaque burden, compared with neurofibrillary tangle density or synaptic loss, to the severity of clinical dementia. There is also weak evidence for linkage of amyloid to putative downstream pathologies, such as apoptosis, oxidative injury, inflammation, and mitochondrial dysfunction. For example, Aβ aggregates, oligomers, and fibrils are neurotoxic, but in vivo evidence is suggestive, and mechanisms, perhaps requiring tau and elevated intracellular Ca^{2+}, remain unclear. There is also poor

```
        Downs              APP turnover
Familial AD mutations          ⬇
     ApoE4 > 3 > 2      Aβ accumulation
          Aging         Aβ oligomers, fibrils   ⬅  low Aβ, high tau
                          amyloid plaques           levels in CSF
                               ⬇
                          neurotoxicity       ⬅  positive amyloid
                       neurofibrillary tangles     imaging scan
                               ⬇
                      mild cognitive impairment   focal
                     microgliosis and astrocytosis  hypometabolism on
     memantine             inflammation           FDG-PET
     donepezil         focal encephalopathy   ⬅
    rivastigmine         neuronal morbidity
    galantamine    synaptic and neurotransmitter loss
                               ⬇
                                              atrophy, white matter
                        neuronal mortality   ⬅ changes on MRI
                          brain atrophy
                      white matter rarefaction
                           dementia
                            death
```

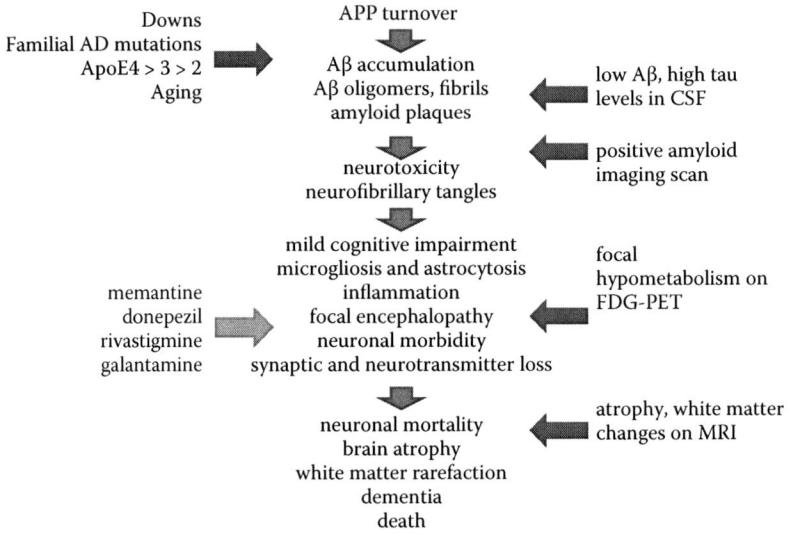

FIGURE 6.3 (See color insert.) The amyloid cascade hypothesis of AD. Similar to most proteins, APP undergoes a rapid and constant turnover in cells throughout life; Aβ is a minor catabolite of normal APP proteolysis, and results from β- and then γ-secretase cleavage of APP. With aging, normal clearance mechanisms of Aβ begin to fail, leading to the progressive accumulation and deposition of neurotoxic Aβ/amyloid aggregates in brain parenchyma of certain regions, causing sporadic AD. Aβ monomers spontaneously alter their predominantly α-helical structure (to a conformation with a greater percentage of β-pleated sheet) and form dimers, trimers, oligomers, fibrils, and finally, the large neuritic plaques found on appropriately stained brain sections under microscopy (and apparent by amyloid PET imaging scans). The accumulation of Aβ oligomers and neuroinflammation result in a neurotoxic milieu that is visible as temporoparietal hypometabolism on FDG-PET imaging, reflecting an underlying focal metabolic encephalopathy. Accelerants of the amyloid cascade include Downs (trisomy 21) and mutations in APP, PS1, or PS2 associated with familial AD (all of which promote Aβ generation or aggregation), and possessing the ApoE4 genotype (which promotes Aβ deposition and impairs neuroplastic responses to brain injury). Current FDA-approved drug therapies for AD target relatively downstream events, thus having only modest, temporary, and palliative (symptomatic) benefits. Newer therapies now in clinical trials include passive and active anti-amyloid immunotherapies designed to promote CNS Aβ/amyloid clearance. Thus, by targeting the putative underlying cause of AD, these therapies may have disease-modifying effects. Abnormal diagnostic studies typically found in individuals with AD are shown on the right. Positive amyloid PET imaging may precede FDG-PET abnormalities and prove useful in detection of AD in the earliest stages.

mechanistic linkage of amyloid plaques to the other major hallmark neuropathology of AD—neurofibrillary tangles that are composed primarily of hyperphosphorylated tau. Studies of mutant human tau and APP double transgenic mice and human mutant tau, PS-1, and APP (triple transgenic) mice support the hypothesis that Aβ pathologies precede and promote tau pathologies in brain (Gotz et al., 2001; Lewis et al., 2001; Oddo et al., 2003). Also in support of this notion, a *PS-1* mutation is associated with a familial Pick-type tauopathy but not β-amyloid plaques, and in this case may reflect loss of γ-secretase activity resulting in neuronal dysfunction and morbidity (Dermaut et al., 2004).

Amyloid is necessary but not sufficient to cause AD. Neurofibrillary tangles, neuronal and synaptic loss, gliosis, inflammation, and other pathologies downstream of CNS Aβ/amyloid accumulation and deposition are equally important in inducing progressive dementia. In fact, AD may be thought of as a focal metabolic encephalopathy, affecting first the medial temporal and parietal lobes, and then spreading to frontal lobes while sparing primary sensory and motor cortices. Tau (*MAPT*) mutations and polymorphisms on chromosome 17 cause different phenotypes, including Pick's disease, collectively referred to as *frontotemporal dementias*. Other familial frontotemporal dementia pedigrees may be linked to progranulin mutations characterized by neuronal aggregates of TDP-43 on appropriately stained brain sections. Similarly, Aβ/amyloid promotes α-synuclein pathologies but mutations in α-*synuclein* on chromosome 4 (or triplication of the α-*synuclein* gene) cause Parkinson's disease and Lewy body dementia.

6.10 GENETIC TESTING

APP, PS-1, and *PS-2* genetic tests are commercially available (Athenadiagnostics. com, 2011) and may be diagnostic for AD in the rare patient with early onset dementia (especially those with age of onset 30 to 55) and a pedigree reflecting possible autosomal-dominant inheritance. Currently, more than 150 different mutations in *PS-1* are known to cause AD (almost all single missense mutations) compared to only a few known missense mutations in *PS-2*. To date *APP, PS-1,* and *PS-2* genetic mutations are the only proven molecular biomarkers of AD. Genetic testing is indicated only for the diagnosis of rare individuals with early-onset AD and a pattern of inheritance consistent with autosomal dominant transmission. Genetic testing should not be obtained in minors. With consenting symptomatic adults (or their legal guardian) testing must be couched by appropriate genetic counseling. Prenatal screening and testing of asymptomatic individuals in affected pedigrees engender ethical debates.

ApoE genotyping is also commercially available (Athenadiagnostics.com, 2011) but its application should be limited to research studies since this information adds little to the predictive value of clinical diagnosis, adds cost, and necessitates genetic counseling for the individual and family members (the Ronald and Nancy Reagan Research Institute of the Alzheimer's Association and the National Institutes on Aging Working Group, 1998). Individuals with ApoE4 may not necessarily develop AD with aging, and approximately 50% of subjects with AD do not carry an *ApoE4* allele. A package of *ApoE* genotyping with tau and Aβ42 levels in cerebrospinal fluid is also marketed as a diagnostic test of AD (Athenadiagnostics.com, 2011), but its clinical utility remains to be determined.

6.11 CURRENT TREATMENTS

A profound cholinergic deficit was discovered in human AD cerebral cortex in 1976. This deficit is partly due to atrophy and loss of cholinergic neurons in the basal forebrain (nucleus basalis of Meynert) that project to the hippocampus and neocortex and play a key role in learning and memory (Davies and Maloney, 1976). This finding led to the notion that supplementing central cholinergic neurotransmission may be effective for the treatment of AD—the cholinergic hypothesis—analogous to dopaminergic supplementation proven effective for individuals with Parkinson's disease. The first drug with proven efficacy for the treatment of cognitive and functional decline in patients with AD was the cholinesterase inhibitor tacrine (Knapp et al., 1994; Doody et al., 2001). However, this medication was limited by its four times a day dosing, multistep titration, and side effects, especially nausea, vomiting, diarrhea, and hepatotoxicity requiring serum alanine aminotransferase monitoring. Thus, second-generation cholinesterase inhibitors without hepatotoxicity eclipsed tacrine—namely, donepezil (Aricept; FDA-approved 1996), rivastigmine (Exelon; approved 2000), and galantamine (Razadyne ER; approved 2001) (Rogers and Friedhoff, 1996). There are few direct comparisons of these drugs, but efficacy in improving or maintaining cognitive, functional, behavioral, and global outcome measures over months to years appears comparable (Doody, 2008). The over-the-counter supplement huperzine is also thought to have benefit for individuals with AD due to inhibition of cholinesterase, but this drug remains unproven in rigorous clinical trials. Other central cholinergic supplementation strategies (cholinergic precursors and muscarinic cholinergic receptor agonists) have so far failed to prove efficacy.

Memantine (Ebixa; Namenda; FDA-approved 2003) is an N-methyl-D-aspartate receptor partial antagonist with proven benefit for patients with moderate to severe dementia due to AD (Reisberg et al., 2003; Tariot et al., 2004). Memantine is thought to protect vulnerable neurons from glutamate-induced excitotoxic morbidity and mortality. This medication is typically prescribed in addition to one of the three widely used cholinesterase inhibitors once dementia has advanced into the moderate or severe stage. The antioxidants α-tocopherol (vitamin E) and selegiline (Deprenyl) delay functional decline and death in subjects with AD (Sano et al., 1997). No cognitive benefits were found in this study, but these were secondary end points. Despite flaws in this study, vitamin E (2000 International Units [IU] daily) was at one time recommended to subjects with AD until a subsequent meta-analysis indicated complications with vitamin E doses exceeding 400 IU daily (Miller et al., 2005). Clinical trials of the over-the-counter supplement *Ginkgo biloba* in subjects with AD remain negative or inconclusive.

In addition to drugs to treat cognitive and functional decline in patients with AD, antidepressants, anxiolytics, antipsychotics, neuroleptics, and anticonvulsants are often prescribed for management of a plethora of behavioral and psychiatric signs and symptoms. These symptoms include apathy, depression, anxiety, hallucinations, delusions, agitation, pacing, shadowing, sleep–wake cycle disturbances, and catastrophic reactions (Doody et al., 2001). Serotonin-modulating antidepressants and atypical antipsychotics are frequently prescribed to individuals with AD, despite the FDA-mandated black box warning of increased adverse events including death when atypical antipsychotics are prescribed to individuals with dementia. There is little guidance in the medical literature on the use of these medications for behavioral management, resulting in empiric treatment trials. The cholinesterase inhibitors and memantine may also have modest benefits on behavioral dysfunction in individuals with AD.

6.12 FUTURE TREATMENTS

To date, drug treatments for AD are presumably symptomatic with no effect on progressive underlying pathogenic processes. In support of this notion, cessation of donepezil (Aricept) results in acute loss of clinical benefits (Rogers and Friedhoff, 1996). The molecular identification of β- and γ-secretases that release Aβ from APP intensified development of small-molecular-weight inhibitors of these proteases as potential drugs for AD. Inhibitors of γ-secretase are now being studied in clinical trials, but a phase III trial (semagacestat) was terminated due to worsening cognition in the treatment group compared to the placebo group. This may have been due to inhibition of Notch processing (an off-target effect) as well as APP; Notch processing plays an important role in regulating neurogenesis in the adult brain. The treatment group also had a higher incidence of skin cancers, perhaps due to increased epidermal growth factor (EGF) receptor (another γ-secretase substrate). The next generation γ-secretase inhibitors and modulators now in preclinical and clinical studies are considered relatively Notch-sparing and thus more specific to APP metabolism (Mangialasche et al., 2010; Citron, 2010).

PS-1 (or PS-2) is the catalytic component of the γ-secretase complex, which also consists of nicastrin, PEN-2, and APH-1. Neither β-secretase nor γ-secretase is specific to APP proteolysis. The γ-secretase complex also cleaves Notch, a protein essential to embryonic development and adult processes such as hematopoiesis and gut epithelial cell differentiation (Selkoe and Kopan, 2003). Underscoring its importance in development, PS-1 knockout (-/-) mice are lethal in utero and resemble the lethal Notch1 -/- phenotype. A potentially more promising approach to AD treatment is inhibition of β-secretase, because BACE1-deficient mice are viable and relatively normal, with the notable exception of developmental hypomyelination. Inhibitors of BACE1 are mostly in preclinical stages of investigation, and this protease has so far proven a less tractable drug target. Due to the lack of substrate specificity of the β- and γ-secretases, however, drugs that inhibit or modulate these proteases may have dose-limiting side effects (Dewachter and Van Leuven, 2002).

Human APP transgenic mice immunized with Aβ develop little or no CNS amyloid deposition, indicating a novel therapeutic strategy (Schenk et al., 1999). Immunization may promote Aβ and amyloid clearance by anti-Aβ immunoglobulin (IgG) complexes and phagocytic cells (microglia) in brain. Peripheral immune-mediated Aβ clearance (a sink) may be an additional therapeutic mechanism. Immunization not only prevents but removes established amyloid plaques in human APP transgenic mouse brain. In support of the amyloid hypothesis, immunization prevents both plaque deposition in transgenic mouse brain and age-dependent decline in learning and memory tasks. The first clinical trial of Aβ42 immunization in patients with dementia due to AD was halted due to the development of aseptic meningoencephalitis in 6% of treated individuals. However, the development of serum anti-Aβ antibodies slows cognitive decline (Hock et al., 2003) and human autopsy data suggest that the immune response generated against the peptide elicits clearance of Aβ plaques in brain (Nicoll et al., 2003). In these few autopsy cases, removal of CNS amyloid plaques did not appear to alter the course of progressive dementia resulting in death, casting doubt on the amyloid hypothesis.

Novel active and passive immunization strategies are now being pursued in transgenic mouse models, nonhuman primates, and in clinical studies of individuals with AD. Phase III clinical trials of passive immunization with humanized anti-Aβ monoclonal antibodies are now underway, each targeting a different Aβ epitope. Preliminary results from the phase II bapineuzumab study suggest CNS amyloid clearance in response to treatment, as detected by amyloid-imaging PET scans (Rinee et al., 2010), but whether this translates into clinical improvements remains to be determined. New active immunization strategies using putative specific B-cell targeted Aβ epitopes, with unique adjuvants and immunization schedules, are in phase II clinical studies. Some older individuals develop little or no detectable titers in response to Aβ immunization. In contrast, excessive neuroinflammation, vasogenic edema, encephalitis, and microhemorrhages may be the dose-limiting side effect of these amyloid-based immunization strategies, and ApoE4-positive individuals may have a higher risk (perhaps due to a greater CNS amyloid burden) (Salloway et al., 2009).

Although epidemiological and pilot data are promising, treatment with estrogens have no benefit in postmenopausal women with AD. Likewise, despite a considerable inflammatory response in AD brain and promising pilot studies of older nonsteroidal anti-inflammatory inhibitors (NSAIDs), drugs inhibiting cyclooxygenase-2 specifically (COX-2 inhibitors) are also ineffective in subjects with AD. Prednisone treatment is also without cognitive benefit. Because retrospective epidemiological studies appear promising, statins that lower serum cholesterol are being explored for potential benefit in prevention or treatment of AD. Estrogenic compounds, NSAIDs, and statins may be effective for the prevention or treatment of AD by inhibiting Aβ42 generation from APP, in addition to their having other therapeutic effects. However, there is currently no evidence to support prescribing these drugs for AD.

Clinical trials are refocusing on more proximate events with the notion that treatment of AD subjects may be "too little, too late" (Aisen et al., 2010). These clinical trials will enroll subjects with prodromal or asymptomatic AD and amnestic MCI, a predementia syndrome with a 5% to 15% annual risk of conversion to dementia and AD (Petersen et al., 2001). A trial of donepezil (Aricept) or vitamin E (2000 IU daily), however, in individuals with MCI found no efficacy in delaying or preventing the onset of dementia and AD at the 3-year end point (Petersen et al., 2005). The exact neuropsychometric and clinical boundaries between normal aging, amnestic MCI, and dementia are now in flux, and redefinitions are being proposed based in part on supportive abnormal molecular biomarkers of disease (Dubois et al., 2007, 2010).

6.13   PERSPECTIVES

The field of AD research is a model of how biochemical pathology and molecular genetics have brought us to the threshold of safe and effective potentially disease-modifying clinical therapies. After decades of anosagnosia writ large and therapeutic nihilism, the identification of rare probands and pedigrees with familial AD led to the discovery of genetic mutations, new hypotheses of pathogenesis, transgenic animal models of disease, and novel therapeutic strategies. The challenge remains, however, to return to the clinic with treatments for familial and sporadic AD based on recent advances in our understanding of this devastating and all-too-common neurodegenerative disorder. The amyloid hypothesis remains unproven, yet remains the main target of ongoing clinical studies.

To accomplish the goal of finding effective means to prevent and treat AD, we will require validated molecular biomarkers to identify individuals in the earliest (preclinical) stages. This will also necessitate redefinition of AD to incorporate those with amnestic MCI and perhaps also those at risk, with prodromal or asymptomatic AD, defined in part by a positive molecular biomarker. The availability of new safe and effective disease-modifying therapies for the treatment and prevention of AD will then shift the cost–benefit equilibrium in favor of widespread population screening efforts. Major questions remain for current and future AD investigators, including: What are these new disease-modifying therapies? Which biomarkers will prove to be valid proxies of clinical disease? And what methods of population screening will be most cost-effective? Progress in all these areas will be essential in thwarting the large and growing international public health threat that is AD.

ACKNOWLEDGMENTS

This work was supported by R01 AG026478 from the National Institute on Aging.

REFERENCES

Aisen, P. S., Petersen, R. C., Donohue, M. C., et al. 2010. Clinical core of the Alzheimer's disease neuroimaging initiative: Progress and plans. *Alzheimer's and Dementia* 6: 239–246.

Alzheimer, A. 1907. Über eine eigenartige Erkrankung der Hirnrinde. *Allg Z Psychiatr* 64: 146–148.

American Psychiatric Association. 1994. *Diagnostic and Statistical Manual of Mental Disorders*. 4th ed. Washington, DC: American Psychiatric Association.

Athena Diagnostics, http://www.athenadiagnostics.com (accessed February 2011).

Bertram, L., McQueen, M., Mullin, K., Blacker, D., and Tanzi, R. 2011. The AlzGene Database. Alzheimer Research Forum, http://www.alzforum.org (accessed February 2011).

Braak, H., and Braak, E. 1991. Neuropathologic staging of Alzheimer-related changes. *Acta Neuropathol* (Berl) 82: 239–259.

Citron, M. 2010. Alzheimer's disease: Strategies for disease modification. *Nat Rev Drug Discov* 9: 387–398.

Cruts, M., and Rademakers, R. n.d. Alzheimer Disease and Frontotemporal Dementia Mutation Database, http://www.molgen.ua.ac.be/ADMutations (accessed February 2011).

Davies, P., and Maloney, A. J. 1976. Selective loss of central cholinergic neurons in Alzheimer's disease. *Lancet* 2: 1403.

Dermaut, B., Kumar-Singh, S., Engelborghs, S., et al. 2004. A novel presenilin 1 mutation associated with Pick's disease but not β–amyloid plaques. *Ann Neurol* 55: 617–626.

Dewachter, I., and Van Leuven, F. 2002. Secretases as targets for the treatment of Alzheimer's disease: The prospects. *Lancet Neurol* 1: 409–416.

Doody, R. S. 2008. Cholinesterase inhibitors and memantine: Best practices. *CNS Spectr* 13: 34–5.

Doody, R. S., Stevens, J. C., Beck, C., et al. 2001. Practice parameter: Management of dementia (an evidence-based review). *Neurology* 56: 1154–1166.

Dubois, B., Feldman, H. H., Jacova, C., et al. 2007. Research criteria for the diagnosis of Alzheimer's disease: Revising the NINCDS-ADRDA criteria. *Lancet Neurol* 6: 734–746.

Dubois, B., Feldman, H. H., Jacova, C., et al. 2010. Revising the definition of Alzheimer's disease: A new lexicon. *Lancet Neurol* 9: 1118–11127.

Evans, D. A., Funkenstein, H. H., Albert, M. S., et al. 1989. Prevalence of Alzheimer's disease in a community population of older persons higher than previously reported. *JAMA* 262: 2551–2556.

Evenhuis, H. M. 1990. The natural history of dementia in Down's syndrome. *Arch Neurol* 47: 263–267.

Games, D., Adams, D., Alessandrini, R., et al. 1995. Alzheimer-type neuropathology in transgenic mice expressing V717F β-amyloid precursor protein. *Nature* 373: 523–527.

Gotz, J., Chen, F., van Dorpe, J., and Nitsch, R. M. 2001. Formation of neurofibrillary tangles in P301L tau transgenic mice induced by Aβ42 fibrils. *Science* 293: 1491–1495.

Haass, C., and Steiner, H. 2001. Protofibrils, the unifying toxic molecule of neurodegenerative disorders? *Nat Neurosci* 4: 859–860.

Hock, C., Konietzko, U., Streffer, J. R., et al. 2003. Antibodies against β-amyloid slow cognitive decline in Alzheimer's disease. *Neuron* 38: 547–554.

Hsiao, K., Chapman, P., Nilsen, S., et al. 1996. Correlative memory deficits, Aβ elevation and amyloid plaques in transgenic mice. *Science* 274: 99–102.

Khachaturian, Z. S. 1985. Diagnosis of Alzheimer's disease. *Arch Neurol* 42: 1097–1105.

Knapp, M. J., Knopman, D. S., Solomon, P. R., Pendlebury, W. W., Davis, C. S., and Gracon, S. I. 1994. A 30-week randomized controlled trial of high-dose tacrine in patients with Alzheimer's disease. *JAMA* 271: 985–991.

Knopman, D. S., DeKosky, S. T., Cummings, J. L., et al. 2001. Practice parameter: Diagnosis of dementia (an evidence-based review). *Neurology* 56: 1143–1153.

Kretzschmar, H. 2009. Brain banking: Opportunities, challenges and meaning for the future. *Nat Rev Neurosci* 10: 70–78.

Lewis, J., Dickson, D. W., Lin, W. L., et al. 2001. Enhanced neurofibrillary degeneration in transgenic mice expressing mutant tau and APP. *Science* 293: 1487–1491.

Mangialasche, F., Solomon, A., Winblad, B., et al. 2010. Alzheimer's disease: Clinical trials and drug development. *Lancet Neurol* 9: 702–716.

Mawuenyega, K. G., Sigurdson, W., Ovod, V., et al. 2010. Decreased clearance of CNS b-amyloid in Alzheimer's disease. *Science* 330: 1774.

Mayeux, R. 2003. Epidemiology of neurodegeneration. *Annu Rev Neurosci* 26: 81–104.

McKhann, G., Drachman, D., Folstein, M., Katzman, R., Price, D., and Stadlan, E. M. 1984. Clinical diagnosis of Alzheimer's disease: Report of the NINCDS-ADRDA Work Group under the auspices of Department of Health and Human Services Task Force on Alzheimer's Disease. *Neurology* 34: 939–944.

Miller, III, E. R., Pastor–Barriuso, R., Dalal, D., Riemersma, R. A., Appel, L. J., and Guallar, E. 2005. Meta-analysis: High-dosage vitamin E supplementation may increase all-cause mortality. *Ann Intern Med* 142: 37–46.

Mirra, S. S., Heyman, A., McKeel, D., et al. 1991. The consortium to establish a registry for Alzheimer's disease (CERAD): Part II. Standardization of the neuropathologic assessment of Alzheimer's disease. *Neurology* 41: 479–486.

National Institute on Aging and Reagan Institute Working Group on Diagnostic Criteria for the Neuropathologic Assessment of Alzheimer's Disease. 1997. Consensus recommendations for the postmortem diagnosis of Alzheimer's disease. *Neurobiol Aging* 18: S1–S2.

Nicoll, J. A., Wilkinson, D., Holmes, C., Steart, P., Markham, H., and Weller, R. O. 2003. Neuropathology of human Alzheimer's disease after immunization with amyloid-β peptide: A case report. *Nat Med* 9: 448–452.

Oddo, S., Caccamo, A., Shepherd, J. D., et al. 2003. Triple-transgenic model of Alzheimer's disease with plaques and tangles: Intracellular Aβ and synaptic dysfunction. *Neuron* 39: 409–421.

Petersen, R. C., Stevens, J. C., Ganguli, M., Tangalos, E. G., Cummings, J. L., and DeKosky, S. T. 2001. Practice parameter-early detection of dementia: Mild cognitive impairment (an evidence-based review). *Neurology* 56: 1133–1142.

Petersen, R. C., Thomas, R. B., Grundman, M., et al. 2005. Vitamin E and donepezil for the treatment of mild cognitive impairment. Alzheimer's Disease Cooperative Study. *N Engl J Med* 352: 2379–2388.

Plassman, B. L., Williams, J. W., Jr., Burke, J. R., et al. 2010. Systematic review: Factors associated with risk for and possible prevention of cognitive decline in later life. *Annals of Int Med* 153: 182–193.

Reisberg, B., Doody, R., Stoffler, A., Schmitt, F., Ferris, S, and Mobius, H. J. 2003. Memantine in moderate-to-severe Alzheimer's disease. *N Engl J Med* 348: 1333–1341.

Rinne, J. O., Brooks, D. J., Rossor, M. N., et al. 2010. 11C-PIB PET assessment of change in fibrillar amyloid-beta load in patients with Alzheimer's disease treated with bapineuzumab: A phase 2, double-blind, placebo-controlled, ascending-dose study. *Lancet Neurol* 9: 363–372.

Rogers, S. L., and Friedhoff, L. T. 1996. The efficacy and safety of donepezil in patients with Alzheimer's disease: Results of a US multicentre, randomized, double-blind, placebo-controlled trial. The Donepezil Study Group. *Dementia* 7: 293–303.

Ronald and Nancy Reagan Research Institute of the Alzheimer's Association and the National Institute on Aging Working Group. 1998. Consensus report of the Working Group on Molecular and biochemical markers of Alzheimer's disease. *Neurobiol Aging* 19: 109–116.

Rovelet-Lecrux, A., Hannequin, D., Raux, G., et al. 2006. APP locus duplication causes autosomal dominant early-onset Alzheimer disease with cerebral amyloid angiopathy. *Nat Genet* 238: 24–26.

Salloway, S., Sperling, R., Gilman, S., et al., 2009. A phase 2 multiple ascending dose trial of bapineuzumab in mild to moderate Alzheimer disease. *Neurology* 73: 2061–2070.

Sano, M., Ernesto, C, Thomas, R. G., et al. 1997. A controlled trial of selegiline, α-tocopherol, or both as treatments for Alzheimer's disease. The Alzheimer's Disease Cooperative Study. *N Engl J Med* 336: 1216–1222.

Savva, G. M., Wharton, S. B., Ince, P. G., et al. 2009. Age, neuropathology, and dementia. *N Engl J Med* 360: 2302–2309.

Schenk, D., Barbour, R., Dunn, W., et al. 1999. Immunization with amyloid-β attenuates Alzheimer-disease-like pathology in the PDAPP mouse. *Nature* 400: 173–177.

Scheuner, D., Eckman, C., Jensen, M., et al. 1996. Secreted amyloid β-protein similar to that in the senile plaques of Alzheimer's disease is increased *in vivo* by the presenilin 1 and 2 and APP mutations linked to familial Alzheimer's disease. *Nat Med* 2: 864–870.

Selkoe, D., and Kopan, R. 2003. Notch and presenilin: Regulated intramembrane proteolysis links development and degeneration. *Annu Rev Neurosci* 26: 565–597.

Selkoe, D. J. 2008a. Biochemistry and molecular biology of amyloid beta-protein and the mechanism of Alzheimer's disease. *Handb Clin Neurol* 89: 245–260.

Selkoe, D. J., 2008b. Soluble oligomers of the amyloid beta-protein impair synaptic plasticity and behavior. *Behav Brain Res* 192: 106–113.

Strittmatter, W. J., Saunders, A. M., Schmechel, D., et al. 1993. Apoliproprotein E: High avidity binding to β–amyloid and increased frequency of type-4 allele in late-onset Alzheimer's disease. *Proc Natl Acad Sci USA* 90: 1977–1981.

Tang, M. X., Jacobs, D., Stern, Y., et al. 1996. Effect of oestrogen during menopause on risk and age at onset of Alzheimer's disease. *Lancet* 348: 429–432.

Tariot, P. N., Farlow, M. R., Grossberg, G. T., Graham, S. M., McDonald, S., and Gergel, I. 2004. Memantine Study Group. Memantine treatment in patients with moderate to severe Alzheimer disease already receiving donepezil: A randomized controlled trial. *JAMA* 291: 317–324.

Theuns, J., Brouwers, N., Engelborghs, S., et al. 2006. Promoter mutations that increase amyloid precursor protein expression are associated with Alzheimer's disease. *Am J Hum Genet* 78: 936–946.

7 Pathogenic Protein Strains as Diagnostic and Therapeutic Targets in Alzheimer's Disease

Lary C. Walker, Rebecca F. Rosen,
and Harry LeVine III

CONTENTS

7.1 PROTEIN AGGREGATION AND NEURODEGENERATIVE DISEASE

The proteopathies comprise numerous diseases of the brain and other organs that are characterized by the aggregation, accumulation, and toxicity of specific proteins (Koo et al., 1999; Walker and LeVine, 2000a, 2000b; Bucciantini et al., 2002). The diversity of proteins that can form pathogenic assemblies is substantial (Chiti and Dobson, 2006); in many instances, the proteins form amyloid, which refers to masses of fibrillar protein that are birefringent under crossed polarizing filters after staining with the dye Congo red. Recently, several amyloid-like protein assemblies have been discovered that serve normal biological functions in a range of species (Chiti and Dobson, 2006; Badtke et al., 2009; Luheshi and Dobson, 2009; Maury, 2009; Wickner et al., 2010; Heinrich and Lindquist, 2011). While it is increasingly clear that aberrant proteinaceous assemblies play a key role in the development of the mammalian proteopathies, little is known about the molecular structure of aggregated proteins in vivo, or about how their misfolding is initiated and propagated in diseased tissue. The development of diagnostic and therapeutic agents will be accelerated by a better understanding of how proteins become corrupted and proliferate their abnormal features in vivo; the mechanistic commonalities among the diseases of protein aggregation suggest the possibility of a unified approach to treatment (Walker and LeVine, 2002).

In Alzheimer's disease (AD), the most prevalent cerebral proteopathy, aggregation of the β-amyloid peptide (Aβ), is an early and critical pathogenic event (Hardy and Selkoe, 2002; Querfurth and LaFerla, 2010). Although the normal function of this ~4-kDa cleavage product of the β-amyloid precursor protein (APP) remains uncertain, in AD, Aβ self-aggregates into β-sheet-rich oligomers, protofibrillar polymers, and fibrils (Kawas and Katzman, 1999; Selkoe, 1999; Hauw and Duyckaerts, 2001; Cummings, 2004; Duyckaerts et al., 2009).

Long, unbranched amyloid fibrils of Aβ comprise the cores of classical senile plaques, which, along with neurofibrillary tangles (below) and cerebral β-amyloid angiopathy, are one of the principal histopathologic attributes of AD (Hauw and Duyckaerts, 2001; Cummings, 2004; Duyckaerts et al., 2009; Querfurth and LaFerla, 2010). Aβ also aggregates into heterogeneous populations of smaller, soluble oligomeric assemblies (e.g., dimers, trimers, tetramers, dodecamers) that can be toxic to neurons (Walker and LeVine, 2000b; Hardy and Selkoe, 2002; Catalano et al., 2006; Lesne et al., 2006), possibly through multiple, distinct mechanisms (Nerelius et al., 2009). Monomers, oligomers, and fibrils are conformationally distinguishable forms, as determined by conformation-specific antibodies (Glabe and Kayed, 2006; Kodali and Wetzel, 2007; Lambert et al., 2009). However, due to their solubility, low abundance, heterogeneous conformational state, and dynamic nature, investigation of oligomeric Aβ in postmortem tissue samples can be problematic (Bitan et al., 2005; Haass and Selkoe, 2007; Walsh and Selkoe, 2007).

Although the evidence implicates the aggregation of Aβ in the initiation of AD, the Alzheimeric brain is beset by other lesions as well. Neurofibrillary tangles, which consist of abnormal, intracellular polymers of hyperphosphorylated microtubule-associated protein tau (Lee et al., 2001), are the second canonical brain lesion in AD (Hauw and Duyckaerts, 2001). The number of tangles correlates strongly with the degree of dementia (Wilcock and Esiri, 1982; Crystal et al., 1988; Giannakopoulos et al., 2007) but, particularly based on genetic evidence, their generation appears to be downstream of Aβ aggregation in the Aβ cascade (Hardy and Selkoe, 2002). The primacy of Aβ aggregation also is supported by experimental analyses, in that tau abnormalities can be induced or exacerbated by aggregated forms of Aβ (Götz et al., 2001; Walker et al., 2002b; Bolmont et al., 2007; Oddo et al., 2008; Clavaguera et al., 2009), but not vice versa (Bolmont et al., 2007). Thus, although tau multimerization is an important component of the AD phenotype, the essential early events that lead to the pathology of AD appear to center around Aβ (Walker and LeVine, 2000b; Hardy and Selkoe, 2002).

7.2 PRION DISEASE

The prion diseases are cerebral proteopathies that are propagated through the corruption of the secondary structure of normal, endogenous prion protein molecules (PrP^C) into a pathogenic conformation of the PrP protein (PrP^{Sc}, or PrP^{Res}) (DeArmond and Prusiner, 1995; Prusiner, 2001; Van Everbroeck et al., 2002; Aguzzi et al., 2007; Collinge and Clarke, 2007; Kovacs and Budka, 2009; Soto and Satani, 2011). Human prion diseases include Creutzfeldt-Jakob disease, kuru, Gerstmann-Sträussler-Scheinker syndrome, and fatal familial insomnia, while the nonhuman prionoses include such ailments as scrapie, transmissible mink encephalopathy, chronic wasting disease, and bovine spongiform encephalopathy (DeArmond and Prusiner, 1995; Johnson, 2005).

The infectivity of prion disease involves an unconventional mechanism whereby misconformed prion protein (i.e., prion protein that is enriched in β-sheet secondary structure) appears to induce the similar misfolding of other prion protein molecules (Prusiner, 1995) by a crystallization-like process that has been called *permissive templating* (Hardy, 2005). Because of their lethality and unorthodox mode of transmission, prion diseases have been the subject of considerable research for many years (Van Everbroeck et al., 2002; Soto and Satani, 2011). The events that initiate prion aggregation and toxicity are becoming increasingly well understood, and the prionoses are a logical prototype for the exogenous induction of proteopathies in general (DeArmond and Prusiner, 1995; Prusiner, 2004; Walker et al., 2006a; Walker et al., 2006b; Collinge and Clarke, 2007; Aguzzi et al., 2008; Caughey et al., 2009; Miller, 2009; Walker et al., 2010; Soto and Satani, 2011).

The particular cross β-sheet structure that is characteristic of many proteins in their disease-causing state has three important characteristics: protease resistance, structural templating, and the potential for transmissibility (Maury, 2009), although protease sensitive seeds exist (Colby and Prusiner, 2011; Langer et al., 2011). The prion diseases were thought to be uniquely transmissible (that is, able to induce disease via corruptive templating), but recent studies indicate that other proteopathies can, at least under experimental conditions, be induced in animal models and cultured cells by pathogenic forms of certain proteins. Like prions, the aggregating proteins in Alzheimer's disease (both Aβ and tau), Parkinson's disease (α-synuclein), and the polyglutamine repeat peptides (as well as various systemic amyloidosis, e.g., serum amyloid A protein) can be induced to misfold and polymerize by the exogenous introduction of multimeric "seeds" of the same protein (Kane et al., 2000; Sigurdsson et al., 2002; Walker et al., 2002a; Walker et al., 2002b; Walker and LeVine, 2002; Meyer-Luehmann et al., 2006; Soto et al., 2006; Walker et al., 2006a; Walker et al., 2006b; Aguzzi and Rajendran, 2009; Caughey et al., 2009; Clavaguera et al., 2009; Desplats et al., 2009; Eisele et al., 2009; Hu et al., 2009; Luk et al., 2009; Miller, 2009; Ren et al., 2009; Brundin et al., 2010; Chia et al., 2010; Cushman et al., 2010; Eisele et al., 2010; Frost and Diamond, 2010; Goedert et al., 2010; Westermark and Westermark, 2010; Hansen et al., 2011; Guo and Lee, 2011; Morales et al., 2011; Rosen et al., 2011a; Watts et al., 2011; Münch et al., 2011).

Furthermore, in some instances there is evidence for cross-seeding of unrelated aggregation-prone proteins, suggesting that a similar corruptive conformational motif may be at least partially shared by disparate proteopathies (Lundmark et al., 2005; Yagi et al., 2005; Bolmont et al., 2007; Yan et al., 2007; Westermark et al., 2009; Morales et al., 2010; Westermark and Westermark, 2010). Cross-seeding among aggregation-prone proteins in vitro generally is less promiscuous than is that in vivo (O'Nuallain et al., 2004), which argues for a potential biological component that can augment heterologous corruptive templating. In addition, protein crowding can promote protein aggregation (Lansbury, 1997), and the loss of proteostasis with age might be one reason that senescence is a prominent risk factor for the development of proteopathies (Ben-Zvi and Goloubinoff, 2001; Balch et al., 2008; Kikis et al., 2010).

7.3 PROTEIN STRAINS

In microbiology, the term *strain* is used to denote structural and/or functional variants of microbes within a particular species. Analogously, the prion protein in mammals can assume distinct pathogenic conformations that also are referred to as strains (Collinge, 2001; Collinge and Clarke, 2007), the molecular features of which can be associated with differences in amino acid sequence, protease sensitivity, conformational stability, and/or glycosylation pattern (Ben-Zvi and Goloubinoff, 2001; McKintosh et al., 2003; Kikis et al., 2010). Prion strains further differ in their pathogenicity and fibrillar morphology, which, in vitro, can be influenced by environmental factors such as temperature, ionic strength, protein concentration (Pedersen and Otzen, 2008), and agitation shear forces (Makarava and Baskakov, 2008; Pedersen and Otzen, 2008). Subtle conformational differences in the prion protein can strongly affect the protein's infectivity and disease phenotype (Peretz et al., 2002; Tanaka et al., 2006). Different prion stains can also interact and/or exert dominance in a host (Nilsson et al., 2010a). As with the reliable transmission of bacterial strain phenotypes, the molecular, structural, and pathogenic characteristics of prion strains are faithfully transmissible to susceptible hosts under the appropriate conditions (Prusiner, 2004; Collinge and Clarke, 2007; Aguzzi et al., 2008; Caughey et al., 2009), although in retransmission studies, host conditions can alter the nature of the prion strain (Chien et al., 2004; Legname et al., 2004; Walker et al., 2006a).

Recently, evidence has emerged that Aβ multimers also may exist as structurally and functionally distinct protein strains (Petkova et al., 2005; Meyer-Luehmann et al., 2006; Nilsson et al., 2007; LeVine and Walker, 2010; Paravastu et al., 2008; Walker et al., 2008; Paravastu et al., 2009; 2011; LeVine and Walker, 2010; Kayed et al., 2010). As with prions, extrinsic factors can drive the in vitro assembly of Aβ into diverse supramolecular structures (Yagi et al., 2007). The resulting fibrillar morphotypes appear to represent variations in molecular packing that can be transmitted to newly formed fibrils in a strain-specific manner (Pedersen and Otzen, 2008; Kodali et al., 2010). It is conceivable that some strains of Aβ are relatively pathogenic, and others relatively benign. Soluble, oligomeric Aβ may also exist in polymorphic forms (Kayed et al., 2010), which could account for different biological activities of oligomers prepared by different means. However, additional tools are required to establish any structure–function relationship between Aβ polymorphs and peptide toxicity, especially for oligomeric proteins. It is important to identify and distinguish among Aβ strains to optimize the diagnosis of AD and cerebral β-amyloid angiopathy, and to provide new insights into the molecular-structural basis of their neurotoxic properties (LeVine and Walker, 2010).

7.4 MOLECULAR PROBES FOR CONFORMATIONAL VARIANTS OF AMYLOIDOGENIC PROTEINS

Much of the evidence for putative mammalian protein strains comes from in vitro studies, in which the characteristics of synthetic protein aggregates can be altered by specific chemical or physical manipulations (Petkova et al., 2006; Makarava and Baskakov, 2008; Caughey et al., 2009; Frost et al., 2009). However, the most pathogenic types of misfolded proteins usually are generated within mammalian tissues, as evidenced by the relative difficulty in transmitting prion disease (Legname et al., 2004; see also Wang et al., 2010) or Aβ-proteopathy (Meyer-Luehmann et al., 2006) using recombinant or synthetic peptides. Variants of protein aggregates that are formed in the complex milieu of the living organism are most rigorously examined in tissues that have undergone little or no processing, as chemical or physical treatment during tissue preparation may artifactually alter the characteristics of the multimeric proteins (a type of uncertainty problem). Newly available probes can mitigate this problem, as they can be applied directly to aggregates that were generated in living tissues, with minimal modification of the samples.

When protein monomers fold into their typical (or atypical) configurations, and as the monomers assemble into multimeric structures, the availability and configuration of binding sites for other molecules can provide experimental clues to molecular structure. Conformation-specific antibodies and single-chain binding proteins are being developed to probe the molecular idiosyncrasies of misfolded proteins (Luheshi and Dobson, 2009; Kayed et al., 2010). In addition, polymeric *luminescent conjugated polythiophenes* (LCPs) and smaller derivatives termed *luminescent conjugated oligothiophenes* (LCOs) are conformation-sensitive amyloid-binding probes that, due to their flexibility, can adjust to small structural differences in the polypeptide backbone of the protein to which they attach (Nilsson et al., 2007; Aslund et al., 2009; Nilsson et al., 2010b). These small differences in conformation of the thiophene polymer twist the planar polythiophene chain, altering the electronic distribution in the conjugated polyaromatic system, which is then reflected in excitation and emission spectral "fingerprints" when the probe–protein complexes are examined via fluorescence microscopy. As a result, the excitation and emission spectra of a polythiophene can reveal the conformation and dynamics of a protein (or protein complex) to which it is bound. Thus far, LCPs and LCOs have been used to differentiate among fibrillar prion strains (Sigurdson et al., 2007; Almstedt et al., 2009; Nilsson et al., 2010a), structural types of systemic amyloidoses (Nilsson et al., 2010b), and morphologically distinct cerebral Aβ deposits as well as regions within deposits (Nilsson et al., 2007; Aslund et al., 2009), which have been hypothesized to consist of structurally polymorphic Aβ strains (Walker et al., 2008). Recent evidence indicates that a particular LCO (pentamer formyl thiophene acetic acid, or p-FTAA) may bind to soluble oligomeric/prefibrillar assemblies of Aβ as well as fibrils (Aslund et al., 2009; Hammarström et al., 2010). These polythiophene compounds and other fluorescent probes (Celej et al., 2009) thus have the potential to serve as instructive experimental tools for the identification and differentiation of proteopathic strains.

7.5 PITTSBURGH COMPOUND B (PIB) AS A MOLECULAR PROBE FOR Aβ

PIB is a brain-penetrant derivative of the benzothiazole Thioflavin-T, a cationic histological dye used to detect amyloid deposits in tissues (Klunk et al., 2001; Klunk et al., 2004; Nordberg, 2008). To assess possible configurational variations in multimeric Aβ, we examined the binding characteristics of PIB to naturally occurring toxic or benign Aβ multimers in autopsy-derived cortical tissue. In vitro, the stoichiometry of high-affinity site binding of PIB to synthetic Aβ fibrils indicates that PIB binds directly to multimeric, insoluble forms of Aβ (Klunk et al., 2005; Lockhart et al., 2005). By contrast, soluble oligomeric forms of synthetic Aβ do not bind significant amounts of PIB with high affinity (LeVine, unpublished data). Carbon-11-radiolabeled PIB efficiently and rapidly crosses the blood–brain barrier; in patients with AD, ^{11}C-PIB is retained in brain regions that are laden with β-amyloid plaques and cerebral β-amyloid angiopathy (CAA), whereas the radioligand rapidly washes out of pathology-free areas (Klunk et al., 2003; Bacskai et al., 2007; Johnson et al., 2007; Leinonen et al., 2008). PIB thus is a promising tool for diagnosing and monitoring β-amyloid deposition in living patients, as demonstrated in a recent analysis of Alzheimer patients receiving the humanized anti-Aβ antibody bapineuzumab (Rinne et al., 2010).

Our interest in PIB as a candidate molecular probe stemmed from the observation by William Klunk and colleagues that, in vitro, PIB binds with high stoichiometry to high-affinity sites on Aβ deposits from AD brain, but with much lower stoichiometry to high-affinity sites on synthetic Aβ fibrils or on Aβ deposits from aged, APP-transgenic mouse brains (Klunk et al., 2005). APP-transgenic mice that express human-sequence Aβ accumulate profuse senile plaques and cerebrovascular β-amyloid with age (Morrissette et al., 2009), yet no transgenic mouse model of cerebral Aβ-amyloidosis has been shown to exhibit the full neuropathological and behavioral spectrum of AD (Götz and Ittner, 2008). In addition to transgenic human Aβ, most mouse models of AD also produce normal, endogenous murine Aβ, which can co-aggregate with human-sequence Aβ in cortical plaques (Jankowsky et al., 2007). Because it differs from human Aβ at 3 amino acid positions, Aβ in mice has a greatly reduced proclivity to self-assemble (Otvos et al., 1993). Additionally, murine Aβ interferes with the binding of PIB when co-assembled with human-sequence Aβ (Ye et al., 2006). Cerebral Aβ deposits in transgenic mice also are more soluble and contain fewer posttranslational modifications than do Aβ lesions in AD (Kuo et al., 2001; Kalback et al., 2002; Maeda et al., 2007). Together, these data suggest that PIB may be an informative experimental and clinical probe that binds specifically to a particularly pathogenic conformation of multimeric Aβ. To test this hypothesis, it is important to investigate PIB binding in a more closely related animal model of naturally occurring, human-sequence Aβ-amyloidosis.

7.6 PIB BINDING IN NONHUMAN PRIMATES

To determine if PIB binds specifically to Aβ multimers in the AD brain, and to obviate potential interference with PIB binding by endogenous murine Aβ in transgenic rodent models, we examined high-affinity PIB binding in cortical tissue samples from normal aged nonhuman primates (Rosen et al., 2011b). As they age, nonhuman primates naturally accumulate copious human-sequence Aβ within senile plaques and as cerebral β-amyloid angiopathy (Walker and Cork, 1999) (Figure 7.1). Unlike humans, however, no nonhuman primate has been shown to manifest the entire behavioral and pathological phenotype of AD (Walker and Cork, 1999; LeVine and Walker, 2006; Rosen et al., 2008; Jucker, 2010; Rosen et al., 2011). Consequently, we proposed that aggregated simian Aβ may differ from that of humans in subtle, yet functionally important, ways. To test this hypothesis, we measured PIB-binding to cortical homogenates and tissue sections using 1 nM ^{3}H-PIB, a ligand concentration comparable to that achieved with ^{11}C-PIB in PET scans, in which only high-affinity PIB binding sites on the Aβ molecule are occupied (Klunk et al., 2003; Klunk et al., 2005; Ye et al., 2005). Despite similarly high levels of Aβ in all species, we found that 1nM ^{3}H-PIB binds with significantly lower stoichiometry to high-affinity sites on simian Aβ than to human Aβ (Rosen et al., 2011) (Figure 7.2), suggesting that PIB specifically recognizes an Aβ polymorph formed uniquely in the AD brain (LeVine and Walker, 2010). Further, because the amino acid sequence of Aβ is the same in the

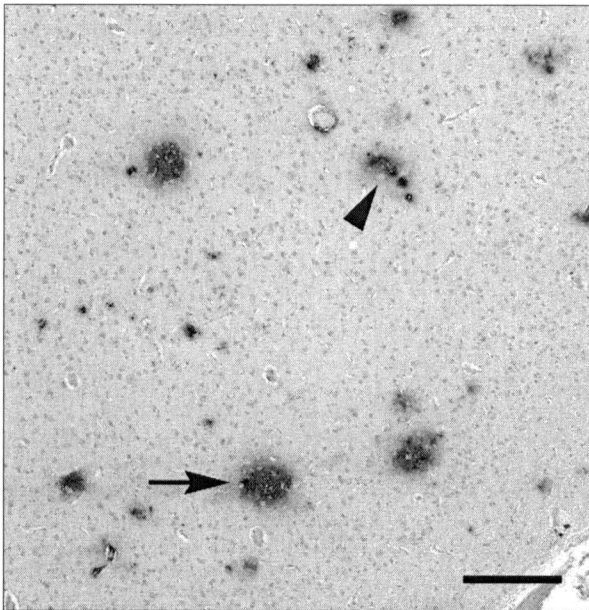

FIGURE 7.1 (See color insert.) Aβ-immunostained senile plaques (one is marked by an arrow) and cerebral β-amyloid angiopathy (arrowhead) in the prefrontal neocortex of a >30-year-old rhesus monkey (*Macaca mulatta*). The Aβ peptide has the same amino acid sequence in humans and all nonhuman primates studied to date. However, cerebral β-amyloid angiopathy is more common in monkeys than in humans, and its incidence varies among species and among individuals within a species (Walker and Cork, 1999). Antibody 6E10 with a hematoxylin counterstain; Bar = 200μm.

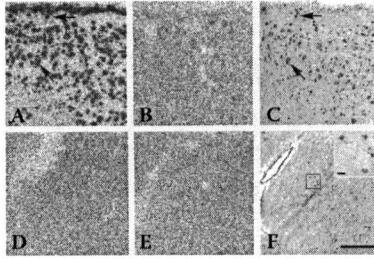

FIGURE 7.2 ³H-PIB binding in neocortical cryosections from a human with AD (top row) and an aged squirrel monkey (*Saimiri sciureus*) with cerebral Aβ-amyloidosis (bottom row). The left column shows specific binding of 1 nM 3H-PIB (black) in the AD case (A) and a relative paucity of specific binding in the squirrel monkey (D). The right column shows the adjacent tissue sections immunostained for Aβ (antibody 6E10) in the human (C) and squirrel monkey (F) (note that the lesions are typically smaller in squirrel monkeys; the inset shows a magnified view of a central region in F). The middle column (B and E) shows sections in which ³H-PIB is mostly (but not entirely) blocked by 1 μM unlabeled PIB in the two species. Bar in F = 1 mm for panels A–F; bar in the inset = 50 μm. (Reprinted from Neurobiology of Aging, March 2009 [Epub ahead of print][Print version published in volume 32:223–234, 2011]; PMID: 19329226, R. F. Rosen, L. C. Walker, and H. LeVine III. "PIB Binding in Aged Primate Brain: Enrichment of High-Affinity Sites in Humans with Alzheimer's Disease." Copyright 2009, with permission from Elsevier.)

four primate species that we examined, these findings imply the existence of a human-specific conformation, or *strain*, of Aβ that may be linked to the neurodegenerative cascade of AD.

7.7   ANOMALOUS PIB BINDING IN ALZHEIMER'S DISEASE

PIB binds with high specificity and sensitivity to Aβ-rich plaques and amyloid angiopathy in the human brain (Klunk et al., 2003; Bacskai et al., 2007; Johnson et al., 2007; Leinonen et al., 2008; Rosen et al., 2011), but some studies in which ¹¹C-PIB binding has been imaged in vivo have found surprisingly high PIB retention in nondemented cases (Rowe et al., 2007), or unexpectedly low retention in clinically diagnosed AD cases (Klunk et al., 2004; Edison et al., 2007; Nelissen et al., 2007; Li et al., 2008; Cairns et al., 2009). Furthermore, in human autopsy-derived brain tissue, autoradiographic analyses have found that some Aβ lesions are relatively refractory to PIB binding (Ikonomovic et al., 2008; Svedberg et al., 2009). These observations collectively imply that PIB binding sites, which differ between humans and nonhuman species (see previous discussion), may be somewhat heterogeneous also among humans. Recently, we discovered a case of idiopathic AD with abundant diffuse and dense-core senile plaques and extraordinarily high levels of Aβ, yet negligible high-affinity binding of PIB (Rosen et al., 2010). In addition to exceptionally large amounts of Aβ40 and Aβ42, this subject was unusual in having relatively profuse cerebral β-amyloid angiopathy, a high ratio of Aβ40:Aβ42, and a distinctive pattern of N- and C-terminally truncated Aβ fragments. While this anomalous case may appear to challenge the hypothesis that PIB recognizes a particularly pathogenic conformation of Aβ, quantitative assessments suggest, rather, that the multimeric Aβ in this instance may have been relatively benign, in that very high amounts of aggregated peptide were needed to precipitate the clinical AD phenotype. Further investigation of this topic is needed, but the findings as a whole imply that, even in humans with AD, there are potentially important variations in the supramolecular structure of Aβ, and that molecular binding agents such as PIB may serve to distinguish among naturally occurring strains of multimeric Aβ.

7.8 CONCLUSIONS

The aberrant conformation and self-assembly of specific proteins is linked to a remarkable variety of disorders of the brain and systemic organs. In Alzheimer's disease (the most prevalent form of cerebral proteopathy), the aggregation of Aβ is an early and critical pathogenic event. Assemblies of Aβ, however, appear not to be uniform, suggesting that Aβ multimers, like prions, can form structurally and functionally heterogeneous strains. Although strain-like variants of Aβ have been demonstrated in vitro, such alternative molecular forms can be difficult to identify in lesions that form in the complex environment of the aging brain. New tools, such as the luminescent conjugated polythiophenes and the PET imaging agent PIB, enable the identification of strain-like structural differences in endogenously generated protein aggregates. These new ligands, and other agents and methods currently under development for both insoluble and soluble protein assemblies, may help to illuminate the region- and species-specific pathogenicity of aggregation-prone proteins. Molecular conformational factors governing the pathogenicity of aggregating proteins could represent new targets for disease-modifying therapies.

ACKNOWLEDGMENTS

We thank Mathias Jucker for helpful comments and Jeromy Dooyema for excellent technical assistance. This work was supported by NIH RR-00165, PO1AG026423, P50AG025688, the Woodruff Foundation, the CART Foundation, a University of Kentucky Faculty University Support Grant 1012101660, and the Emory University Research Committee.

REFERENCES

Aguzzi, A., Heikenwalder, M., and Polymenidou, M. 2007. Insights into prion strains and neurotoxicity. *Nat Rev Mol Cell Biol* 8: 552–561.
Aguzzi, A., and Rajendran, L. 2009. The transcellular spread of cytosolic amyloids, prions, and prionoids. *Neuron* 64: 783–790.
Aguzzi, A., Sigurdson, C., and Heikenwaelder, M. 2008. Molecular mechanisms of prion pathogenesis. *Annu Rev Pathol* 3: 11–40.
Almstedt, K., Nyström, S., Nilsson, K. P., and Hammarström, P. 2009. Amyloid fibrils of human prion protein are spun and woven from morphologically disordered aggregates. *Prion* 3: 224–235.

Aslund, A., Nilsson, K. P., and Konradsson, P. 2009. Fluorescent oligo and poly-thiophenes and their utilization for recording biological events of diverse origin—When organic chemistry meets biology. *J Chem Biol* 2: 161–175.

Bacskai, B. J., Frosch, M. P., Freeman, S. H., Raymond, S. B., Augustinack, J. C., Johnson, K. A., Irizarry, M. C., Klunk, W. E., Mathis, C. A., DeKosky, S. T., Greenberg, S. M., Hyman, B. T., and Growdon, J. H. 2007. Molecular imaging with Pittsburgh Compound B confirmed at autopsy: A case report. *Arch Neurol* 64(3): 431–434.

Badtke, M. P., Hammer, N. D., and Chapman, M. R. 2009. Functional amyloids signal their arrival. *Sci Signal* 2(80): pe43.

Balch, W. E., Morimoto, R. I., Dillin, A., and Kelly, J. W. 2008. Adapting proteostasis for disease intervention. *Science* 319: 916–919.

Ben-Zvi, A. P., and Goloubinoff, P. 2001. Review: Mechanisms of disaggregation and refolding of stable protein aggregates by molecular chaperones. *J Struct Biol* 135: 84–93.

Bitan, G., Fradinger, E. A., Spring, S. M., and Teplow, D. B. 2005. Neurotoxic protein oligomers: What you see is not always what you get. *Amyloid* 12: 88–95.

Bolmont, T., Clavaguera, F., Meyer-Luehmann, M., Herzig, M. C., Radde, R., Staufenbiel, M., Lewis, J., Hutton, M., Tolnay, M., and Jucker, M. 2007. Induction of tau pathology by intracerebral infusion of amyloid-beta-containing brain extract and by amyloid-beta deposition in APP x Tau transgenic mice. *Am J Pathol* 171: 2012–2020.

Brundin, P., Melki, R., and Kopito, R. 2010. Prion-like transmission of protein aggregates in neurodegenerative diseases. *Nat Rev Mol Cell Biol* 11: 301–307.

Bucciantini, M., Giannoni, E., Chiti, F., Baroni, F., Formigli, L., Zurdo, J., Taddei, N., Ramponi, G., Dobson, C. M., and Stefani, M. 2002. Inherent toxicity of aggregates implies a common mechanism for protein misfolding diseases. *Nature* 416: 507–511.

Cairns, N. J., Ikonomovic, M. D., Benzinger, T., Storandt, M., Fagan, A. M., Shah, A. R., Reinwald, L. T., Carter, D., Felton, A., Holtzman, D. M., Mintun, M. A., Klunk, W. E., and Morris, J. C. 2009. Absence of Pittsburgh compound B detection of cerebral amyloid beta in a patient with clinical, cognitive, and cerebrospinal fluid markers of Alzheimer disease: A case report. *Arch Neurol* 66: 1557–1562.

Catalano, S. M., Dodson, E. C., Henze, D. A., Joyce, J. G., Krafft, G. A., and Kinney, G. G. 2006. The role of amyloid-beta derived diffusible ligands (ADDLs) in Alzheimer's disease. *Curr Top Med Chem* 6: 597–608.

Caughey, B., Baron, G. S., Chesebro, B., and Jeffrey, M. 2009. Getting a grip on prions: Oligomers, amyloids, and pathological membrane interactions. *Annu Rev Biochem* 78: 177–204.

Celej, M. S., Caarls, W., Demchenko, A. P., and Jovin, T. M. 2009. A triple emission fluorescent probe reveals distinctive amyloid fibrillar polymorphism of wild-type-synuclein and its familial Parkinsons disease-mutants. *Biochemistry* 48: 7465–72.

Chia, R., Tattum, M. H., Jones, S., Collinge, J., Fisher, E. M., and Jackson, G. S. 2010. Superoxide dismutase 1 and tgSOD1 mouse spinal cord seed fibrils, suggesting a propagative cell death mechanism in amyotrophic lateral sclerosis. *PLoS One* 5(5): e10627.

Chien, P., Weissman, J. S., and DePace, A. H. 2004. Emerging principles of conformation-based prion inheritance. *Annu Rev Biochem* 73: 617–656.

Chiti, F., and Dobson, C. M. 2006. Protein misfolding, functional amyloid, and human disease. *Annu Rev Biochem* 75: 333–366.

Clavaguera, F., Bolmont, T., Crowther, R. A., Abramowski, D., Frank, S., Probst, A., Fraser, G., Stalder, A. K., Beibel, M., Staufenbiel, M., Jucker, M., Goedert, M., and Tolnay, M. 2009. Transmission and spreading of tauopathy in transgenic mouse brain. *Nat Cell Biol* 11: 909–913.

Colby, D. W., and Prusiner, S. B. 2011. Prions. *Cold Spring Harb Perspect Biol.*

Collinge, J. 2001. Prion diseases of humans and animals: Their causes and molecular basis. *Annu Rev Neurosci* 24: 519–550.

Collinge, J., and Clarke, A. R. 2007. A general model of prion strains and their pathogenicity. *Science* 318: 930–936.

Crystal, H., Dickson, D., Fuld, P., Masur, D., Scott, R., Mehler, M., Masdeu, J., Kawas, C., Aronson, M., and Wolfson, L. 1988. Clinico-pathologic studies in dementia: Nondemented subjects with pathologically confirmed Alzheimer's disease. *Neurology* 38: 1682–1687.

Cummings, J. L. 2004. Alzheimer's disease. *New Engl J Med* 351: 56–67.

Cushman, M., Johnson, B. S., King, O. D., Gitler, A. D., and Shorter, J. 2010. Prion-like disorders: Blurring the divide between transmissibility and infectivity. *J Cell Sci* 123: 1191–1201.

DeArmond, S. J., and Prusiner, S. B. 1995. Etiology and pathogenesis of prion diseases. *Am J Pathol* 146: 785–811.

Desplats, P., Lee, H. J., Bae, E. J., Patrick, C., Rockenstein, E., Crews, L., Spencer, B., Masliah, E., and Lee, S. J. 2009. Inclusion formation and neuronal cell death through neuron-to-neuron transmission of alpha-synuclein. *Proc Natl Acad Sci USA* 106: 13010–13015.

Duyckaerts, C., Delatour, B., and Potier, M. C. 2009. Classification and basic pathology of Alzheimer disease. *Acta Neuropath* 118: 5–36.

Edison, P., Archer, H. A., Hinz, R., Hammers, A., Pavese, N., Tai, Y. F., Hotton, G., Cutler, D., Fox, N., Kennedy, A., Rossor, M., and Brooks, D. J. 2007. Amyloid, hypometabolism, and cognition in Alzheimer disease: An [11C]PIB and [18F]FDG PET study. *Neurology* 68: 501–508.

Eisele, Y. S., Bolmont, T., Heikenwalder, M., Langer, F., Jacobson, L. H., Yan, Z. X., Roth, K., Aguzzi, A., Staufenbiel, M., Walker, L. C., and Jucker, M. 2009. Induction of cerebral beta-amyloidosis: Intracerebral versus systemic Abeta inoculation. *Proc Natl Acad Sci USA* 106: 12926–12931.

Eisele, Y. S., Obermuller, U., Heilbronner, G., Baumann, F., Kaeser, S. A., Wolburg, H., Walker, L. C., Staufenbiel, M., Heikenwalder, M., and Jucker, M. 2010. Peripherally applied Aβ-containing inoculates induce cerebral β-amyloidosis. *Science* 330: 980–982.

Frost, B., and Diamond, M. I. 2010. Prion-like mechanisms in neurodegenerative diseases. *Nat Rev Neurosci* 11: 155–159.

Frost, B., Ollesch, J., Wille, H., and Diamond, M. I. 2009. Conformational diversity of wild-type Tau fibrils specified by templated conformation change. *J Biol Chem* 284: 3546–3551.

Giannakopoulos, P., Gold, G., Kovari, E., von Gunten, A., Imhof, A., Bouras, C., and Hof, P. R. 2007. Assessing the cognitive impact of Alzheimer disease pathology and vascular burden in the aging brain: The Geneva experience. *Acta Neuropathol* 113: 1–12.

Glabe, C. G., and Kayed, R. 2006. Common structure and toxic function of amyloid oligomers implies a common mechanism of pathogenesis. *Neurology* 66(2 Suppl 1): S74–78.

Goedert, M., Clavaguera, F., and Tolnay, M. 2010. The propagation of prion-like protein inclusions in neurodegenerative diseases. *Trends Neurosci* 33: 317–325.

Götz, J., Chen, F., van Dorpe, J., and Nitsch, R. M. 2001. Formation of neurofibrillary tangles in P301l tau transgenic mice induced by Abeta 42 fibrils. *Science* 293: 1491–1495.

Götz, J., and Ittner, L. M. 2008. Animal models of Alzheimer's disease and frontotemporal dementia. *Nat Rev Neurosci* 9: 532–544.

Guo, J. L., and Lee, V. M. 2011. Seeding of normal Tau by pathological Tau conformers drives pathogenesis of Alzheimer-like tangles. *J Biol Chem* 286: 15317–15331.

Haass, C., and Selkoe, D. J. 2007. Soluble protein oligomers in neurodegeneration: Lessons from the Alzheimer's amyloid beta-peptide. *Nat Rev Mol Cell Biol* 8: 101–112.

Hammarström, P., Simon, R., Nyström, S., Konradsson, P., Aslund, A., and Nilsson, K. P. 2010. A fluorescent pentameric thiophene derivative detects in vitro-formed prefibrillar protein aggregates. *Biochemistry* 49: 6838–6845.

Hansen, C., Angot, E., Bergström, A.L., Steiner, J. A., Pieri, L., Paul, G., Outeiro, T. F., Melki, R., Kallunki, P., Fog, K., Li, J. Y., and Brundin, P. 2011. α-Synuclein propagates from mouse brain to grafted dopaminergic neurons and seeds aggregation in cultured human cells. *J Clin Invest* 121: 715–725.

Hardy, J. 2005. Expression of normal sequence pathogenic proteins for neurodegenerative disease contributes to disease risk: "Permissive templating" as a general mechanism underlying neurodegeneration. *Biochem Soc Trans* 33: 578–581.

Hardy, J., and Selkoe, D. J. 2002. The amyloid hypothesis of Alzheimer's disease: Progress and problems on the road to therapeutics. *Science* 297: 353–356.

Hauw, J. J., and Duyckaerts, C. 2001. Alzheimer's disease. In *Pathology of the aging human nervous system*, ed. S. Duckett and J. C. de la Torre, 207–263. New York: Oxford University Press.

Heinrich, S. U., and Lindquist, S. 2011. Protein-only mechanism induces self-perpetuating changes in the activity of neuronal Aplysia cytoplasmic polyadenylation element binding protein (CPEB). *Proc Natl Acad Sci USA* 108: 2999–3004.

Hu, X., Crick, S. L., Bu, G., Frieden, C., Pappu, R. V., and Lee, J. M. 2009. Amyloid seeds formed by cellular uptake, concentration, and aggregation of the amyloid-beta peptide. *Proc Natl Acad Sci USA* 106: 20324–20329.

Ikonomovic, M. D., Klunk, W. E., Abrahamson, E. E., Mathis, C. A., Price, J. C., Tsopelas, N. D., Lopresti, B. J., Ziolko, S., Bi, W., Paljug, W. R., Debnath, M. L., Hope, C. E., Isanski, B. A., Hamilton, R. L., and DeKosky, S. T. 2008. Post-mortem correlates of in vivo PIB-PET amyloid imaging in a typical case of Alzheimer's disease. *Brain* 131: 1630–1645.

Jankowsky, J. L., Younkin, L. H., Gonzales, V., Fadale, D. J., Slunt, H. H., Lester, H. A., Younkin, S. G., and Borchelt, D. R. 2007. Rodent A beta modulates the solubility and distribution of amyloid deposits in transgenic mice. *J Biol Chem* 282: 22707–22720.

Johnson, K. A., Gregas, M., Becker, J. A., Kinnecom, C., Salat, D. H., Moran, E. K., Smith, E. E., Rosand, J., Rentz, D. M., Klunk, W. E., Mathis, C. A., Price, J. C., DeKosky, S. T., Fischman, A. J., and Greenberg, S. M. 2007. Imaging of amyloid burden and distribution in cerebral amyloid angiopathy. *Ann Neurol* 62: 229–234.

Johnson, R. T. 2005. Prion diseases. *Lancet Neurol* 4: 635–642.

Jucker, M. 2010. The benefits and limitations of animal models for translational research in neurodegenerative diseases. *Nat Med* 16: 1210–1214.

Kalback, W., Watson, M. D., Kokjohn, T. A., Kuo, Y. M., Weiss, N., Luehrs, D. C., Lopez, J., Brune, D., Sisodia, S. S., Staufenbiel, M., Emmerling, M., and Roher, A. E. 2002. APP transgenic mice Tg2576 accumulate Abeta peptides that are distinct from the chemically modified and insoluble peptides deposited in Alzheimer's disease senile plaques. *Biochemistry* 41: 922–928.

Kane, M. D., Lipinski, W. J., Callahan, M. J., Bian, F., Durham, R. A., Schwarz, R. D., Roher, A. E., and Walker, L. C. 2000. Evidence for seeding of beta-amyloid by intracerebral infusion of Alzheimer brain extracts in beta-amyloid precursor protein-transgenic mice. *J Neurosci* 20: 3606–3611.

Kawas, C., and Katzman, R. 1999. Epidemiology of dementia and Alzheimer disease. In *Alzheimer Disease*, ed. R. D. Terry, R. Katzman, K. L. Bick, and S. S. Sisodia, 95–116. Philadelphia: Lippincott Williams & Wilkins.

Kayed, R., Canto, I., Breydo, L., Rasool, S., Lukacsovich, T., Wu, J., Albay, R., III, Pensalfini, A., Yeung, S., Head, E., Marsh, J. L., and Glabe, C. 2010. Conformation dependent monoclonal antibodies distinguish different replicating strains or conformers of prefibrillar Aβ oligomers. *Mol Neurodegener* 5: 57.

Kikis, E. A., Gidalevitz, T., and Morimoto, R. I. 2010. Protein homeostasis in models of aging and age-related conformational disease. *Adv Exp Med Biol* 694: 138–159.

Klunk, W. E., Engler, H., Nordberg, A., Bacskai, B. J., Wang, Y., Price, J. C., Bergstrom, M., Hyman, B. T., Langstrom, B., and Mathis, C. A. 2003. Imaging the pathology of Alzheimer's disease: Amyloid-imaging with positron emission tomography. *Neuroimaging Clin N Am* 13: 781–789, ix.

Klunk, W. E., Engler, H., Nordberg, A., Wang, Y., Blomqvist, G., Holt, D. P., Bergstrom, M., Savitcheva, I., Huang, G. F., Estrada, S., Ausen, B., Debnath, M. L., Barletta, J., Price, J. C., Sandell, J., Lopresti, B. J., Wall, A., Koivisto, P., Antoni, G., Mathis, C. A., and Langstrom, B. 2004. Imaging brain amyloid in Alzheimer's disease with Pittsburgh Compound-B. *Ann Neurol* 55: 306–319.

Klunk, W. E., Lopresti, B. J., Ikonomovic, M. D., Lefterov, I. M., Koldamova, R. P., Abrahamson, E. E., Debnath, M. L., Holt, D. P., Huang, G. F., Shao, L., DeKosky, S. T., Price, J. C., and Mathis, C. A. 2005. Binding of the positron emission tomography tracer Pittsburgh compound-B reflects the amount of amyloid-beta in Alzheimer's disease brain but not in transgenic mouse brain. *J Neurosci* 25: 10598–10606.

Klunk, W. E., Wang, Y., Huang, G. F., Debnath, M. L., Holt, D. P., and Mathis, C. A. 2001. Uncharged thioflavin-T derivatives bind to amyloid-beta protein with high affinity and readily enter the brain. *Life Sci* 69: 1471–1484.

Kodali, R., and Wetzel, R. 2007. Polymorphism in the intermediates and products of amyloid assembly. *Curr Opinion Struct Biol* 17: 48–57.

Kodali, R., Williams, A. D., Chemuru, S., and Wetzel, R. 2010. Abeta(1-40) forms five distinct amyloid structures whose beta-sheet contents and fibril stabilities are correlated. *J Mol Biol* 401: 503–517.

Koo, E. H., Lansbury, P. T., Jr., and Kelly, J. W. 1999. Amyloid diseases: Abnormal protein aggregation in neurodegeneration. *Proc Natl Acad Sci USA* 96: 9989–9990.

Kovacs, G. G., and Budka, H. 2009. Molecular pathology of human prion diseases. *Int J Mol Sci* 10: 976–999.

Kuo, Y. M., Kokjohn, T. A., Beach, T. G., Sue, L. I., Brune, D., Lopez, J. C., Kalback, W. M., Abramowski, D., Sturchler-Pierrat, C., Staufenbiel, M., and Roher, A. E. 2001. Comparative analysis of amyloid-beta chemical structure and amyloid plaque morphology of transgenic mouse and Alzheimer's disease brains. *J Biol Chem* 276: 12991–12998.

Lambert, M. P., Velasco, P. T., Viola, K. L., and Klein, W. L. 2009. Targeting generation of antibodies specific to conformational epitopes of amyloid beta-derived neurotoxins. *CNS Neurol Disord Drug Targets* 8: 65–81.

Langer, F., Eisele, Y. S., Fritschi, S. K., et al. 2011. Soluble Aβ seeds are potent inducers of cerebral β-amyloid deposition. *J Neurosci* 31: 14488–14495.

Lansbury, P. T., Jr. 1997. Structural neurology: Are seeds at the root of neuronal degeneration? *Neuron* 19: 1151–1154.

Lee, V. M-Y., Goedert, M., and Trojanowski, J. Q. 2001. Neurodegenerative tauopathies. *Annu Rev Neurosci* 24: 1121–1159.

Legname, G., Baskakov, I. V., Nguyen, H. O., Riesner, D., Cohen, F. E., DeArmond, S. J., and Prusiner, S. B. 2004. Synthetic mammalian prions. *Science* 305: 673–676.

Leinonen, V., Alafuzoff, I., Aalto, S., Suotunen, T., Savolainen, S., Nagren, K., Tapiola, T., Pirttila, T., Rinne, J., Jaaskelainen, J. E., Soininen, H., and Rinne, J. O. 2008. Assessment of {beta}-amyloid in a frontal cortical brain biopsy specimen and by positron emission tomography with carbon 11-labeled Pittsburgh Compound B. *Arch Neurol* 65: 1304–1309.

Lesne, S., Koh, M. T., Kotilinek, L., Kayed, R., Glabe, C. G., Yang, A., Gallagher, M., and Ashe, K. H. 2006. A specific amyloid-beta protein assembly in the brain impairs memory. *Nature* 440: 352–357.

LeVine, H., III, and Walker, L. C. 2006. Models of Alzheimer's disease. In *Handbook of models for human aging*, ed. P. M. Conn, 121–134. Burlington, MA: Academic Press.

LeVine, H., III, and Walker, L. C. 2010. Molecular polymorphism of Abeta in Alzheimer's disease. *Neurobiol Aging* 31: 542–548.

Li, Y., Rinne, J. O., Mosconi, L., Pirraglia, E., Rusinek, H., Desanti, S., Kemppainen, N., Nagren, K., Kim, B. C., Tsui, W., and de Leon, M. J. 2008. Regional analysis of FDG and PIB-PET images in normal aging, mild cognitive impairment, and Alzheimer's disease. *Eur J Nuc Med Mol Imaging* 35: 2169–2181.

Lockhart, A., Ye, L., Judd, D. B., Merritt, A. T., Lowe, P. N., Morgenstern, J. L., Hong, G., Gee, A. D., and Brown, J. 2005. Evidence for the presence of three distinct binding sites for the thioflavin T class of Alzheimer's disease PET imaging agents on beta-amyloid peptide fibrils. *J Biol Chem* 280: 7677–7684.

Luheshi, L. M., and Dobson, C. M. 2009. Bridging the gap: From protein misfolding to protein misfolding diseases. *FEBS Lett* 583: 2581–2586.

Luk, K. C., Song, C., O'Brien, P., Stieber, A., Branch, J. R., Brunden, K. R., Trojanowski, J. Q., and Lee, V. M. 2009. Exogenous alpha-synuclein fibrils seed the formation of Lewy body-like intracellular inclusions in cultured cells. *Proc Natl Acad Sci USA* 106: 20051–20056.

Lundmark, K., Westermark, G. T., Olsen, A., and Westermark, P. 2005. Protein fibrils in nature can enhance amyloid protein A amyloidosis in mice: Cross-seeding as a disease mechanism. *Proc Natl Acad Sci USA* 102: 6098–6102.

Maeda, J., Ji, B., Irie, T., Tomiyama, T., Maruyama, M., Okauchi, T., Staufenbiel, M., Iwata, N., Ono, M., Saido, T. C., Suzuki, K., Mori, H., Higuchi, M., and Suhara, T. 2007. Longitudinal, quantitative assessment of amyloid, neuroinflammation, and anti-amyloid treatment in a living mouse model of Alzheimer's disease enabled by positron emission tomography. *J Neurosci* 27: 10957–10968.

Makarava, N., and Baskakov, I. V. 2008. The same primary structure of the prion protein yields two distinct self-propagating states. *J Biol Chem* 283: 15988–15996.

Maury, C. P. 2009. The emerging concept of functional amyloid. *J Intern Med* 265(3): 329–334.

McKintosh, E., Tabrizi, S. J., Collinge, J. 2003. Prion diseases. *J Neurovirol* 9: 183–193.

Meyer-Luehmann, M., Coomaraswamy, J., Bolmont, T., Kaeser, S., Schaefer, C., Kilger, E., Neuenschwander, A., Abramowski, D., Frey, P., Jaton, A. L., Vigouret, J. M., Paganetti, P., Walsh, D. M., Mathews, P. M., Ghiso, J., Staufenbiel, M., Walker, L. C., and Jucker, M. 2006. Exogenous induction of cerebral beta-amyloidogenesis is governed by agent and host. *Science* 313: 1781–1784.

Miller, G. 2009. Neurodegeneration. Could they all be prion diseases? *Science* 326: 1337–1339.

Morales, R., Estrada, L. D., Diaz-Espinoza, R., Morales-Scheihing, D., Jara, M. C., Castilla, J., and Soto, C. 2010. Molecular cross talk between misfolded proteins in animal models of Alzheimer's and prion diseases. *J Neurosci* 30: 4528–4535.

Morales, R., Duran-Aniotz, C., Castilla, J., et al. 2011. De novo induction of amyloid-β deposition in vivo. *Mol Psychiatry*. [Epub ahead of print]

Morrissette, D. A., Parachikova, A., Green, K. N., and LaFerla, F. M. 2009. Relevance of transgenic mouse models to human Alzheimer disease. *J Biol Chem* 284: 6033–6037.

Münch, C., O'Brien, J., and Bertolotti, A. 2011. Prion-like propagation of mutant superoxide dismutase-1 misfolding in neuronal cells. *Proc Natl Acad Sci USA* 108: 3548–3553.

Nelissen, N., Vandenbulcke, M., Fannes, K., Verbruggen, A., Peeters, R., Dupont, P., Van Laere, K., Bormans, G., and Vandenberghe, R. 2007. Abeta amyloid deposition in the language system and how the brain responds. *Brain* 130: 2055–2069.

Nerelius, C., Johansson, J., and Sandegren, A. 2009. Amyloid beta-peptide aggregation. What does it result in and how can it be prevented? *Front Biosci* 14: 1716–1729.

Nilsson, K. P., Aslund, A., Berg, I., Nyström, S., Konradsson, P., Herland, A., Inganas, O., Stabo-Eeg, F., Lindgren, M., Westermark, G. T., Lannfelt, L., Nilsson, L. N., and Hammarström, P. 2007. Imaging distinct conformational states of amyloid-beta fibrils in Alzheimer's disease using novel luminescent probes. *ACS Chem Biol* 2: 553–560.

Nilsson, K. P., Ikenberg, K., Aslund, A., Fransson, S., Konradsson, P., Röcken, C., Moch, H., and Aguzzi, A. 2010b. Structural typing of systemic amyloidoses by luminescent-conjugated polymer spectroscopy. *Am J Pathol* 176: 563–574.

Nilsson, K. P., Joshi-Barr, S., Winson, O., and Sigurdson, C. J. 2010a. Prion strain interactions are highly selective. *J Neurosci* 30: 12094–12102.

Nordberg, A. 2008. Amyloid plaque imaging in vivo: Current achievement and future prospects. *Eur J Nuc Med Mol Imaging* 35 Suppl 1: S46–50.

O'Nuallain, B., Williams, A. D., Westermark, P., and Wetzel, R. 2004. Seeding specificity in amyloid growth induced by heterologous fibrils. *J Biol Chem* 279: 17490–17499.

Oddo, S., Caccamo, A., Tseng, B., Cheng, D., Vasilevko, V., Cribbs, D. H., and LaFerla, F. M. 2008. Blocking Abeta42 accumulation delays the onset and progression of tau pathology via the C terminus of heat shock protein70-interacting protein: A mechanistic link between Abeta and tau pathology. *J Neurosci* 28: 12163–12175.

Otvos Jr, L., Szendrei, G. I., Lee, V. M-Y., and Mantsch, H. H. 1993. Human and rodent Alzheimer beta-amyloid peptides acquire distinct conformations in membrane-mimicking solvents. *Eur J Biochem* 211: 249–257.

Paravastu, A. K., Leapman, R. D., Yau, W. M., and Tycko, R. 2008. Molecular structural basis for polymorphism in Alzheimer's beta-amyloid fibrils. *Proc Natl Acad Sci USA* 105: 18349–18354.

Paravastu, A. K., Qahwash, I., Leapman, R. D., Meredith, S. C., and Tycko, R. 2009. Seeded growth of beta-amyloid fibrils from Alzheimer's brain-derived fibrils produces a distinct fibril structure. *Proc Natl Acad Sci USA* 106: 7443–7448.

Pedersen, J. S., and Otzen, D. E. 2008. Amyloid-a state in many guises: Survival of the fittest fibril fold. *Protein Sci* 17: 2–10.

Peretz, D., Williamson, R. A., Legname, G., Matsunaga, Y., Vergara, J., Burton, D. R., DeArmond, S. J., Prusiner, S. B., and Scott, M. R. 2002. A change in the conformation of prions accompanies the emergence of a new prion strain. *Neuron* 34: 921–932.

Petkova, A. T., Leapman, R. D., Guo, Z., Yau, W. M., Mattson, M. P., and Tycko, R. 2005. Self-propagating, molecular-level polymorphism in Alzheimer's beta-amyloid fibrils. *Science* 307: 262–265.

Petkova, A. T., Yau, W. M., and Tycko, R. 2006. Experimental constraints on quaternary structure in Alzheimer's beta-amyloid fibrils. *Biochemistry* 45: 498–512.

Prusiner, S. B. 1995. The prion diseases. *Sci Am* 272: 48–51, 54–47.

Prusiner, S. B. 2001. Shattuck lecture: Neurodegenerative diseases and prions. *New Engl J Med* 344: 1516–1526.

Prusiner, S. B. 2004. *Prion biology and diseases*. Cold Spring Harbor, NY: CSHL Press.

Querfurth, H. W., and LaFerla, F. M. 2010. Alzheimer's disease. *New Engl J Med* 362: 329–344.

Ren, P. H., Lauckner, J. E., Kachirskaia, I., Heuser, J. E., Melki, R., and Kopito, R. R. 2009. Cytoplasmic penetration and persistent infection of mammalian cells by polyglutamine aggregates. *Nat Cell Biol* 11: 219–225.

Rinne, J. O., Brooks, D. J., Rossor, M. N., Fox, N. C., Bullock, R., Klunk, W. E., Mathis, C. A., Blennow, K., Barakos, J., Okello, A. A., Rodriguez Martinez de Liano, S., Liu, E., Koller, M., Gregg, K. M., Schenk, D., Black, R., and Grundman, M. 2010. 11C-PiB PET assessment of change in fibrillar amyloid-beta load in patients with Alzheimer's disease treated with bapineuzumab: A phase 2, double-blind, placebo-controlled, ascending-dose study. *Lancet Neurol* 9: 363–372.

Rosen, R. F., Ciliax, B. J., Wingo, T. S., Gearing, M., Dooyema, J., Lah, J. J., Ghiso, J. A., LeVine, H., III, and Walker, L. C. 2010. Deficient high-affinity binding of Pittsburgh compound B in a case of Alzheimer's disease. *Acta Neuropathol* 119: 221–233.

Rosen, R. F., Farberg, A. S., Gearing, M., Dooyema, J., Long, P. M., Anderson, D. C., Davis-Turak, J., Coppola, G., Geschwind, D. H., Pare, J. F., Duong, T. Q., Hopkins, W. D., Preuss, T. M., and Walker, L. C. 2008. Tauopathy with paired helical filaments in an aged chimpanzee. *J Comp Neurol* 509: 259–270.

Rosen, R. F., Fritz, J. J., Dooyema, J., et al. 2011a. Exogenous seeding of cerebral β-amyloid deposition in βAPP-transgenic rats. *J Neurochem.* [Epub ahead of print]

Rosen, R. F., Walker, L. C., and LeVine, H., III. 2011b. PIB binding in aged primate brain: Enrichment of high-affinity sites in humans with Alzheimer's disease. *Neurobiol Aging* 32: 223–234.

Rowe, C. C., Ng, S., Ackermann, U., Gong, S. J., Pike, K., Savage, G., Cowie, T. F., Dickinson, K. L., Maruff, P., Darby, D., Smith, C., Woodward, M., Merory, J., Tochon-Danguy, H., O'Keefe, G., Klunk, W. E., Mathis, C. A., Price, J. C., Masters, C. L., and Villemagne, V. L. 2007. Imaging beta-amyloid burden in aging and dementia. *Neurology* 68: 1718–1725.

Selkoe, D. J. 1999. Biology of beta-amyloid precursor protein and the mechanism of Alzheimer disease. In *Alzheimer Disease*, ed. R. D. Terry, R. Katzman, K. L. Bick, and S. S. Sisodia, 293–310. Philadelphia: Lippincott Williams & Wilkins.

Sigurdson, C. J., Nilsson, K. P., Hornemann, S., Manco, G., Polymenidou, M., Schwarz, P., Leclerc, M., Hammarström, P., Wuthrich, K., and Aguzzi, A. 2007. Prion strain discrimination using luminescent conjugated polymers. *Nat Methods* 4: 1023–1030.

Sigurdsson, E. M., Wisniewski, T., and Frangione, B. 2002. Infectivity of amyloid diseases. *Trends Mol Med* 8: 411–413.

Soto, C., Estrada, L., and Castilla, J. 2006. Amyloids, prions and the inherent infectious nature of misfolded protein aggregates. *Trends Biochem Sci* 31: 150–155.

Soto, C., and Satani, N. 2011. The intricate mechanisms of neurodegeneration in prion diseases. *Trends Mol Med* 17: 14–24.

Svedberg, M. M., Hall, H., Hellstrom-Lindahl, E., Estrada, S., Guan, Z., Nordberg, A., and Langstrom, B. 2009. [(11)C]PIB-amyloid binding and levels of Abeta40 and Abeta42 in postmortem brain tissue from Alzheimer patients. *Neurochem Int* 54: 347–357.

Tanaka, M., Collins, S. R., Toyama, B. H., and Weissman, J. S. 2006. The physical basis of how prion conformations determine strain phenotypes. *Nature* 442: 585–589.

Van Everbroeck, B., Pals, P., Martin, J. J., and Cras, P. 2002. Transmissible spongiform encephalopathies: The story of a pathogenic protein. *Peptides* 23: 1351–1359.

Walker, L. C., Bian, F., Callahan, M. J., Lipinski, W. J., Durham, R. A., and LeVine, H., III. 2002a. Modeling Alzheimer's disease and other proteopathies in vivo: Is seeding the key? *Amino Acids* 23: 87–93.

Walker, L. C., Callahan, M. J., Bian, F., Durham, R. A., Roher, A. E., and Lipinski, W. J. 2002b. Exogenous induction of cerebral beta-amyloidosis in betaAPP-transgenic mice. *Peptides* 23: 1241–1247.

Walker, L. C., and Cork, L. C. 1999. The neurobiology of aging in nonhuman primates. In *Alzheimer Disease*, ed. R. D. Terry, R. Katzman, K. L. Bick, and S. S. Sisodia, 233–243. Philadelphia: Lippincott Williams & Wilkins.

Walker, L. C., and LeVine, H., III. 2000a. Protein conformational diseases: The case for new semantic currency. *Neurobiol Aging* 21: 567.

Walker, L. C., and LeVine, H., III. 2000b. The cerebral proteopathies. *Neurobiol Aging* 21: 559–561.

Walker, L. C., and LeVine, H., III. 2002. Proteopathy: The next therapeutic frontier? *Curr Opin Investig Drugs* 3: 782–787.

Walker, L., LeVine, H., III, and Jucker, M. 2006a. Koch's postulates and infectious proteins. *Acta Neuropathol* 112: 1–4.

Walker, L. C., LeVine, H., III, Mattson, M. P., and Jucker, M. 2006b. Inducible proteopathies. *Trends Neurosci* 29: 438–443.

Walker, L. C., Rosen, R. F., and LeVine, H., III, 2008. Diversity of Abeta deposits in the aged brain: A window on molecular heterogeneity? *Rom J Morphol and Embryol* 49: 5–11.

Walker, L. C., Rosen, R. F., Fritz, J. J., Betarbet, R., Lah, J. J., LeVine, H., III, and Jucker, M. 2010. Prion-like induction of Alzheimer-type proteopathy in transgenic rodents. In *Prion 2010*, 1–6. Pianoro, Italy: Medimond International Proceedings.

Walsh, D. M., and Selkoe, D. J. 2007. Abeta oligomers—a decade of discovery. *J Neurochem* 101: 1172–1184.

Wang, F., Wang, X., Yuan, C. G., and Ma, J. 2010. Generating a prion with bacterially expressed recombinant prion protein. *Science* 327: 1132–1135.

Watts, J. C., Giles, K., Grillo, S. K., Lemus, A., DeArmond, S. J., and Prusiner, S. B. 2011. Bioluminescence imaging of Abeta deposition in bigenic mouse models of Alzheimer's disease. *Proc Natl Acad Sci USA* 108: 2528–2533.

Westermark, G. T., and Westermark, P. 2010. Prion-like aggregates: Infectious agents in human disease. *Trends Mol Med* 16: 501–507.

Westermark, P., Lundmark, K., and Westermark, G. T. 2009. Fibrils from designed non-amyloid-related synthetic peptides induce AA-amyloidosis during inflammation in an animal model. *PLoS One* 4(6): e6041, doi:10.1371/journal.pone.0006041.

Wickner, R. B., Shewmaker, F., Edskes, H., Kryndushkin, D., Nemecek, J., McGlinchey, R., Bateman, D., and Winchester, C. L. 2010. Prion amyloid structure explains templating: How proteins can be genes. *FEMS Yeast Res* 10: 980–991.

Wilcock, G. K., and Esiri, M. M. 1982. Plaques, tangles and dementia. A quantitative study. *J Neurol Sci* 56: 343–356.

Yagi, H., Ban, T., Morigaki, K., Naiki, H., and Goto, Y. 2007. Visualization and classification of amyloid beta supramolecular assemblies. *Biochemistry* 46: 15009–15017.

Yagi, H., Kusaka, E., Hongo, K., Mizobata, T., and Kawata, Y. 2005. Amyloid fibril formation of alpha-synuclein is accelerated by preformed amyloid seeds of other proteins: Implications for the mechanism of transmissible conformational diseases. *J Biol Chem* 280: 38609–38616.

Yan, J., Fu, X., Ge, F., Zhang, B., Yao, J., Zhang, H., Qian, J., Tomozawa, H., Naiki, H., Sawashita, J., Mori, M., and Higuchi, K. 2007. Cross-seeding and cross-competition in mouse apolipoprotein A-II amyloid fibrils and protein A amyloid fibrils. *Am J Pathol* 171: 172–180.

Ye, L., Morgenstern, J. L., Gee, A. D., Hong, G., Brown, J., and Lockhart, A. 2005. Delineation of positron emission tomography imaging agent binding sites on beta-amyloid peptide fibrils. *J Biol Chem* 280: 23599–23604.

Ye, L., Morgenstern, J. L., Lamb, J. R., and Lockhart, A. 2006. Characterisation of the binding of amyloid imaging tracers to rodent Abeta fibrils and rodent-human Abeta co-polymers. *Biochem Biophys Res Comm* 347: 669–677.

8 Traumatic Brain Injury in the Development of Alzheimer's Disease: Risk Factors, Diagnosis, and Treatment Strategies

Mark P. Burns

CONTENTS

8.1 TRAUMATIC BRAIN INJURY: THE STATISTICS

According to the Centers for Disease Control, each year 1.7 million people receive a traumatic brain injury (TBI) severe enough to result in an emergency room visit. Of this number, 1.3 million will be treated and released, 275,000 will be hospitalized, and 52,000 will die. In the United States, it is estimated that 5 million Americans are living with a TBI-related disability, costing an estimated $60 billion a year (Faul et al., 2010).

These numbers, however, may underestimate the impact of TBI as they only represent hospital-reported injuries. Up to 75% of emergency room TBIs that occur each year are concussions or other forms of "mild" TBI. However, it is known that the majority of mild TBIs, especially sports-related concussions and subconcussive blows, go unreported. Estimates of the actual number of TBIs that occur each year are as high as 3.8 million (Langlois, Rutland-Brown, and Wald, 2006).

There are a number of at-risk age groups. Those under the age of 4, teenagers aged 15 to 19, and the elderly aged over 65. Males have a threefold greater incidence of TBI than females, and once an initial TBI has occurred, the relative risk of a recurrent TBI is three times that of the normal population. Adults aged 75 and older have the highest rate of TBI-related emergency room visits and deaths.

What makes studying the long-term effects of brain trauma a difficult process is that there are so many variations of brain trauma. The term *TBI* is an all-encompassing term that includes all severities of TBI (mild, moderate, and severe). The wide variety of TBI causes and clinical manifestations that may occur afterward are apparent when studying the TBI literature. TBI can occur with and without loss of consciousness, fractures, hemorrhages, or lacerations. It can occur as a result of a blow (a fall, car crash, or strike to the head). It can occur without any impact, such as the acceleration and deceleration injuries seen in whiplash. And it can occur in multiple phases, such as in blast injury (consists of 4 different phases of possible head injury). As each type of injury involves different patterns of cell stress and death, extrapolating the long-term outcomes in these very diverse categories is extremely difficult. The purpose of this chapter is to discuss the latest epidemiological, pathological, biochemical, and behavioral studies that may shed some light on the risk of developing Alzheimer's disease (AD) and similar dementias after TBI.

8.2 EPIDEMIOLOGY OF A DISEASE: SINGLE TBI AND THE RISK OF AD

Given that TBI alone can result in significant cognitive impairment, resolving the relative risk of TBI causing dementia later in life is a difficult prospect. The detrimental consequences of repeat TBI in sports, such as that reported with dementia pugilistica in boxers, has been well documented and will be discussed at the end of the chapter. In this section we will discuss the epidemiological data that argues for and against a role of a single head trauma in the development of AD.

Several retrospective and prospective trials have been conducted, and a significant number report that there is no effect of TBI on the development of AD (Shalat et al., 1987; Katzman et al., 1989; Broe et al., 1990; Fratiglioni et al., 1993; Tsolaki et al., 1997). Conversely, there are many reports that find a positive interaction between brain trauma and AD, with reported relative risk (RR) increasing from two-fold (O'Meara et al., 1997) to fourteen-fold (Rasmusson et al., 1995).

To help understand the implications of these studies, two in-depth meta-analyses have been conducted. The first analyzed 11 case-controlled studies (Mortimer et al., 1991). Alone, these studies found that TBI increased the risk of developing AD with odds ratios from 0.6 to 6.0. However, none of the published studies had a more than 41% chance of detecting an odds ratio of 2.0. In contrast, the meta-analysis of the pooled data from these studies had a power of 97% to identify a similar odds ratio. Analysis of this pooled data revealed a relative risk of 1.82 (95% confidence interval [CI]: 1.26–2.67). Further analysis of the data revealed a slightly higher risk of developing sporadic AD after TBI (RR: 2.31; CI: 1.17–4.84) compared to familial AD after TBI (RR: 1.42; CI: 0.76–2.71). Unlike earlier reports, the authors did not reveal a significant effect of TBI on the age of onset of dementia, with those developing

AD under the age of 70 being very similar to those developing AD over 70. The time between TBI and the onset of disease was also a significant factor (Mortimer et al., 1991). As first reported by Graves et al., the estimated risk of AD increased as the time between the last brain injury event and the onset of disease symptoms diminished (Graves et al., 1990). This trend remained statistically significant when head injuries occurring within 5 years of onset of the disease were excluded from the analysis. This was upheld in the meta-analysis with head trauma occurring less than 10 years prior to disease onset increasing relative risk to 5.33. For those with the TBI occurring more than 10 years prior to disease the risk was only 1.63 (Mortimer et al., 1991). Another robust finding from the meta-analysis was the very different outcome between the sexes. Women are already much less likely to succumb to TBI than men; however, they also appear to be much less likely to develop AD after TBI than men. Males have a relative risk of 2.67 (CI: 1.64–4.41), while for females the risk is only 0.85 (CI: 0.43–1.70) (Mortimer et al., 1991).

More than a decade later, another group undertook a similar project and performed another meta-analysis (Fleminger et al., 2003). This study required that studies meet seven criteria to be included:

1. Head trauma with loss of consciousness
2. Matching of case and control subjects
3. National Institute of Neurological Disorders and Stroke /Alzheimer's Disease and Related Disorders Association (NINDS-ADRDA) criteria for diagnosis of AD
4. Inclusion criteria for controls
5. Symmetrical data collection from cases and controls
6. Recruitment of controls had to be outside of psychiatric departments
7. TBI must have occurred prior to the onset of AD

Fleminger and colleagues ended up with 15 studies that met their initial criteria: 8 predated, and 7 postdated, Mortimer et al. (1991). A separate analysis of the 7 postdated studies found no significant·interaction between TBI and AD. However, a full analysis of all 15 studies found a risk of 1.58 (CI: 1.21–2.06). Again, the sex differences were upheld, with the excess risk of head trauma in those with AD found only in males (RR: 2.29; CI: 1.47–2.06) and not in females (RR: 0.91; CI 0.56–1.47). The difference between males and females found in these studies helped spark renewed interest in the role of female sex hormones for the treatment of TBI. The neuroprotective effects of progesterone in animal models of TBI have been well documented (Roof et al., 1994; Roof et al., 1996), and recent early-stage clinical trials have found that progesterone can reduce mortality and improve recovery after TBI (Wright et al., 2007; Xiao et al., 2008). Progesterone had just entered a stage III clinical trial for the treatment of brain injury (ProTECT III: Progesterone for Traumatic Brain Injury, Experimental Clinical Treatment). At this stage it is too early to determine if progesterone will also reduce the risk of developing AD after TBI.

The epidemiology of both AD and TBI are also dominated by one genetic risk factor: APOE genotype. APOE encodes for a protein, apolipoprotein E (apoE). ApoE is a polymorphic protein that is primarily a lipid transport molecule in the brain and periphery. Three different isoforms exist in humans: apoE2, apoE3, and apoE4. These are the end products of three alleles that are encoded on a single gene locus on chromosome 19 (e2, e3, and e4). ApoE genotype changes the risk of developing late-onset AD from 20% in non-E4 people to over 90% in apoE4 homozygotes (Corder et al., 1993). Not only does the apoE genotype act as a risk factor for developing the disease, but it also has an impact on the age of disease onset. The average age of onset for AD decreases from 84 in non-E4 carriers to 68 years in apoE4 homozygotes (Corder et al., 1993). ApoE genotype is also strongly predictive of outcome in patients with severe TBI. The presence of an apoE4 allele is linked to a poor recovery from extended coma (Sorbi et al., 1995), and the odds of a poor prognosis (suboptimal functional recovery) increased by fourteen-fold (Friedman et al., 1999). In a study of 236 community-dwelling elderly persons, Mayeux and colleagues found that TBI did not alter the odds of developing AD, but the presence of an apoE4 allele increased the risk of developing AD by two. The combination of TBI and apoE4 together increased the risk of developing AD by ten (Mayeux et al., 1995). This interaction was not upheld in a recent study of a Seattle-based population aged 60 or older (O'Meara et al., 1997). O'Meara and colleagues found an elevated risk of AD in male (RR = 4.2), but not female (RR = 1.1), TBI patients. They did not, however, find any interaction of the apoE4 allele with susceptibility to AD (O'Meara et al., 1997).

Another important mediator of AD risk involves the concept of cognitive reserve. This concept is based on the idea that having increased neurons or synapses allows the brain to maintain function for a longer period of time before succumbing to AD. The protective effect of the cognitive reserve may be observed in the increased risk of developing AD in those with low levels of education (high education 1.0; medium education 1.44; low education 1.80 [Caamano-Isorna et al., 2006]). Cognitive decline after TBI is also linked to poor pre-injury cognitive testing ability. In a study of Vietnam veterans with a history of penetrating injury suffered more than 30 years before, the authors found that TBI exacerbated long-term cognitive decline, but this did not lead to a clinical diagnosis of dementia (Raymont et al., 2008). They did find that pre-injury intelligence was predictive of cognitive decline after penetrating head trauma. A higher baseline score before injury acted in a protective manner and predicted a higher intelligence score more than 30 years after injury (Raymont et al., 2008).

The final note on the risk of developing AD after TBI focuses on injury severity. In most of the analysis mentioned preciously, the inclusion criterion was loss of consciousness. In studies where the criteria are more broadly defined, we can analyze the relative risk from head trauma of differing severity. In a study of World War II Navy and Marine (male) veterans, the authors characterized three severities of injury: mild (loss of consciousness/amnesia less than 30 minutes with no skull fracture), moderate (loss of consciousness/amnesia more than 30 minutes but less than 24 hours, and/or skull fracture), or severe (loss of consciousness/amnesia greater than 24 hours) (Plassman et al., 2000). The injuries were sustained in 1944–1945, and were found in the military medical records to avoid recall bias. Participants were followed up in 1996–1997 and assessed for AD or other dementias. 548 veterans with head injury and 1228 without head injury (but with either pneumonia or non-head-injury wounds) completed the multistage procedure. The authors found that moderate head trauma (RR: 2.32; CI: 1.04–5.17) and severe head trauma (RR: 4.51; CI: 1.77–11.47) increased the risk of developing AD, but mild TBI did not. An interesting point to note is that the authors also found a very similar risk of developing non-AD-type dementia. Moderate (RR: 2.39; CI: 1.24–4.58) and severe (RR: 4.28; CI 2.09–9.63) TBI increased the risk of developing dementia, but mild TBI did not. The data are very similar for both AD and dementia, suggesting that TBI increases the risk of all dementias, not just dementia of the Alzheimer's type.

In conclusion, the data seems to support a role for TBI in the development of dementias, including AD. As the epidemiological studies listed do not include postmortem confirmation of pathology, it is impossible to determine the type of dementia suffered by patients who previously suffered TBI, and therefore the data should be interpreted with caution. However, what is apparent is that the risk of developing dementia after TBI is dependent on injury severity, and may only affect males. Risk factors important in AD also appear to be important for TBI-induced dementia, including APOE genotype and cognitive reserve at time of injury.

8.3 SINGLE TBI CAUSES AD-LIKE PATHOLOGY

Epidemiological evidence shows that TBI is a risk-factor for the development of AD, and certainly there is a large amount of information available that suggests that AD-related pathways are activated immediately after TBI. This section will examine the pathological and biochemical data that hint at the etiology of this risk.

AD is a progressive neurodegenerative disease, which can only be fully diagnosed at autopsy. It is characterized histologically by the presence of amyloid plaques and neurofibrillary tangles in the brain. The amyloid plaques consist of aggregated proteinaceous material, a major component of which is Aβ. The neurofibrillary tangles are composed of paired helical filaments (PHF) of the microtubule-associated phosphoprotein, tau. For almost two decades, the amyloid cascade hypothesis has focused on how Aβ is generated, how it impacts cellular function, and how it promotes the pathobiology of tau.

Aβ is produced by sequential cleavage of the amyloid precursor protein (APP) by two enzymes, β- and γ-secretase. Depending on the cleavage point of γ-secretase, Aβ peptides of different amino acid length are produced. The two most closely linked to AD are Aβ40 and Aβ42. The accumulation of Aβ peptides is thought to be a major initiating event in AD pathogenesis.

In humans, the first studies to examine Aβ deposition after a severe TBI occurred in 1991 (Roberts et al. 1991). Roberts and colleagues examined the brains of 16 patients who died within 18 days of TBI and found that 38% of the patients had Aβ deposits. While most of these deposits were diffuse plaques, some classic and vascular deposits were also noted. The ages of the patients with Aβ deposition were 45 to 63. Three years later, the same group published a more in-depth study of amyloid pathology in 152 TBI patients (Roberts et al. 1994). They found that 30% of subjects had Aβ deposits after TBI, the youngest of which was just 10 years old. A detailed look at the published data yields interesting results: No control cases under the age of 60 had amyloid plaques. In TBI cases under 40 years old, only 20% had plaques. This increased to 27% in the 41–50 age group, and 60% in the 51–60 age group. In the 60–80 age category, 50%

of controls had plaques, and this increased to 70% after TBI. Similar to the authors' earlier study, it was noted that the majority of amyloid plaques were diffuse plaques, with neuritic plaques restricted to the oldest cases. The group noticed that falling was the most common type of injury associated with Aβ deposition, and did not notice a significant effect of skull fracture, diffuse axonal injury (DAI), hypoxia, sex, degree of coma, intracranial pressure (ICP), blood pressure, or survival time (Roberts et al. 1994). Later studies noted that Aβ42 appeared to be the predominant form of amyloid deposited after TBI (Gentleman et al. 1997).

These groundbreaking postmortem studies were the first to note that the TBI process was causing the accumulation of amyloid peptides after injury. In an elegant 2004 study, a group from the University of Pittsburgh demonstrated just how rapidly this event could occur in living survivors of TBI (Ikonomovic et al. 2004). Their sample set was 18 patients who had severe TBI and had a Glasgow Coma Score of less than 9. The patients underwent decompressive craniotomy to relieve intractable swelling or to remove severely damaged brain tissue. For most of the patients, this surgery was performed between 2 and 19 hours after injury. Showing remarkable similarity to earlier studies, the authors found that 33% of patients had Aβ deposits, again primarily consisting of the Aβ42 peptide. Plaques were once again diffuse, with most being negative for Thioflavin S. The investigators in this study did not restrict themselves to extracellular Aβ deposits, but also examined intracellular Aβ staining. They found that neuronal or glial intracellular Aβ staining occurred in more than 80% of cases (Ikonomovic et al. 2004). A later follow-up study of the same sample set showed that soluble Aβ (measured by enzyme-linked immunosorbent assay [ELISA]) was increased in the TBI group, but the plaque-positive group had significantly higher levels of Aβ42 (DeKosky et al. 2007).

Excess axonal APP immunoreactivity occurs very quickly after death in DAI, and is used as a primary measure of DAI in postmortem tissue. This accumulation is thought to be due to the disruption of fast axonal transport, the mechanism by which APP is transported in the neuronal axon. In a study designed to examine Aβ production in relation to axonal injury, Uryu and colleagues examined 18 cases of human TBI (time of death: 4 hours to 5 weeks after TBI) (Uryu et al. 2007). The authors found axonal injury was recognizable by the accumulation of APP or neurofilament, and immunohistochemical detection of Aβ showed that this peptide was accumulating in damaged axons. The number of axonal profiles increased with survival time. Also, many of the axonal bulbs stained positive for Aβ42, but not for Aβ40. Aβ staining was seen in both young and old patients, and the investigators were able to localize APP, β-secretase, and γ-secretase proteins in the same axonal swellings.

As mentioned in the previous section, ApoE4 genotype is an important risk factor for the development of AD after TBI (Mayeux et al. 1995). ApoE genotype is also a factor for the development of amyloid plaques after TBI. The presence of the apoE4 allele has a gene dose effect, with only 10% of patients with no apoE4 alleles having amyloid plaques. This increases to 35% with one apoE4 allele, and 100% of cases with 2 apoE4 alleles with all cases having amyloid plaques (Nicoll, Roberts, and Graham 1995).

Although amyloid pathology has been well documented after cases of severe TBI, there is not much data describing changes in tau pathology in humans. In two of the studies outlined above (Ikonomovic et al. 2004; Uryu et al. 2007) tau pathology was looked for at the same time as amyloid pathology. Ikonomovic et al. found evidence of PHF-1 positive immunoreactive axons in the white matter of almost all TBI subjects; however, they only saw somatodendritic PHF-1 staining in 2 out of 18 cases, both of which were amyloid plaque negative (Ikonomovic et al. 2004). Both of these cases were of advanced age, and the inclusions were ThioS positive. In the second study, Uryu and colleagues also found PHF-1 positive immunoreactivity in 2 out of 18 cases. The tau staining was observed in axons and in clusters of neuronal cell bodies in the cerebral cortex. They also noted the existence of tau-positive reactive astrocytes (Uryu et al. 2007), a pathology that is not usually observed in AD.

There are multiple types of in vivo mechanical injury paradigms that model TBI in animals. These models have been used to examine the production, aggregation, and accumulation of Aβ after injury. The most commonly used type of injury is a contusion injury directly on the cortex, and has been employed in both mice and rats. The simpler version of this protocol involves the controlled release of a fixed weight onto the skull of an anesthetized rodent. The more complex controlled cortical impact (CCI) model involves a very regulated and reproducible injury administered via a computer-controlled pneumatic device, usually onto the exposed brain of a rodent.

Due to methodological constraints, many of the early studies relied on immunohistochemistry to look for amyloid accumulation after injury. The major constraint with this approach is that many of the antibodies available at that time were either human Aβ specific with no cross-reactivity to rodent Aβ, or antibodies that detected both human and mouse Aβ, but also cross-reacted with full length APP. As such, many of the early papers should be interpreted with care. Many of these issues have been resolved as cleavage site–specific antibodies have become available, and with the introduction of APP transgenic and knock-in mice, as well as human- and mouse-specific ELISAs.

Despite a streamlining of methodological techniques, the data from transgenic mice has provided somewhat erratic results. While almost all show that Aβ levels are elevated after TBI, the timeline of these changes is variable. CCI in a type of APP transgenic mouse (PDAPP) causes a brief spike in Aβ40 and Aβ42, peaking at 2 h post injury and returning to baseline by 6 h (Smith et al. 1998). Longer studies in PDAPP mice have shown that CCI can actually decrease deposition of Aβ in the ipsilateral cortex and hippocampus 4–8 months after injury compared to the uninjured side of the brain (Nakagawa et al. 1999; Nakagawa et al. 2000). The same group also reported that CCI injuries in a different type of APP transgenic mouse (Tg2576) cause elevated soluble and insoluble cortical Aβ40 and Aβ42, and amyloid plaque deposition (Uryu et al. 2002). Finally, studies in the APP$^{NLh/NLh}$ mice, a gene-targeted mouse that expresses normal levels of human APP, showed elevated Aβ40 only through the first 24 h after CCI, while Aβ42 levels remain elevated through 14 days (Abrahamson et al. 2006).

Consistent with a role for apoE in influencing amyloid deposition in humans, apoE4 also increases amyloid plaque formation in mice. Using PDAPP mice crossed with apoE3- and apoE4-expressing mice, the authors found that 56% of apoE4:PDAPP mice had amyloid plaques 3 months after TBI, compared to only 20% of apoE3:PDAPP mice. Mature plaques were only found in apoE4:PDAPP mice

(Hartman et al. 2002). ApoE4 mice are also more likely to die after a closed head injury, and surviving mice have poorer outcomes than apoE3 mice with a similar injury (Sabo et al. 2000).

With the availability of Aβ ELISA kits sensitive enough to detect rodent Aβ, newer studies have reported Aβ levels in wild-type mice. Profiles of APP, β-secretase, and γ-secretase protein changes after TBI have been reported in C57/Bl6 mice, and the resulting change in Aβ40 and Aβ42 after injury. APP and the APP secretases all accumulate after TBI, peaking at 1 to 3 days and returning to baseline levels by 7 days postinjury. This profile is exactly mirrored by changes in Aβ40 and Aβ42, which also peak within the 3-day time frame and return to normal levels by 7 days (Loane et al. 2009; Loane et al. 2011). Unfortunately, using wild-type mice has limitations as rodent Aβ differs from human Aβ at 3 amino acid sites (arginine 5, tyrosine 10, and histidine 13; Yamada et al. 1987), and rodent Aβ does not deposit as amyloid plaques in wild-type mice. It is able to form beta-sheet fibrils in vitro (Fraser et al. 1992; Boyd-Kimball et al. 2004), albeit not as aggressively as human Aβ (Boyd-Kimball et al. 2004). These changes are thought to reduce the ability of rodent Aβ to reduce Cu (II) to Cu (I), and thus rodent Aβ is perceived to lack oxidative stress properties. However, rodent Aβ can still induce protein oxidation and lipid peroxidation in primary neurons, and can trigger apoptosis and cell death, although at a slower rate than human Aβ (Boyd-Kimball et al. 2004).

The CCI model of TBI is designed to mimic contusional impacts, and as such produces limited white matter damage. Also, because of the short axonal pathways found in rodents, CCI in mice and rats is a poor model of DAI. One model that has been developed to study DAI is rotational acceleration in miniature swine (Smith et al. 1997). As pigs have a large gyrencephalic brain with substantial white matter domains, they are more susceptible to DAI than rodents. By utilizing nonimpact inertial loading, the investigators are able to replicate the shear, tensile, and compressive strains that often result in human DAI. As mentioned earlier, DAI in humans produces hotspots of Aβ production in axonal bulbs and swellings, and the pig model of DAI has also been examined for accumulation of β- and γ-secretase proteins, as well as Aβ accumulation (Chen et al. 2004). Short-term (3 hours, 3 days, and 7 days) and long-term (6 month) profiles were examined using Aβ and APP secretase–specific antibodies, and Thioflavin S (for detection of β-sheet conformation-specific proteins). The authors found that rotational acceleration in pigs led to a high density of axonal bulbs and swellings throughout the brain at 3 and 7 days post-trauma, which remained high through 6 months after injury. Aβ-containing plaque-like profiles were detected in about half the animals at short- and long-term time points, and Aβ also accumulated in axonal bulbs along with APP secretase proteins (Chen et al. 2004). Positive staining for Thioflavin S was observed in axonal bulbs of the subcortical white matter at 3 days, 7 days, and 6 months after injury, suggesting the formation of Aβ fibrils in subcortical white matter compartments. The authors also found that levels of soluble and insoluble frontal lobe white matter Aβ42 was elevated by almost threefold 3 hours postinjury, and by almost eightfold at 7 days postinjury, as measured by ELISA (Chen et al. 2004).

In conclusion, there is overwhelming evidence that there is a sudden and sharp increase in Aβ levels after TBI, to such an extent that amyloid plaques begin to form in approximately 30% of severe cases. What is unclear is if these early pathological changes are contributing to, or causing, the development of AD in later life. Much more work needs to be done to understand the changes in Aβ dynamics immediately after trauma, and the long-term consequences of these changes.

8.4   Aβ AS A BIOMARKER OF TBI

Because of the reported increases in amyloid and tau in animals and humans after TBI, it is no surprise that attempts have been made to harness these proteins as biomarkers of TBI. The first such study measured Aβ40 and Aβ42 in cerebrospinal fluid (CSF) of TBI patients on consecutive days for up to 3 weeks (Raby et al. 1998). It was found that both species of Aβ increased in the first week after injury before returning to baseline levels. Overall, Aβ42 levels were three times higher than noninjured control CSF samples (Raby et al. 1998). However, five years later, two very similar studies were published that refuted this claim. In one, the authors found that Aβ42 levels were significantly lower in TBI patients compared to controls (dementia patients or headache patients), and that the levels of CSF Aβ42 were directly correlated with clinical outcome as quantified by the Glasgow Coma Scale (GCS; Franz et al. 2003). In the other study, Kay et al. found that CSF levels of both Aβ40 and Aβ42 were significantly decreased in the first 5 days posttrauma, and that there was a significant inverse correlation between Aβ40 levels and injury severity, as measured by the Glasgow Coma Scale (Kay et al. 2003).

In more recent times, interest has shifted to brain interstitial fluid (ISF), which can be sampled with the placement of microdialysis probes, usually at the same time as placement of probes for measuring intracranial pressure. In 2008, Brody and colleagues used this technique to sample ISF from 18 patients with severe TBI. They found a strong positive correlation between changes in ISF Aβ levels and neurological status, with Aβ levels increasing as neurological status improved (Brody et al. 2008). Several case studies were used to demonstrate this point, including a patient that made a rapid recovery over 48 hours with a GCS score beginning at 5 and recovering to 15. Aβ levels in this patient increased about threefold over the 48-hour period. A second case study showed that a patient remaining in a coma had no changes in Aβ levels over a 160-hour period. Finally, a patient that suffered a secondary insult during the monitoring period (ischemia) had a sudden drop-off in Aβ levels as his GCS dropped. These cases support earlier hypotheses that extracellular Aβ levels are dictated by neuronal activity (Cirrito et al. 2008; Cirrito et al. 2005), with the increased neuronal activity causing Aβ release as the patient emerges from coma. A second, similar study published at the same time also used in vivo microdialysis probes to measure Aβ levels after both focal TBI and DAI in humans (Marklund et al. 2009). The authors report the highest levels of Aβ early after TBI, and trending higher in DAI cases compared to the focal TBI cases. Interestingly, the authors provided 3 case studies. In the first case study, the patient presented with a GCS of 4, and did not improve above this score on follow-up. This patient's Aβ42 levels were low and remained stable throughout the monitoring period. In the second case study, the patient presented with a GCS of 4, improving to 6 over time. This patient had high Aβ42 levels when monitoring began, and this increased further over the 124-hour monitoring period. In the final case study, the patient presented with a GCS of 14–15, but rapidly deteriorated to 5–6 and finally died. From the moment of probe placement to the end of the monitoring period, Aβ levels were below the detection threshold in this patient. The individual case records from both ISF microdialysis studies appear very similar, and would seem to conclude that ISF Aβ levels recover as patients emerge from coma.

The CSF and ISF data from the human studies is confusing, and in many ways contradicts what is observed in postmortem tissue after TBI. Much more work still needs to be done to characterize the intracellular and extracellular pools of Aβ after injury, to determine the rate of Aβ accumulation into oligomers and fibrils, and to measure if Aβ clearance rates are altered after injury. Until we have this data, interpreting data involving snapshots of Aβ levels from both human and animal studies will be difficult. Currently there are attempts being made to track Aβ in real time after TBI using novel amyloid imaging agents that have shown viability in AD diagnostic testing. Compounds such as Pittsburgh Compound B (PiB) (Mathis et al. 2003) have shown the ability to detect amyloid plaques in living patients, and may be able to predict the future decline of a patient prior to a diagnosis of mild cognitive impairment or AD (Morris et al. 2009; Storandt et al. 2009). This has led to speculation that amyloid imaging agents may be helpful in the detection of TBI. However, several technical problems need to be examined before this possibility can be fully explored.

- While 30% of severe TBI cases accumulate amyloid plaques after TBI, this still means that 70% do not. In TBI patients under the age of 40, the rate of Aβ plaques drops to 20%. This leads to a very large chance of false negatives.
- It is apparent that 30% of *severe* TBIs result in amyloid accumulation, but it is unclear if amyloid accumulates after mild and moderate TBI as well.
- Most of the amyloid diagnostics currently being evaluated for use in AD are designed for detecting the presence of mature, β-sheet conformation plaques. The PiB compound, and many similar compounds, are derived from Thioflavin T (Mathis et al. 2003), and as such will only detect mature amyloid plaques. Unfortunately, it is the diffuse, immature plaques that accumulate after TBI, not the mature type. This means that any detection agent will have to detect amyloid aggregates prior to final conformational changes, such as oligomers, protofibrils, and early-stage fibrils.

Despite these issues, there may be a role of existing amyloid imaging agents for TBI patients. Given the propensity of moderate to severe TBI patients to progress to AD, imaging compounds could be used as part of a battery of tests to assess if the patient is healing, or is developing AD.

8.5   TREATMENT STRATEGIES: TARGETING Aβ AFTER TBI

It is obvious from the AD field that Aβ peptides are detrimental to numerous cell types in the CNS. In vitro, Aβ is toxic to neurons (Yankner et al. 1989), glial cells (Brera, Serrano, and de Ceballos 2000; Xu et al. 2001), and endothelial cells (Davis-Salinas et al. 1995). Aβ induces the production of cytokines and reactive oxygen species in microglial cells (Combs et al. 2001), increases sensitivity of neurons to excitotoxic damage (Mark et al. 1995; Mattson et al. 1992), and Aβ-mediated cell death demonstrates morphological and molecular features of apoptosis (Imaizumi et al. 1999).

As TBI causes large increases in Aβ, it is possible that Aβ may be involved in the cascade of neuronal, glial, and endothelial cell death caused by brain injury. There are no studies that directly target Aβ after TBI in preclinical models, but there are a number of reports that have shown that beneficial preclinical therapies reduce Aβ after injury. Abrahamson and colleagues used the pan-caspase inhibitor BAF to prevent caspase-induced cleavage of APP into Aβ following injury (Abrahamson et al. 2006). They successfully reduced Aβ levels 24 hours after TBI, and reduced lesion volume 7 days following injury. Other studies have examined the effects of an apoE-mimetic compound on Aβ and behavior following closed head injury in rodents (Wang et al. 2007). Their drug reduced trauma-induced Aβ42, and ameliorated motor deficits following trauma. More recently it has been shown that simvastatin administered 3 hours after injury can reduce Aβ levels in an APP mouse model (Abrahamson et al. 2009).

Using a more direct approach, it has been reported that targeting the APP secretases after TBI can improve functional recovery, prevent hippocampal neurodegeneration, and reduce lesion volume (Loane et al. 2009). In those experiments, lesion volume, functional recovery, and spatial learning were examined in β-secretase knockout mice. The authors found that the knockout mice had reduced hippocampal cell loss following TBI. This resulted in improved spatial learning and improved fine motor coordination. Inhibitors of γ-secretase were also used to reduce Aβ production after injury. This inhibitor is able to completely block the TBI-induced Aβ response at 24 hours (Burns, unpublished data), and long-term treatment improved fine motor coordination and completely abolished learning deficits in TBI mice. On the cellular level, γ-secretase inhibition after injury resulted in less neuronal cell death in the CA1 region of the hippocampus, and overall lesion volume was reduced by 70% (Loane et al. 2009).

Aβ homeostasis is maintained by balancing production (APP processing) and clearance (Aβ degradation). Clearance of Aβ is positively enhanced by activity of the cholesterol efflux transporter ABCA1 (ATP binding cassette protein A1). The degradation of Aβ involves a complex pathway by which ABCA1 enhances lipidation of apoE. Lipidated apoE binds to Aβ and delivers it to microglia for degradation by neprilysin (Fitz et al. 2010; Jiang et al. 2008), with the amount of Aβ destined for degradation being proportional to the lipidation status of apoE. ABCA1 is the primary factor in the brain that regulates apoE lipidation (Fitz et al. 2010; Jiang et al. 2008), and ABCA1 levels are increased after TBI—but only starting at 3 days postinjury (Loane et al., 2011). Pharmacologically increasing ABCA1 immediately after TBI enhances clearance of Aβ and prevents TBI-induced increases in Aβ40 and Aβ42. These changes in Aβ are accompanied by improvements in fine motor coordination and a reduction in brain lesion volume (Loane et al., 2011).

The caveat of all of the previously discussed research is that Aβ itself has not been directly targeted. Even studies targeting the APP secretases cannot rule out an effect mediated by secretase substrates other than Aβ. However, there is evidence that cleavage products of APP are playing a role in secondary injury after TBI.

Intracerebroventricular infusion of antibodies directed against the N-terminus of APP reduced glial activation and apoptotic cell death in a rat model of TBI, leading to improved functional recovery and reduced lesion volume (Itoh et al. 2009), suggesting that APP or its cleavage products are involved in detrimental downstream pathways after brain injury. Production of Aβ through the β-secretase pathway also comes at the expense of α-cleaved secreted APP (sAPPα). sAPPα has a known neuroprotective role, and reduces cell loss and improve functional recovery after TBI (Corrigan et al. 2011; Thornton et al. 2006), again suggesting that APP processing fragments play an important role after TBI.

In conclusion, it appears that APP and the APP secretases are partial mediators of injury cascades after TBI, and strategies that target the processing of APP after TBI may have therapeutic value after trauma. In order to determine the exact role of Aβ after trauma, more preclinical studies are needed that target Aβ directly.

8.6 REPETITIVE BRAIN INJURY AND CHRONIC TRAUMATIC ENCEPHALOPATHY (CTE)

All of the pathological changes described up to this point have focused mainly on a single, severe TBI. In this section the detrimental neurological effects of repetitive mild TBI, and the resultant pathological changes that occur, will be discussed. In recent years, there has been a surge in public focus on the effects of repeat concussions in contact sports. The pursuit of sporting activity has, and continues to be, one of the biggest risk factors for mild TBI (Carroll et al. 2004). Up to 4 million sports-related concussions occur annually in the United States (Langlois, Rutland-Brown, and Wald 2006), and repetitive concussions are known to occur in a wide variety of sports such as boxing, American football, rugby, and ice hockey. Within the medical literature the phenomenon of repeat concussions in boxing has been the best documented. The terminology has changed over the years: punch-drunk symptoms were first described in 1928 in the *Journal of the American Medical Association* (Martland, 1928). Martland is the first to have described the mental and physical problems suffered by boxers, including clumsiness, ataxia, and disorientation. While most cases were mild, severe cases were described with what we would now call Parkinsonism-type symptoms and dementia (Martland 1928). The commonly used term *dementia pugilistica* was first used in 1937 (Millspaugh 1937). In 1927 a study of over 100 clinical cases was published where the authors proposed that those suffering from postconcussion neurosis should be considered to be suffering traumatic encephalitis (Osnato and Giliberti 1927), and today we use the phrase *chronic traumatic encephalopathy* (CTE) to describe the neurological sequelae and neuropathological changes that occur as a result of repeat concussive or subconcussive blows to the head.

There are published manuscripts on at least 50 CTE cases, spanning the 1950s to the 2000s. These data are very nicely summarized in a recent review article from Boston University in which the authors also add 3 new cases to the literature (McKee et al. 2009). The pathology of CTE is now established primarily as a tauopathy, a class of neurodegenerative disease caused by the pathological aggregation of tau protein. Other tauopathies include AD, Pick's disease, corticobasal degeneration (CBD), and progressive supranuclear palsy (PSP).

By comparing the known pathological profile of CTE to the other tauopathies, we can begin to elucidate the biochemical basis of this disease. Each tauopathy can be identified as a distinct disease based mainly on their neuropathological and biochemical profile postmortem. AD inclusions are made up of PHFs that are densely packed into the neuronal cell body. CBD inclusions resemble AD; however, the inclusions are made up of single twisted ribbons of tau instead of PHFs, and the accumulation of inclusions cause neurons to swell up like balloons. Astrocytes also accumulate tau in CBD, and the cells then tend to group into localized areas known as *astrocytic plaques*. Pick's disease inclusions are called Pick bodies—single tau filaments forming round inclusions in neuronal soma. And in PSP the characteristic pathology is tau-filled astrocytes called *tufted astrocytes*.

In CTE, the neuronal inclusions are morphologically most similar to those found in AD, with pyramidal neurons maintaining their shape. However, there is much more astrocytic tau found in CTE compared to AD. Another distinct difference between AD and CTE is the distribution of neocortical tangles. The tau immunoreactive profile of CTE is characteristically very patchy and irregular, with preferential deposition in layers II and II of the cortex compared to the preference for layers V and VI in AD (Hof et al., 1992).

Tau isoform distribution is also an important factor in the different tauopathies. In humans there are six isoforms of tau that are generated from a single gene. The different splice variants can have exon 10 included or excluded, making a tau protein with three or four C-terminus microtubule binding domains (called 3R or 4R) and 0, 1, or 2 N-terminal inserts (called 0N, 1N, or 2N). In normal brain, the ratio of 3R:4R tau is approximately 1:1, however the ratio is altered in other tauopathies such as corticobasal degeneration, progressive supranuclear palsy (where 4R is the predominant isoform), or Pick's disease (where 3R is the predominant isoform). In AD the ratio of 3R:4R remains 1:1, with both isoforms being similarly hyperphosphorylated in the disease. CTE bears most resemblance to AD in that both 3R and 4R tau are hyperphosphorylated in a similar manner (Schmidt et al., 2001).

Although there are distinct differences between AD and CTE, there remain many morphological, biochemical, and pathophysiological similarities. Thus it is conceivable that the tau hyperphosphorylation and aggregation in AD and CTE begin with common pathological pathways. However, we can conclude that CTE is a stand-alone disease in the family of tauopathies and, like the other tauopathies, can present with a broad spectrum of behavioral abnormalities. Because of this, it is likely that CTE is often misdiagnosed as a similar disease, such as AD or Parkinson's disease. In fact, a careful look at the data presented in the CTE review by McKee and colleagues (McKee et al., 2009) shows that 69% of cases reported cognitive changes including memory loss or dementia, and 41% presented with movement abnormalities including gait problems or Parkinsonism. Out of 18 patients with reported Parkinsonism, 17 had concurrent memory loss. This mixed pathology presents a challenge to a diagnosing neurologist, but it also is a challenge to epidemiologists who study dementia. Should epidemiologists be focusing solely on AD, mild cognitive impairment, movement disorders, or a combination of symptoms?

One retrospective study that has been conducted on repeat concussion and the odds of developing AD involves a interview follow-up of professional American football players (Guskiewicz et al. 2005). A general health questionnaire was completed by 2,552 retired professionals, with a second questionnaire completed by 758 players. The study was designed to investigate the association between concussion and mild cognitive impairment and AD. Sixty-one percent of the football players reported having sustained at least one concussion during their professional career, and 24% sustained three or more concussions. Players with no concussion had a Mental Component Score (MCS) of 54.35 (CI: 53.77–54.94), which dropped to 50.31 (CI: 49.35–51.27) for those with three or more concussions. The key finding of the study was that players with a history of three or more concussions were five times more likely to be physician diagnosed with mild cognitive impairment. Finally, the authors could find no association between repeat concussion and the development of AD, but they did find a higher prevalence of AD in retired footballer players, especially in men aged 70 and under (Guskiewicz et al. 2005).

Naturally, the Guskiewicz study could not include postmortem confirmation to ensure that the AD cases are pathologically distinct from CTE. However, the data gives credence to the idea that repeat concussions can affect long-term cognitive decline.

8.7 AD PATHOLOGY IN ANIMAL MODELS OF REPETITIVE BRAIN TRAUMA

In order to understand the basic biology underlying CTE, we require an animal model that can recapitulate the disease after repeat trauma. Unfortunately, such a model does not yet exist. Here we will examine the existing literature that has questioned the effects of repeat trauma on the brain.

Repeat injury is known to cause cumulative damage both in vitro and in vivo. In hippocampal cell cultures, exposure to a single stretch injury causes release of neuron-specific enolase (NSE) and S-100b, two common clinical markers of CNS damage. Exposing cells to a repeat stretch injury in the space of one hour significantly increases the release of these two markers (Slemmer et al. 2002), with both neurons and glial cells exhibiting signs of cumulative damage after repeat injury. In vivo, mice exposed to mild TBI on two consecutive days show delayed recovery from fine motor coordination deficits and have evidence of enhanced blood–brain barrier breakdown and axonal injury (Laurer et al. 2001).

Using two different animal models of AD—one amyloid, one tau—the Trojanowski laboratory has come closest to seeing the effects of repeat trauma in mice (Uryu et al. 2002; Yoshiyama et al. 2005). In the first set of experiments the authors used Tg2576 mice (Uryu et al. 2002): 9-month-old mice were anesthetized and impacted on their exposed skull. A subset of these mice received a second mild TBI consisting of the same surgery and same impact site 24 hours after the first surgery. The mice were left for either 9 or 16 weeks after injury and then had their spatial learning and amyloid burden quantified. At 16 weeks postinjury, single mTBI mice behaved similarly to their sham counterparts, however mice injured twice had impaired learning ability in the test. Amyloid burden was quantified by immunohistochemistry, and the authors found that 16 weeks after injury there was a significant increase in Aβ deposition in single mild TBI mice, but this was further enhanced by repetitive mild TBI (Uryu et al. 2002).

In a similarly designed study, the group followed this work with an analysis of tau transgenic mice (Yoshiyama et al. 2005). However, in the tau study the mice were given four mild TBIs per day, one day a week for four weeks (a total of 16 impacts over 4 weeks). The mice were sacrificed 9 months later, and only one mouse demonstrated advanced tau pathology above and beyond that seen in sham controls. It is unclear why only one mouse of twelve showed accelerated pathology (Yoshiyama et al. 2005).

Recapitulating the pathology of repetitive mild TBI in animals is no easy task. It is unclear if an impact has to be above a certain velocity, in a specific brain region, or if a certain number of impacts are required to begin the destructive cascade that results in amyloid or tau accumulation. Other practical issues such as skin deflection, tissue necrosis, and repeat anesthesia complicate matters. Until an animal model of repeat trauma is designed, we will not be able to determine the underlying causes and risk factors associated with CTE.

8.8 CONCLUSIONS

While the data concerning TBI as a risk factor for AD is often confusing and contradictory, a pattern is emerging that appears to confirm the damaging effects of brain trauma on long-term cognition. While many of the studies have focused on the detrimental effect of TBI on AD, it is apparent that trauma is just as much of a risk factor for other dementias. There is a tendency to focus more on the AD field as there are multiple human and animal studies that show amyloid-producing pathways are acutely activated after TBI. However, it remains difficult to determine whether these pathways are involved in the increased levels of AD and dementia after trauma.

It is not hard to imagine that TBI immensely stresses the brain and leaves it vulnerable and primed for endogenous and exogenous stressors in later life. Much more work needs to be done to characterize Aβ dynamics following injury, and to determine the exact role of Aβ and other APP cleavage products following injury. Studies examining Aβ as a biomarker of injury have yielded surprising results that may help us understand how Aβ is released into the extracellular space after injury, but the therapeutic or diagnostic potential of these remain unclear at this time. Similarly, the diagnostic potential of amyloid imaging agents requires careful selection of imaging tools and test subjects before any conclusions can be drawn.

As a therapeutic target, there does appear to be merit in targeting Aβ and other APP cleavage products after injury. While we do not know how this would impact long-term outcome and the risk of dementia, it is clear that amyloid pathways have an important role in secondary injury and acute cell death after trauma. Thanks to the explosion of AD research over the past 20 years, there are many investigative tools that can be used to determine the role of amyloid pathways in acute cell death after brain trauma.

This remains an active and rapidly moving field, with good reason. The incidence of TBI in the US remains high, and the number of AD cases is predicted to rise to over 13 million by the year 2050 (Hebert et al. 2003). We need to continue studying why TBI and repeat concussions are leading to AD and other dementias, we need to understand the molecular mechanisms underlying these events, and we need to design better animal models to mimic the behavioral and pathological changes observed. Only then will we be able to test new therapeutic agents that may intervene in the disease process.

ACKNOWLEDGMENTS

This publication was made possible by a grant from KPB Corporation, and by grant number R03NS67417 from the National Institute of Neurological Disorders and Stroke (NINDS), a component of the National Institutes of Health (NIH). Its contents are solely the responsibility of the author and do not necessarily represent the official view of the NIH.

REFERENCES

Abrahamson, E. E., Ikonomovic, M. D., Ciallella, J. R., Hope, C. E., Paljug, W. R., Isanski, B. A., Flood, D. G., Clark, R. S., and DeKosky, S. T. 2006. Caspase inhibition therapy abolishes brain trauma-induced increases in Abeta peptide: Implications for clinical outcome. *Exp Neurol* 197: 437–450.

Abrahamson, E. E., Ikonomovic, M. D., Dixon, C. E., and Dekosky, S. T. 2009. Simvastatin therapy prevents brain trauma-induced increases in beta-amyloid peptide levels. *Ann Neurol* 66: 407–414.

Boyd-Kimball, D., Sultana, R., Mohmmad-Abdul, H., and Butterfield, D. A. 2004. Rodent Abeta(1-42) exhibits oxidative stress properties similar to those of human Abeta(1-42): Implications for proposed mechanisms of toxicity. *J Alzheimers Dis* 6: 515–525.

Brera, B., Serrano, A., and de Ceballos, M. L. 2000. Beta-amyloid peptides are cytotoxic to astrocytes in culture: A role for oxidative stress. *Neurobiol Dis.* 7: 395–405.

Brody, D. L., Magnoni, S., Schwetye, K. E., Spinner, M. L., Esparza, T. J., Stocchetti, N., Zipfel, G. J., and Holtzman, D. M. 2008. Amyloid-beta dynamics correlate with neurological status in the injured human brain. *Science* 321: 1221–1224.

Broe, G. A., Henderson, A. S., Creasey, H., McCusker, E., Korten, A. E., Jorm, A. F., Longley, W., and Anthony, J. C. 1990. A case-control study of Alzheimer's disease in Australia. *Neurology* 40: 1698–1707.

Caamano-Isorna, F., Corral, M., Montes-Martinez, A., and Takkouche, B. 2006. Education and dementia: A meta-analytic study. *Neuroepidemiology* 26: 226–232.

Carroll, L. J., Cassidy, J. D., Holm, L., Kraus, J., and Coronado, V. G. 2004. Methodological issues and research recommendations for mild traumatic brain injury: The WHO Collaborating Centre Task Force on Mild Traumatic Brain Injury. *J Rehabil Med*: 113–125.

Chen, X. H., Siman, R., Iwata, A., Meaney, D. F., Trojanowski, J. Q., and Smith, D. H. 2004. Long-term accumulation of amyloid-beta, beta-secretase, presenilin-1, and caspase-3 in damaged axons following brain trauma. *Am J Pathol* 165: 357–371.

Cirrito, J. R., Kang, J. E., Lee, J., Stewart, F. R., Verges, D. K., Silverio, L. M., Bu, G., Mennerick, S., and Holtzman, D. M. 2008. Endocytosis is required for synaptic activity-dependent release of amyloid-beta in vivo. *Neuron* 58: 42–51.

Cirrito, J. R., Yamada, K. A., Finn, M. B., Sloviter, R. S., Bales, K. R., May, P. C., Schoepp, D. D., Paul, S. M., Mennerick, S., and Holtzman, D. M. 2005. Synaptic activity regulates interstitial fluid amyloid-beta levels in vivo. *Neuron* 48: 913–922.

Combs, C. K., Karlo, J. C., Kao, S. C., and Landreth, G. E. 2001. beta-Amyloid stimulation of microglia and monocytes results in TNFalpha-dependent expression of inducible nitric oxide synthase and neuronal apoptosis. *J Neurosci* 21: 1179–1188.

Corder, E. H., Saunders, A. M., Strittmatter, W. J., Schmechel, D. E., Gaskell, P. C., Small, G. W., Roses, A. D., Haines, J. L., and Pericak-Vance, M. A. 1993. Gene dose of apolipoprotein E type 4 allele and the risk of Alzheimer's disease in late onset families. *Science* 261: 921–923.

Corrigan, F., Pham, C. L., Vink, R., Blumbergs, P. C., Masters, C. L., van den Heuvel, C., and Cappai, R. 2011. The neuroprotective domains of the amyloid precursor protein, in traumatic brain injury, are located in the two growth factor domains. *Brain Res* 1378: 137–143.

Davis-Salinas, J., Saporito-Irwin, S. M., Cotman, C. W., and Van Nostrand, W. E. 1995. Amyloid beta-protein induces its own production in cultured degenerating cerebrovascular smooth muscle cells. *J Neurochem* 65: 931–934.

DeKosky, S. T., Abrahamson, E. E., Ciallella, J. R., Paljug, W. R., Wisniewski, S. R., Clark, R. S., and Ikonomovic, M. D. 2007. Association of increased cortical soluble abeta42 levels with diffuse plaques after severe brain injury in humans. *Arch Neurol* 64: 541–544.

Faul, M., Xu, L., Wald, M. M., Coronado, V. G. 2010. Traumatic brain injury in the United States: Emergency department visits, hospitalizations, and deaths. Atlanta (GA): Centers for Disease Control and Prevention, National Center for Injury Prevention and Control.

Fitz, N. F., Cronican, A., Pham, T., Fogg, A., Fauq, A. H., Chapman, R., Lefterov, I., and Koldamova, R. 2010. Liver X receptor agonist treatment ameliorates amyloid pathology and memory deficits caused by high-fat diet in APP23 mice. *J Neurosci* 30: 6862–6872.

Fleminger, S., Oliver, D. L., Lovestone, S., Rabe-Hesketh, S., and Giora, A. 2003. Head injury as a risk factor for Alzheimer's disease: The evidence 10 years on: A partial replication. *J Neurol Neurosurg Psychiatry* 74: 857–862.

Franz, G., Beer, R., Kampfl, A., Engelhardt, K., Schmutzhard, E., Ulmer, H., and Deisenhammer, F. 2003. Amyloid beta 1-42 and tau in cerebrospinal fluid after severe traumatic brain injury. *Neurology* 60: 1457–1461.

Fraser, P. E., Nguyen, J. T., Inouye, H., Surewicz, W. K., Selkoe, D. J., Podlisny, M. B., and Kirschner, D. A. 1992. Fibril formation by primate, rodent, and Dutch-hemorrhagic analogues of Alzheimer amyloid beta-protein. *Biochemistry* 31: 10716–10723.

Fratiglioni, L., Ahlbom, A., Viitanen, M., and Winblad, B. 1993. Risk factors for late-onset Alzheimer's disease: a population-based, case-control study. *Ann Neurol* 33: 258–266.

Friedman, G., Froom, P., Sazbon, L., Grinblatt, I., Shochina, M., Tsenter, J., Babaey, S., Yehuda, B., and Groswasser, Z. 1999. Apolipoprotein E-epsilon4 genotype predicts a poor outcome in survivors of traumatic brain injury. *Neurology* 52: 244–248.

Gentleman, S. M., Greenberg, B. D., Savage, M. J., Noori, M., Newman, S. J., Roberts, G. W., Griffin, W. S., and Graham, D. I. 1997. A beta 42 is the predominant form of amyloid beta-protein in the brains of short-term survivors of head injury. *Neuroreport* 8: 1519–1522.

Graves, A. B., White, E., Koepsell, T. D., Reifler, B. V., van Belle, G., Larson, E. B., and Raskind, M. 1990. The association between head trauma and Alzheimer's disease. *Am J Epidemiol* 131: 491–501.

Guskiewicz, K. M., Marshall, S. W., Bailes, J., McCrea, M., Cantu, R. C., Randolph, C., and Jordan, B. D. 2005. Association between recurrent concussion and late-life cognitive impairment in retired professional football players. *Neurosurgery* 57: 719–726.

Hartman, R. E., Laurer, H., Longhi, L., Bales, K. R., Paul, S. M., McIntosh, T. K., and Holtzman, D. M. 2002. Apolipoprotein E4 influences amyloid deposition but not cell loss after traumatic brain injury in a mouse model of Alzheimer's disease. *J Neurosci* 22: 10083–10087.

Hebert, L. E., Scherr, P. A., Bienias, J. L., Bennett, D. A., and Evans, D. A. 2003. Alzheimer disease in the US population: Prevalence estimates using the 2000 census. *Arch Neurol* 60: 1119–11122.

Hof, P. R., Bouras, C., Buee, L., Delacourte, A., Perl, D. P., and Morrison, J. H. 1992. Differential distribution of neurofibrillary tangles in the cerebral cortex of dementia pugilistica and Alzheimer's disease cases. *Acta Neuropathol* 85: 23–30.

Ikonomovic, M. D., Uryu, K., Abrahamson, E. E., Ciallella, J. R., Trojanowski, J. Q., Lee, V. M., Clark, R. S., Marion, D. W., Wisniewski, S. R., and Dekosky, S. T. 2004. Alzheimer's pathology in human temporal cortex surgically excised after severe brain injury. *Exp Neurol* 190: 192–203.

Imaizumi, K., Morihara, T., Mori, Y., Katayama, T., Tsuda, M., Furuyama, T., Wanaka, A., Takeda, M., and Tohyama, M. 1999. The cell death-promoting gene DP5, which interacts with the BCL2 family, is induced during neuronal apoptosis following exposure to amyloid beta protein. *J Biol Chem* 274: 7975–7981.

Itoh, T., Satou, T., Nishida, S., Tsubaki, M., Hashimoto, S., and Ito, H. 2009. Improvement of cerebral function by anti-amyloid precursor protein antibody infusion after traumatic brain injury in rats. *Mol Cell Biochem* 324: 191–199.

Jiang, Q., Lee, C. Y., Mandrekar, S., Wilkinson, B., Cramer, P., Zelcer, N., Mann, K., Lamb, B., Willson, T. M., Collins, J. L., Richardson, J. C., Smith, J. D., Comery, T. A., Riddell, D., Holtzman, D. M., Tontonoz, P., and Landreth, G. E. 2008. ApoE promotes the proteolytic degradation of Abeta. *Neuron* 58: 681–693.

Katzman, R., Aronson, M., Fuld, P., Kawas, C., Brown, T., Morgenstern, H., Frishman, W., Gidez, L., Eder, H., and Ooi, W. L. 1989. Development of dementing illnesses in an 80-year-old volunteer cohort. *Ann Neurol* 25: 317–324.

Kay, A. D., Petzold, A., Kerr, M., Keir, G., Thompson, E., and Nicoll, J. A. 2003. Alterations in cerebrospinal fluid apolipoprotein E and amyloid beta-protein after traumatic brain injury. *J Neurotrauma* 20: 943–952.

Langlois, J. A., Rutland-Brown, W., and Wald, M. M. 2006. The epidemiology and impact of traumatic brain injury: A brief overview. *J Head Trauma Rehabil* 21: 375–378.

Laurer, H. L., Bareyre, F. M., Lee, V. M., Trojanowski, J. Q., Longhi, L., Hoover, R., Saatman, K. E., Raghupathi, R., Hoshino, S., Grady, M. S., and McIntosh, T. K. 2001. Mild head injury increasing the brain's vulnerability to a second concussive impact. *J Neurosurg* 95: 859–870.

Loane, D. J., Pocivavsek, A., Moussa, C. E., Thompson, R., Matsuoka, Y., Faden, A. I., Rebeck, G. W., and Burns, M. P. 2009. Amyloid precursor protein secretases as therapeutic targets for traumatic brain injury. *Nat Med* 15: 377–379.

Loane, D. J., Washington, P. M., Vardanian, L., Pocivavsek, A., Hoe, H. S., Duff, K. E., Cernak, I., Rebeck, G. W., Faden, A. I., and Burns, M. P. 2011. Modulation of ABCA1 by an LXR agonist reduces beta-amyloid levels and improves outcome after traumatic brain injury. *J Neurotrauma* 28: 225–236.

Mark, R. J., Hensley, K., Butterfield, D. A., and Mattson, M. P. 1995. Amyloid beta-peptide impairs ion-motive ATPase activities: evidence for a role in loss of neuronal Ca2+ homeostasis and cell death. *J Neurosci* 15: 6239–6249.

Marklund, N., Blennow, K., Zetterberg, H., Ronne-Engstrom, E., Enblad, P., and Hillered, L. 2009. Monitoring of brain interstitial total tau and beta amyloid proteins by microdialysis in patients with traumatic brain injury. *J Neurosurg* 110: 1227–1237.

Martland, Harrison S. 1928. Punch drunk. *JAMA* 91: 1103–1107.

Mathis, C. A., Wang, Y., Holt, D. P., Huang, G. F., Debnath, M. L., and Klunk, W. E. 2003. Synthesis and evaluation of 11C-labeled 6-substituted 2-arylbenzothiazoles as amyloid imaging agents. *J Med Chem* 46: 2740–2754.

Mattson, M. P., Cheng, B., Davis, D., Bryant, K., Lieberburg, I., and Rydel, R. E. 1992. Beta-amyloid peptides destabilize calcium homeostasis and render human cortical neurons vulnerable to excitotoxicity. *J Neurosci* 12: 376–389.

Mayeux, R., Ottman, R., Maestre, G., Ngai, C., Tang, M. X., Ginsberg, H., Chun, M., Tycko, B., and Shelanski, M. 1995. Synergistic effects of traumatic head injury and apolipoprotein-epsilon 4 in patients with Alzheimer's disease. *Neurology* 45: 555–557.

McKee, A. C., Cantu, R. C., Nowinski, C. J., Hedley-Whyte, E. T., Gavett, B. E., Budson, A. E., Santini, V. E., Lee, H. S., Kubilus, C. A., and Stern, R. A. 2009. Chronic traumatic encephalopathy in athletes: progressive tauopathy after repetitive head injury. *J Neuropathol Exp Neurol* 68: 709–735.

Millspaugh, H. S. 1937. Dementia pugilistica. *US Med Bull* 35: 297–303.

Morris, J. C., Roe, C. M., Grant, E. A., Head, D., Storandt, M., Goate, A. M., Fagan, A. M., Holtzman, D. M., and Mintun, M. A. 2009. Pittsburgh compound B imaging and prediction of progression from cognitive normality to symptomatic Alzheimer disease. *Arch Neurol* 66: 1469–1475.

Mortimer, J. A., van Duijn, C. M., Chandra, V., Fratiglioni, L., Graves, A. B., Heyman, A., Jorm, A. F., Kokmen, E., Kondo, K., Rocca, W. A., et al. 1991. Head trauma as a risk factor for Alzheimer's disease: A collaborative re-analysis of case-control studies. EURODEM Risk Factors Research Group. *Int J Epidemiol* 20 Suppl 2: S28–35.

Nakagawa, Y., Nakamura, M., McIntosh, T. K., Rodriguez, A., Berlin, J. A., Smith, D. H., Saatman, K. E., Raghupathi, R., Clemens, J., Saido, T. C., Schmidt, M. L., Lee, V. M., and Trojanowski, J. Q. 1999. Traumatic brain injury in young, amyloid-beta peptide overexpressing transgenic mice induces marked ipsilateral hippocampal atrophy and diminished Abeta deposition during aging. *J Comp Neurol* 411: 390–398.

Nakagawa, Y., Reed, L., Nakamura, M., McIntosh, T. K., Smith, D. H., Saatman, K. E., Raghupathi, R., Clemens, J., Saido, T. C., Lee, V. M., and Trojanowski, J. Q. 2000. Brain trauma in aged transgenic mice induces regression of established Abeta deposits. *Exp Neurol* 163: 244–252.

Nicoll, J. A., Roberts, G. W., and Graham, D. I. 1995. Apolipoprotein E epsilon 4 allele is associated with deposition of amyloid beta-protein following head injury. *Nat Med* 1: 135–137.

O'Meara, E. S., Kukull, W. A., Sheppard, L., Bowen, J. D., McCormick, W. C., Teri, L., Pfanschmidt, M., Thompson, J. D., Schellenberg, G. D., and Larson, E. B. 1997. Head injury and risk of Alzheimer's disease by apolipoprotein E genotype. *Am J Epidemiol* 146: 373–384.

Osnato, M., and Giliberti, V. 1927. Postconcussion neurosis-traumatic encephalitis: A conception of postconcussion phenomena. *Arch Neurol Psychiatry* 18: 181–214.

Plassman, B. L., Havlik, R. J., Steffens, D. C., Helms, M. J., Newman, T. N., Drosdick, D., Phillips, C., Gau, B. A., Welsh-Bohmer, K. A., Burke, J. R., Guralnik, J. M., and Breitner, J. C. 2000. Documented head injury in early adulthood and risk of Alzheimer's disease and other dementias. *Neurology* 55: 1158–1166.

Raby, C. A., Morganti-Kossmann, M. C., Kossmann, T., Stahel, P. F., Watson, M. D., Evans, L. M., Mehta, P. D., Spiegel, K., Kuo, Y. M., Roher, A. E., and Emmerling, M. R. 1998. Traumatic brain injury increases beta-amyloid peptide 1-42 in cerebrospinal fluid. *J Neurochem* 71: 2505–2509.

Rasmusson, D. X., Brandt, J., Martin, D. B., and Folstein, M. F. 1995. Head injury as a risk factor in Alzheimer's disease. *Brain Inj* 9: 213–219.

Raymont, V., Greathouse, A., Reding, K., Lipsky, R., Salazar, A., and Grafman, J. 2008. Demographic, structural and genetic predictors of late cognitive decline after penetrating head injury. *Brain* 131: 543–558.

Roberts, G. W., Gentleman, S. M., Lynch, A., and Graham, D. I. 1991. Beta A4 amyloid protein deposition in brain after head trauma. *Lancet* 338: 1422–1423.

Roberts, G. W., Gentleman, S. M., Lynch, A., Murray, L., Landon, M., and Graham, D. I. 1994. Beta amyloid protein deposition in the brain after severe head injury: implications for the pathogenesis of Alzheimer's disease. *J Neurol Neurosurg Psychiatry* 57: 419–425.

Roof, R. L., Duvdevani, R., Braswell, L., and Stein, D. G. 1994. Progesterone facilitates cognitive recovery and reduces secondary neuronal loss caused by cortical contusion injury in male rats. *Exp Neurol* 129: 64–69.

Roof, R. L., Duvdevani, R., Heyburn, J. W., and Stein, D. G. 1996. Progesterone rapidly decreases brain edema: Treatment delayed up to 24 hours is still effective. *Exp Neurol* 138: 246–251.

Sabo, T., Lomnitski, L., Nyska, A., Beni, S., Maronpot, R. R., Shohami, E., Roses, A. D., and Michaelson, D. M. 2000. Susceptibility of transgenic mice expressing human apolipoprotein E to closed head injury: The allele E3 is neuroprotective whereas E4 increases fatalities. *Neuroscience* 101: 879–884.

Schmidt, M. L., Zhukareva, V., Newell, K. L., Lee, V. M., and Trojanowski, J. Q. 2001. Tau isoform profile and phosphorylation state in dementia pugilistica recapitulate Alzheimer's disease. *Acta Neuropathol* 101: 518–524.

Shalat, S. L., Seltzer, B., Pidcock, C., and Baker, E. L., Jr. 1987. Risk factors for Alzheimer's disease: A case-control study. *Neurology* 37: 1630–1633.

Slemmer, J. E., Matser, E. J., De Zeeuw, C. I., and Weber, J. T. 2002. Repeated mild injury causes cumulative damage to hippocampal cells. *Brain* 125: 2699–2709.

Smith, D. H., Chen, X. H., Xu, B. N., McIntosh, T. K., Gennarelli, T. A., and Meaney, D. F. 1997. Characterization of diffuse axonal pathology and selective hippocampal damage following inertial brain trauma in the pig. *J Neuropathol Exp Neurol* 56: 822–834.

Smith, D. H., Nakamura, M., McIntosh, T. K., Wang, J., Rodriguez, A., Chen, X. H., Raghupathi, R., Saatman, K. E., Clemens, J., Schmidt, M. L., Lee, V. M., and Trojanowski, J. Q. 1998. Brain trauma induces massive hippocampal neuron death linked to a surge in beta-amyloid levels in mice overexpressing mutant amyloid precursor protein. *Am J Pathol* 153: 1005–1010.

Sorbi, S., Nacmias, B., Piacentini, S., Repice, A., Latorraca, S., Forleo, P., and Amaducci, L. 1995. ApoE as a prognostic factor for post-traumatic coma. *Nat Med* 1: 852.

Storandt, M., Mintun, M. A., Head, D., and Morris, J. C. 2009. Cognitive decline and brain volume loss as signatures of cerebral amyloid-beta peptide deposition identified with Pittsburgh compound B: cognitive decline associated with Abeta deposition. *Arch Neurol* 66: 1476–1481.

Thornton, E., Vink, R., Blumbergs, P. C., and Van Den, Heuvel C. 2006. Soluble amyloid precursor protein alpha reduces neuronal injury and improves functional outcome following diffuse traumatic brain injury in rats. *Brain Res* 1094: 38–46.

Tsolaki, M., Fountoulakis, K., Chantzi, E., and Kazis, A. 1997. Risk factors for clinically diagnosed Alzheimer's disease: A case-control study of a Greek population. *Int Psychogeriatr* 9: 327–341.

Uryu, K., Chen, X. H., Martinez, D., Browne, K. D., Johnson, V. E., Graham, D. I., Lee, V. M., Trojanowski, J. Q., and Smith, D. H. 2007. Multiple proteins implicated in neurodegenerative diseases accumulate in axons after brain trauma in humans. *Exp Neurol* 208: 185–192.

Uryu, K., Laurer, H., McIntosh, T., Pratico, D., Martinez, D., Leight, S., Lee, V. M., and Trojanowski, J. Q. 2002. Repetitive mild brain trauma accelerates Abeta deposition, lipid peroxidation, and cognitive impairment in a transgenic mouse model of Alzheimer amyloidosis. *J Neurosci* 22: 446–454.

Wang, H., Durham, L., Dawson, H., Song, P., Warner, D. S., Sullivan, P. M., Vitek, M. P., and Laskowitz, D. T. 2007. An apolipoprotein E-based therapeutic improves outcome and reduces Alzheimer's disease pathology following closed head injury: Evidence of pharmacogenomic interaction. *Neuroscience* 144: 1324–1333.

Wright, D. W., Kellermann, A. L., Hertzberg, V. S., Clark, P. L., Frankel, M., Goldstein, F. C., Salomone, J. P., Dent, L. L., Harris, O. A., Ander, D. S., Lowery, D. W., Patel, M. M., Denson, D. D., Gordon, A. B., Wald, M. M., Gupta, S., Hoffman, S. W., and Stein, D. G. 2007. ProTECT: A randomized clinical trial of progesterone for acute traumatic brain injury. *Ann Emerg Med* 49: 391–402.

Xiao, G., Wei, J., Yan, W., Wang, W., and Lu, Z. 2008. Improved outcomes from the administration of progesterone for patients with acute severe traumatic brain injury: A randomized controlled trial. *Crit Care* 12: R61.

Xu, J., Chen, S., Ahmed, S. H., Chen, H., Ku, G., Goldberg, M. P., and Hsu, C. Y. 2001. Amyloid-beta peptides are cytotoxic to oligodendrocytes. *J Neurosci* 21: RC118.

Yamada, T., Sasaki, H., Furuya, H., Miyata, T., Goto, I., and Sakaki, Y. 1987. Complementary DNA for the mouse homolog of the human amyloid beta protein precursor. *Biochem Biophys Res Commun* 149: 665–671.

Yankner, B. A., Dawes, L. R., Fisher, S., Villa-Komaroff, L., Oster-Granite, M. L., and Neve, R. L. 1989. Neurotoxicity of a fragment of the amyloid precursor associated with Alzheimer's disease. *Science* 245: 417–420.

Yoshiyama, Y., Uryu, K., Higuchi, M., Longhi, L., Hoover, R., Fujimoto, S., McIntosh, T., Lee, V. M., and Trojanowski, J. Q. 2005. Enhanced neurofibrillary tangle formation, cerebral atrophy, and cognitive deficits induced by repetitive mild brain injury in a transgenic tauopathy mouse model. *J Neurotrauma* 22: 1134–1141.

Index

A